# ADVANCES IN
# HUMAN GENETICS 10

# CONTRIBUTORS TO THIS VOLUME

**D. Bernard Amos**
Division of Immunology
Duke University Medical Center
Durham, North Carolina

**P. Michael Conneally**
Department of Medical Genetics
Indiana University School of Medicine
Indianapolis, Indiana

**Charlotte P. Dougherty**
Division of Genetics and Mental Retardation
  Center
Children's Hospital Medical Center and the
  Department of Pediatrics
Harvard Medical School
Boston, Massachusetts

**Kaye R. Fichman**
Department of Pediatrics, Divisions of
Pediatric Endocrinology and Pediatric
  Genetics
The Johns Hopkins University
School of Medicine and Hospital
Baltimore, Maryland

**D. D. Kostyu**
Division of Immunology
Duke University Medical Center
Durham, North Carolina

**Samuel A. Latt**
Division of Genetics and Mental Retardation
  Center
Children's Hospital Medical Center and the
  Department of Pediatrics
Harvard Medical School
Boston, Massachusetts

**Kenneth S. Loveday**
Division of Genetics and Mental Retardation
  Center
Children's Hospital Medical Center and the
  Department of Pediatrics
Harvard Medical School
Boston, Massachusetts

**Barbara R. Migeon**
Department of Pediatrics, Divisions of
Pediatric Endocrinology and Pediatric
  Genetics
The Johns Hopkins University
School of Medicine and Hospital
Baltimore, Maryland

**Claude J. Migeon**
Department of Pediatrics, Divisions of
Pediatric Endocrinology and Pediatric
  Genetics
The Johns Hopkins University
School of Medicine and Hospital
Baltimore, Maryland

**Marian L. Rivas**
Neurological Sciences Institute
Good Samaritan Hospital and
  Medical Center
Portland, Oregon

**Rhona R. Schreck**
Division of Genetics and Mental Retardation
  Center
Children's Hospital Medical Center and the
  Department of Pediatrics
Harvard Medical School
Boston, Massachusetts

**Charles F. Shuler**
Division of Genetics and Mental Retardation
  Center
Children's Hospital Medical Center and the
  Department of Pediatrics
Harvard Medical School
Boston, Massachusetts

**Winifred M. Watkins**
Division of Immunochemical Genetics
MRC Clinical Research Centre
Harrow, Middlesex, England

A Continuation Order Plan is available for this series. A continuation order will bring
delivery of each new volume immediately upon publication. Volumes are billed only upon
actual shipment. For further information please contact the publisher.

# ADVANCES IN HUMAN GENETICS 10

Edited by

## Harry Harris

*Harnwell Professor of Human Genetics*
*University of Pennsylvania, Philadelphia*

and

## Kurt Hirschhorn

*Arthur J. and Nellie Z. Cohen Professor of Genetics and Pediatrics*
*Mount Sinai School of Medicine of The City University of New York*

**PLENUM PRESS • NEW YORK AND LONDON**

The Library of Congress cataloged the first volume of this title as follows:

Advances in human genetics. 1-
    New York, Plenum Press, 1970-

    (1) v. illus. 24-cm.

    Editors: v. 1- H. Harris and K. Hirschhorn.

    1. Human genetics—Collected works. I. Harris, Harry, ed. II. Hirschhorn, Kurt,
1926-     joint ed.
        QH431.A1A32                         573.2'1                         77-84583

Library of Congress Card Catalog Number 77-84583

ISBN-13: 978-1-4615-8290-8    e-ISBN-13: 978-1-4615-8288-5
DOI: 10.1007/978-1-4615-8288-5

A Division of Plenum Publishing Corporation
227 West 17th Street, New York, N.Y. 10011

# ARTICLES PLANNED FOR FUTURE VOLUMES:

# CONTENTS OF EARLIER VOLUMES:

# Preface to Volume 1

During the last few years the science of human genetics has been expanding almost explosively. Original papers dealing with different aspects of the subject are appearing at an increasingly rapid rate in a very wide range of journals, and it becomes more and more difficult for the geneticist and virtually impossible for the nongeneticist to keep track of the developments. Furthermore, new observations and discoveries relevant to an overall understanding of the subject result from investigations using very diverse techniques and methodologies and originating in a variety of different disciplines. Thus, investigations in such various fields as enzymology, immunology, protein chemistry, cytology, pediatrics, neurology, internal medicine, anthropology, and mathematical and statistical genetics, to name but a few, have each contributed results and ideas of general significance to the study of human genetics. Not surprisingly it is often difficult for workers in one branch of the subject to assess and assimilate findings made in another. This can be a serious limiting factor on the rate of progress.

Thus, there appears to be a real need for critical review articles which summarize the positions reached in different areas, and it is hoped that "Advances in Human Genetics" will help to meet this requirement.

Each of the contributors has been asked to write an account of the position that has been reached in the investigations of a specific topic in one of the branches of human genetics. The reviews are intended to be critical and to deal with the topic in depth from the writer's own point of view. It is hoped that the articles will provide workers in other branches of the subject, and in related disciplines, with a detailed account of the results so far obtained in the particular area, and help them to assess the relevance of these discoveries to aspects of their own work, as well as to the science as a whole. The reviews are also intended to give the reader some idea of the nature of the technical and methodological problems involved, and to indicate new directions stemming from recent advances.

The contributors have not been restricted in the arrangement or organization of their material or in the manner of its presentation, so that the reader should be able to appreciate something of the individuality of approach which goes to make up the subject of human genetics, and which, indeed, gives it much of its fascination.

HARRY HARRIS
*The Galton Laboratory*
*University College London*

KURT HIRSCHHORN
*Division of Medical Genetics*
*Department of Pediatrics*
*Mount Sinai School of Medicine*

# Preface to Volume 10

This is the tenth volume of *Advances in Human Genetics* and some fifty different reviews covering a very wide range of topics have now appeared. Many of the earlier articles still stand as valuable sources of reference. But the subject continues to move forward at an increasing speed and its vitality is indicated by its remarkable recruitment of young investigators. New areas of research which could hardly have been envisaged only a few years ago have emerged, and quite unexpected discoveries have been made in parts of the subject which only recently had come to be thought of as fully explored. So there continues to be a need for authoritative and critical reviews intended to keep workers in the various branches of this seemingly ever-expanding subject fully informed about the progress that is being made and also, of course, to provide a ready and accessible account of new developments in human genetics for those whose primary interests are in other fields of biological and medical research.

We see no reason to alter the general policy which was outlined in the preface to the first volume. We believe that it has served our readers well. The subject seems to us to be just as exciting and intellectually stimulating and rewarding as it did when this series was first started. We expect the next decade of research in human genetics to be as innovative and productive as the last and our aim is to record its progress in *Advances in Human Genetics*.

HARRY HARRIS
*University of Pennsylvania, Philadelphia*

KURT HIRSCHHORN
*Mount Sinai School of Medicine
of the City University of New York*

# Contents

*Chapter 2*

**HLA—A Central Immunological Agency of Man**

*D. Bernard Amos and D. D. Kostyu*

*Chapter 3*

**Linkage Analysis in Man**

*P. Michael Conneally and Marian L. Rivas*

*Chapter 4*

**Sister Chromatid Exchanges**

*Samuel A. Latt, Rhona R. Schreck, Kenneth S. Loveday,
Charlotte P. Dougherty, and Charles F. Shuler*

*Chapter 5*

**Genetic Disorders of Male Sexual Differentiation**

*Kaye R. Fichman, Barbara R. Migeon, and Claude J. Migeon*

*Chapter 1*

# Biochemistry and Genetics of the ABO, Lewis, and P Blood Group Systems

Winifred M. Watkins

*Division of Immunochemical Genetics*
*MRC Clinical Research Centre*
*Harrow, Middlesex, England*

## INTRODUCTION

Many inherited polymorphisms in plasma proteins and in enzyme activities of red blood cells are now available as genetic markers to differentiate bloods within a species (see Giblett, 1969, and Harris, 1975). However, the term "blood groups" is still usually retained to describe antigenic differences detected on the red cell surface by means of specific antibodies. Macromolecules occurring in secretions of the same or different species which carry serological specificities related to the red cell antigens are called blood group substances; these substances are designated by the letter or symbol assigned to the corresponding antigen on the red cell surface. In man fifteen well-defined independent blood group systems are recognized, each comprising antigens believed to be the products of alleles at one gene locus or of closely linked gene loci. In addition, there are some very frequent ("public") and infrequent ("private") antigens which may belong to established systems or may be parts of new systems (see Race and Sanger, 1975). For only three blood group systems, namely ABO, Lewis, and P, is the chemical nature of the antigens unequivocally established, and this review will be primarily concerned with these systems. The recognition sites of some of the heterogeneous group of cold agglutinins collectively termed anti-I (Wiener *et al.*, 1956) are now known to be directed toward structures present in the glycosphingolipid (see Koscielak, 1977; Hakomori *et al.*, 1977*a*) and glycoprotein (see Feizi, 1977) molecules that also carry the determinants associated with the ABO and Lewis blood group systems. The I determinants will be briefly considered in this context.

The involvement of sialic acid residues in both M and N specificities in the MNS system has been known for 20 years, as has also the fact that the specific structures are associated with glycoprotein molecules (Springer and Ansell, 1958; Mäkelä and Cantell, 1958; Romanowska, 1959). More recently it was established that the glycoprotein carrying M and N specificities is the major sialoglycoprotein constituent of the human erythrocyte membrane (Marchesi *et al.*, 1972). However, whether M and N are the products of allelic genes and whether the genes code for the amino acid sequence of the protein core of the sialoglycoprotein or for different glycosyltransferases that add sialic acid residues to the oligosaccharide chains is still controversial (Springer *et al.*, 1977; Dahr *et al.*, 1977; Wasniowska *et al.*, 1977). Detailed consideration of the MNS  system is therefore best deferred until these fundamental differences are resolved. Similarly the chemical nature of the antigens in the Rhesus blood group system is still only partially elucidated. Although the association of Rh(D) activity with membrane protein is strongly indicated by the observations of Green (1968*a,b*, 1972) and Lorusso *et al.* (1977), the relevant protein component has yet to be identified.

## THE ABO SYSTEM

Since the discovery by von Dungern and Hirszfeld (1910) that the human ABO groups are inherited characters, the antigens associated with this system have been widely used in genetic and anthropological investigations. The observation that human red cells can be classified into groups on the basis of antigenic substances on their surfaces was made at the beginning of the century by Landsteiner (1900, 1901). Despite the ever increasing number of variant forms of human genes that are being discovered it is still probably true that more people throughout the world have been accurately classified for the *ABO* genes than for any other polymorphic character. The usefulness of the ABO system as a genetic marker was increased even further by the observation of Schiff and Sasaki (1932) that secretion of A and B substances in saliva and other body fluids is a dimorphic character dependent upon a pair of allelic genes situated at a different locus from the *ABO* genes. The next major genetic landmark associated with the ABO system was the elucidation of the chemical nature of the determinant structures (see Morgan, 1960); this step enabled pathways for the biosynsthesis of the antigens to be proposed. The explanation of these pathways and the characterization of the enzymes believed to be the primary protein products of the blood group genes have opened a new phase for the further genetic analysis of the subgroups and rare variants in the ABO system and for fundamental investigations into the primary gene products.

## Serology and Genetics

*A, B,* and *O* are the three major alleles at the *ABO* locus (Bernstein, 1924). This locus is linked to the loci for the nail-patella syndrome (Np) (Renwick and Lawler, 1955) and for adenylate kinase $AK_1$ (Weitkamp *et al.,* 1969). Experiments with man–Chinese hamster somatic cell hybrids provided evidence for the localization of the gene for $AK_1$ on chromosome 9 (Westerveld *et al.,* 1976). A significant increase in $AK_1$ activity in a patient with duplication of the terminal band of the long arm of chromosome 9 confirmed the assignment of the *ABO:Np-1:$AK_1$* linkage group to this chromosome and suggested a precise location in the region 9q34-qter at the distal end of the long arm (Ferguson-Smith *et al.,* 1976).

There is now ample evidence that the *O* gene does not give rise to an antigenic product on the red cell surface and that the two functional alleles at the *ABO* locus are *A* and *B.* Many rare variant forms of both A and B antigens are detectable serologically (see Race and Sanger, 1975) but the major subdivision is that of A into $A_1$ and $A_2$. The three allele theory of Bernstein (1924) was extended by Thomsen *et al.* (1930) to include the four alleles $A^1$, $A^2$, *B* and *O.* A child receives one of these four genes from each parent, giving ten possible genotypes (Table I). With the commonly available antisera, anti-A, anti-$A_1$ and anti-B, six phenotypes are distinguished. Without the information that may be disclosed by family studies, the genotypes $A^1A^1$ and $A^1O$ cannot be distinguished, nor can *BB* and *BO* or $A^2A^2$ and $A^2O$. The genotype $A^1A^2$ was also formerly indistinguishable from $A^1A^1$ and $A^1O$ but may now be differentiated by means of glycosyltransferase assays (see below).

**TABLE I. The ABO Blood Group System**

| Red cells | | Serum | |
|---|---|---|---|
| Genotypes | Phenotypes[a] | Antibodies | Glycosyltransferases |
| $A^1A^1$ $A^1A^2$ $A^1O$ | $A_1$ | Anti-B | $\alpha$-3-$N$-Acetyl-D-galactosaminyl |
| $A^2A^2$ $A^2O$ | $A_2$ | Anti-B[b] | $\alpha$-3-$N$-Acetyl-D-galactosaminyl |
| $BB$ $BO$ | B | Anti-A | $\alpha$-3-D-Galactosyl |
| $A^1B$ $A^2B$ | $A_1B$ $A_2B$ | − −[b] | $\alpha$-3-$N$-Acetyl-D-galactosaminyl and $\alpha$-3-D-Galactosyl |
| $OO$ | O | Anti-A + anti-B | − |

[a] Defined by antisera anti-A, anti-B, and anti-$A_1$.
[b] Anti-$A_1$ sometimes present in serum of $A_2$ and $A_2B$ people.

Many reagents of human, animal, and plant origin react more strongly with group O red cells than with cells of other ABO groups. At one time these agglutinins were thought to be detecting a product of the $O$ gene but this idea had to be abandoned when it became clear that red cells from persons not carrying an $O$ gene, that is, those homozygous for the $A$ gene or the $B$ gene, or heterozygous for $A$ and $B$ genes, may be agglutinated by these serological reagents. The term H was introduced to describe the antigen on the red cell and the agglutinins were called anti-H (Morgan and Watkins, 1948). H substance is a product of a gene $H$ at a locus independent of $ABO$ but it is the substrate which is modified by the enzymic products of the $A$ or $B$ genes. Thus when A or B specificities are formed in group A, B, or AB individuals there is a complete or partial elimination of H reactivity whereas in group O individuals the H specificity on the red cells is unchanged (Watkins and Morgan, 1955a). The gene $h$ is a rare, silent allele of $H$.

A, B, and H antigenic specificities are not confined to red cells. They occur as cell surface antigens on probably all endothelial cells and many epithelial cells (Szulman, 1960, 1962, 1966; Holborow et al., 1960; Kent,

1964; Sanders and Kent, 1970). In addition, in many individuals substances which specifically combine with anti-A, anti-B, or anti-H agglutinins, and thereby inhibit the agglutination of A, B, or O cells, respectively, occur in a water soluble form in secretions (Yamakami 1926; Yosida, 1928; Lehrs, 1930; Putkonen, 1930). The capacity to secrete ABH substances is a dimorphic character (Schiff and Sasaki, 1932) determined by a pair of allelic genes now referred to as *Se* and *se*. The secretor (*Se*) locus is linked to the Lutheran blood group locus (see Race and Sanger, 1975) but this linkage group has not yet been assigned to a chromosome (Edwards and McKusick, 1978). An individual carrying an *Se* allele, whether homozygous *SeSe* or heterozygous *Sese*, is a "secretor," whereas an individual homozygous for the alternative allele *se* is a "nonsecretor." Among Europeans about 80% are secretors and about 20% nonsecretors. The proportion of secretors and nonsecretors is different in some other ethnic groups (see Race and Sanger, 1975). The proposed function of the secretor gene is that of regulation of the expression of the *H* gene; since H structures are the precursors of the A and B structures the absence of H results in the absence of A and B even when individuals are carrying the appropriate blood group genes (Watkins, 1966). The role of the secretor gene *Se* will be discussed in more detail in the section describing the *H*-gene-specified glycosyltransferase.

I and i specificities are defined by cold agglutinins which most frequently are associated with autoimmune disease. Those antibodies that react more strongly with normal adult red cells than with cord cells are designated as anti-I (Wiener *et al.*, 1956) while those that react more strongly with cord cells and rare adult i cells are designated anti-i (Marsh and Jenkins, 1960). The change from i to I specificity occurs gradually during the first year of life and there is no evidence that i and I antigens are the products of allelic genes (see Giblett, 1969). The extreme heterogeneity of anti-I reagents has been commented on by many workers (see Race and Sanger, 1975) both with regard to their agglutinating capacity with a given panel of red cells and to their inhibitability by a range of different substances. The determinants detected by these reagents are carbohydrates (Feizi *et al.*, 1971a; Cooper and Brown, 1973; Gardas and Koscielak, 1974b; Zopf *et al.*, 1977) and some of the structures available for reactivity on the red cells appear to correspond to structures that normally constitute inner portions of the carbohydrate chains in the secreted blood-group-specific glycoproteins (Feizi *et al.*, 1971b). For this reason A, B, H, Lewis, and I specificities are now frequently linked together but it has to be borne in mind that I does not constitute a discrete entity definable in the same precise genetic and chemical terms as the A, B, H, and Lewis determinants.

## Chemistry of A, B, and H Substances

Early investigations revealed that of the normal human body fluids, saliva, gastric juice, bile, and seminal fluid were the most potent sources of blood-group-specific substances (see Kabat, 1956). Blood group activity was reported by Yosida (1928) in the pathological fluid from ovarian cysts, and subsequently these fluids have proved to be the richest sources of the soluble A, B, H, and Lewis blood group substances (Morgan and van Heyningen, 1944; Morgan, 1960). Earlier workers encountered considerable difficulties in obtaining any quantity of active material from red cells and reports on the chemical nature of the isolated substances were conflicting (see Kabat, 1956). The greater availability of the blood group substances in secretions, and especially of the substances isolated from ovarian cyst fluids, resulted in the pioneering chemical work being carried out on the soluble blood group substances; indeed, all the determinant structures associated with the ABO and Lewis systems were established on fragments isolated from the acid or alkaline degradation products of blood group substances purified from human ovarian cyst fluids (see Morgan and Watkins, 1969 and Kabat, 1970). Substances with serological specificities closely related to human A, B, and H are widely distributed in nature and are found in many animal species (see Kabat, 1956), in microorganisms, and in certain plants (see Springer, 1958). However although much early chemical work was carried out on blood group substances of animal origin, especially the A substance from pig gastric mucosa and B substance from horse gastric mucosa, the nature of the A and B determinants in these materials was not elucidated until after this information was available for the human blood group substances.

### Structure of the A, B, and H Antigenic Determinants

Before the isolation and characterization of the antigenic determinants, various indirect approaches had implicated carbohydrate structures in A, B, and H specificity both on the red cell surface and in the secreted glycoproteins (see Kabat, 1956). Moreover, inhibition of blood group lectin-mediated agglutination of human red cells pointed to the role of L-fucose in H specificity and of N-acetylgalactosamine in A specificity (Morgan and Watkins, 1953). Inhibition of specific precipitation (Kabat and Leskowitz, 1955) and of enzymic decomposition (Watkins and Morgan, 1955b) of blood-group-specific glycoproteins supported the role of these two sugars in H and A specificity and indicated the importance of D-galactose in B specificity. These three sugars were subsequently termed the immunodominant sugars in the respective determinants.

Two types of carbohydrate chain endings may form the basis of the A, B, and H determinants (Rege et al., 1963). The Type 1 chain ending has a β-galactosyl residue joined by a 1→3 linkage to N-acetylglucosamine whereas the Type 2 chain ending has a 1→4 linkage between these two sugars (Fig. 1). The unsubstituted Type 1 chain ending has no known serological specificity but the Type 2 chain ending is responsible for the cross reactivity of partially degraded blood group substances with horse anti-Type XIV pneumococcal serum (Watkins and Morgan, 1956). For many years a somewhat anomalous aspect of this finding was that β-Gal (1→4)GlcNAc had not been shown to constitute a structural unit in the pneumococcus Type XIV capsular polysaccharide (How et al., 1964). Recently, however, the structure has been reinvestigated (Lindberg et al., 1977) and β-Gal(1→4)GlcNAc has for the first time been unequivo-

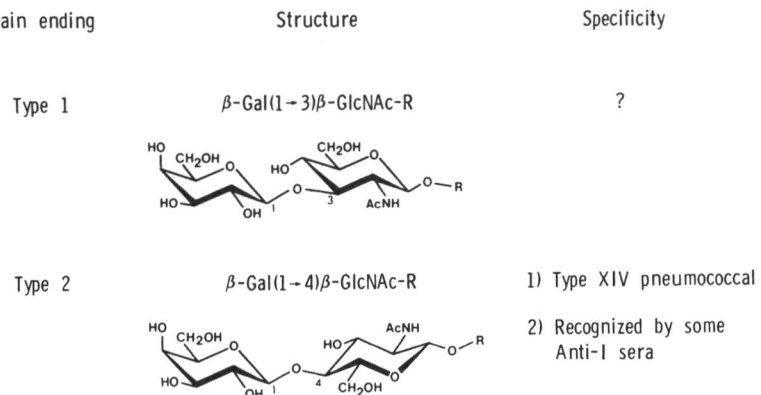

| Chain ending | Structure | Specificity |
|---|---|---|
| Type 1 | β-Gal(1→3)β-GlcNAc-R | ? |
| Type 2 | β-Gal(1→4)β-GlcNAc-R | 1) Type XIV pneumococcal<br>2) Recognized by some Anti-I sera |

Fig. 1. Two types of carbohydrate chain endings which form the basis of A, B, and H determinants. Abbreviations: Gal, D-galactose; GlcNAc, N-acetyl-D-glucosamine; R, remainder of molecule.

cally established as part of the tetrasaccharide repeating unit constituting the polysaccharide. Inhibition of precipitation assays has shown that the Type 2 chain is involved in the specificity of two anti-I sera (Feizi *et al.*, 1971*b*; Kabat *et al.*, 1978; Feizi *et al.*, 1978; Zdebska and Koscielak, 1978). These sera are representative of only a minority of anti-I specificities, but the recognition sites of these two cold agglutinins share features in common with the Type XIV pneumococcal antibody.

The structures of the H (Rege *et al.*, 1964*a*; Lloyd *et al.*, 1966), A, and B (Painter *et al.*, 1965; Lloyd *et al.*, 1966) determinants based on the Type 1 and Type 2 chain endings are shown in Fig. 2. The two H trisaccharides each have an L-fucosyl residue joined by an α-anomeric linkage of the C-2 position of the terminal β-galactosyl unit. The A- and B-active structures differ from H only in the nature of the terminal nonreducing sugar; *N*-acetyl-D-galactosamine in A or D-galactose in B.

The structures of these determinants were ascertained by the classical methods of carbohydrate chemistry, periodate oxidation, methylation, etc. However, the information had to be wrested from milligram quantities of materials painstakingly isolated from degradation products containing complex mixtures of closely related oligosaccharides. Recently, remarkable advances in synthetic carbohydrate chemistry have permitted the synthesis in gram amounts of complex oligosaccharides with the variety of sugars and anomeric and positional linkages found in the blood group determinants (Lemieux *et al.*, 1975*a*; David and Veyrieres, 1975; Jacquinet and Sinäy, 1975; Lemieux, 1978). The terminal nonreducing trisaccharide portion of the B determinant was synthesized by Lemieux and Driguez (1975*a*) and the Type 2 H trisaccharide (Fig. 2) by Jacquinet and Sinäy (1976). The synthetic trisaccharides had chemical and biological properties identical with those of the corresponding trisaccharides of natural origin (Lemieux and Driguez, 1975*a*; Cartron *et al.*, 1976*a*).

From conformational analysis of the Type 1 and Type 2 disaccharides Lemieux (1978) concludes that these are vastly different molecular structures and that they must, therefore, present very different profiles to antibodies and enzymes. He has also suggested that in the A and B terminal tetrasaccharide units the *N*-acetyl-α-D-galactosamine and α-D-galactose residues are expected to be far removed from the *N*-acetyl-β-D-glucosamine residues in both the Type 1 and the Type 2 forms and, therefore, speculates that the combining sites for anti-A and anti-B antibodies would be directed mainly, if not entirely, towards the terminal trisaccharide units. If this is true then the H determinant would be more accurately represented as α-Fuc(1→2)β-Gal-R and the A and B determinants as α-GalNAc(1→3)[α-Fuc(1→2)] β-Gal-R and α-Gal(1→3)[α-Fuc(1→2)]β-Gal-R, respectively. Now that methods are available for the chemical synthesis of these structures many possibilities are opened up for detailed investigations of the binding sites of the blood group antibodies. At least insofar as the primary blood group gene products, the glycosyltransferases, are concerned, the nature of R appears to play only a limited role in the acceptor requirements of the enzymes (see section on glycosyltransferase products of *H*, *A*, and *B* genes).

The A, B, and H determinants constitute the terminal nonreducing sequences of the carbohydrate chains in a variety of different types of molecule. In secretions they are carried by macromolecular glycoproteins; on the surface of red cells they are part of both glycosphingolipid and glycoprotein molecules; and in milk and urine they occur as part of free oligosaccharides.

## Secreted Blood Group Substances with A, B, and H Specificity

The A, B, and H activities in the secretions of the goblet and mucous glands of the gastrointestinal tract, genital tract, and respiratory tract are associated with the glycoprotein molecules which are the main carbohydrate-containing constituents of epithelial mucin. The glycoproteins secreted by the cells in the inner linings of ovarian cyst walls are of the same type. These glycoproteins have been extensively reviewed both as carriers of blood group specificity (Morgan, 1960, 1970; Kabat, 1970, 1973; Watkins, 1972, 1974) and as macromolecules with a role to play in the structure and function of mucin (Clamp *et al.*, 1978; Creeth, 1978; Carlson, 1977). Only a few salient points will, therefore, be mentioned here.

Purified specimens of human blood group A, B, and H substances isolated from ovarian cyst fluids are macromolecules having molecular weight averages ranging from $2 \times 10^5$ to several millions. Even the most highly purified preparations usually show a considerable degree of polydispersity and it is now recognized that the blood-group-specific glycoproteins do not represent a single molecular species but a family of closely related macromolecules. The exact ratio of carbohydrate to peptide varies in different preparations but an average figure for the carbohydrate content is about 85%. The qualitative composition of the glycoproteins is given in Table II. The analytical figures for any one sugar

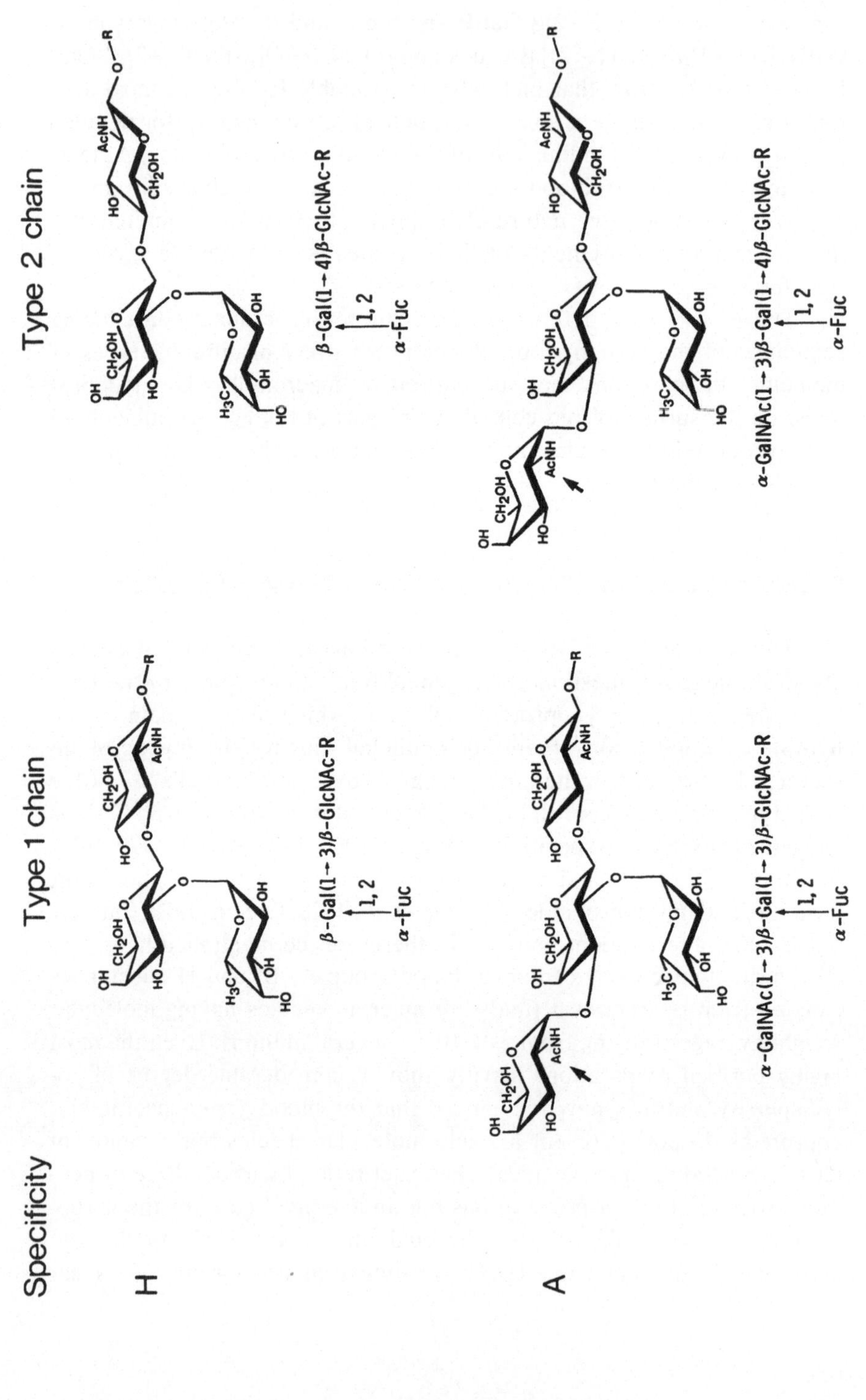
Specificity
Type 1 chain
Type 2 chain
H
β-Gal(1→3)β-GlcNAc-R
1,2
α-Fuc
β-Gal(1→4)β-GlcNAc-R
1,2
α-Fuc
A
α-GalNAc(1→3)β-Gal(1→3)β-GlcNAc-R
1,2
α-Fuc
α-GalNAc(1→3)β-Gal(1→4)β-GlcNAc-R
1,2
α-Fuc

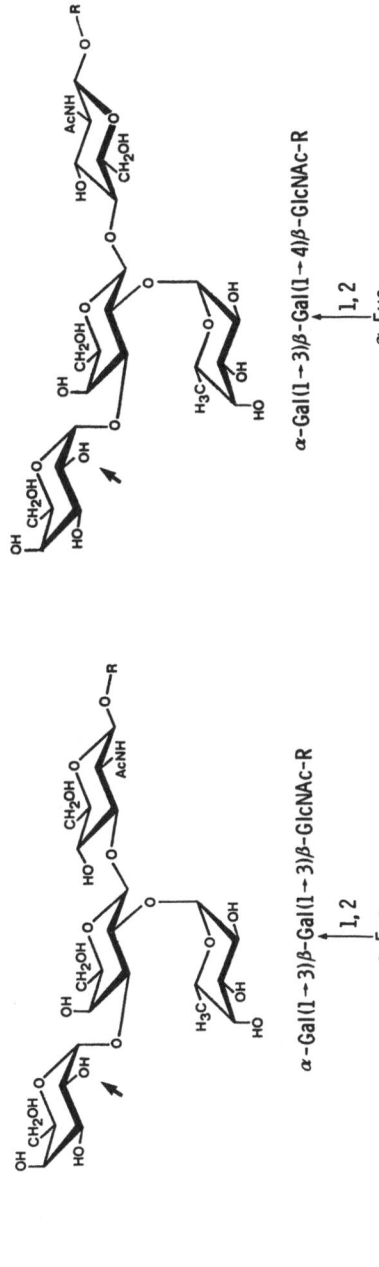

α-Gal(1 → 3)β-Gal(1 → 4)β-GlcNAc-R

1, 2
α-Fuc

α-Gal(1 → 3)β-Gal(1 → 3)β-GlcNAc-R

1, 2
α-Fuc

Fig. 2. Structures of H. A, and B determinants based on Type 1 and Type 2 carbohydrate chains. The arrows indicate the position in the terminal sugar ring where there is a difference between the A and B structures. Abbreviations: GalNAc, N-acetyl-D-galactosamine: Fuc, L-fucose; others as in Fig. 1.

TABLE II. Qualitative Composition of Blood-Group-Specific Glycoproteins
Isolated from Ovarian Cyst Fluids

| Sugars | Amino acids | | |
|---|---|---|---|
| L-Fucose | Aspartic acid | Leucine | |
| D-Galactose | Threonine | Arginine | |
| N-Acetyl-D-glucosamine | Serine | Histidine | |
| N-Acetyl-D-galactosamine | Glutamic acid | Lysine | |
| N-Acetylneuraminic acid | Proline | Tyrosine | |
| | Glycine | Phenylalanine | Trace amounts |
| | Alanine | Cystine | |
| | Valine | Methionine | |
| | Isoleucine | | |

component vary among preparations with the same blood group specificity owing to the heterogeneity of the carbohydrate chains and variations in the total amount of carbohydrate in the molecules. Hence the differences in composition between specimens of differing blood group activity can be regarded as significant only if they fall outside this range. The trend toward a higher $N$-acetylgalactosamine figure for A preparations than for B or H preparations is frequently observed, as is also a higher galactose figure for B preparations than for A or H preparations. In general, however, it would be hazardous to infer the blood group specificity of these glycoproteins from their analytical composition.

The overall similarity of the glycoproteins, irrespective of their blood group activities, was one of the first intimations that the specific structures were carried on common precursor molecules and that the determinants comprised only a small part of the complete macromolecule (Watkins and Morgan, 1959). That this is indeed true was borne out by the many carbohydrate fragments, apart from the determinant structures, that have been isolated and characterized from the acid and alkaline degradation products of the blood-group-specific glycoproteins from ovarian cyst fluids (see Morgan, 1970; Kabat, 1973; Watkins, 1972; Rovis $et\ al.$, 1973; Maisonrouge-McAuliffe and Kabat, 1976). The isolation of a branched pentasaccharide fragment:

$$\begin{array}{c} \beta\text{-Gal}(1\to4)\beta\text{-GlcNAc}(1\to6) \\ \searrow \\ \beta\text{-Gal}(1\to3)\beta\text{-GlcNAc}(1\to3) \nearrow \end{array} \text{galactitol}$$

from the alkaline-borohydride degradation products of blood group substances (Lloyd *et al.*, 1968) revealed that both Type 1 and Type 2 chain endings (Fig. 1) may occur as branches on a single carbohydrate chain. On the basis of this oligosaccharide, and other characterized carbohydrate fragments, Lloyd *et al.* (1968) proposed the structure shown in Fig. 3a for the basic carbohydrate chains in the blood-group-specific glycoproteins. Even this complex structure does not encompass all the serologically inactive oligosaccharide sequences that have been isolated from the blood-group-specific glycoproteins (see Watkins, 1972). However, it has been pointed out by Kabat (1970) that the formula is essentially a statistical average and is intended as a representation of the majority of the chains in the blood group substances and not as the definitive structure of every carbohydrate chain. The A, B, and H determinants can be accommodated on the Type 1 and Type 2 chain endings of the branched oligosaccharide (Fig. 3b), and may also be found on the Type 2 chain ending which occurs on the branch shown as proximal to the *N*-acetylgalactosamine-peptide

(a) Proposed basic chain in blood group specific glycoproteins

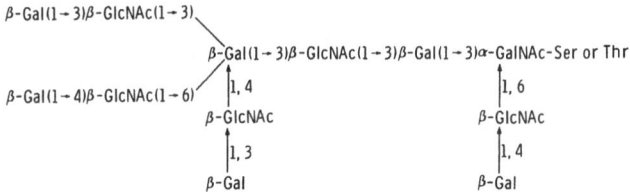

(b) A-active structures on each of the Type 1 and 2 chain endings of the basic chain

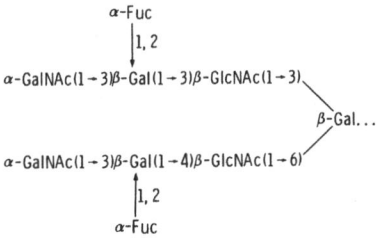

Fig. 3. Branched carbohydrate chains in blood group specific glycoproteins. (a) Basic chain proposed by Lloyd *et al.* (1968). (b) A-active structures on both branches of the basic chain. Abbreviations as in Figs. 1 and 2.

linkage in Fig. 3a (Maisonrouge-McAuliffe and Kabat, 1976). Irrespective of length and complexity, all the carbohydrate chains are thought to be $O$-glycosidically linked via $N$-acetylgalactosamine to the hydroxy amino acids serine and threonine in the peptide core (Anderson *et al.*, 1963; Kabat *et al.*, 1965; Donald *et al.*, 1969). Hence irrespective of blood group specificity $N$-acetylgalactosamine is always a constituent of these glycoprotein molecules.

In the secretions from group AB persons, A and B specificities are carried on the same macromolecules (Morgan and Watkins, 1956). As is to be expected from the precursor–product relationship of H to A and B, H-active structures may occur on the same molecules as A- or B-active structures (Watkins and Morgan, 1957*a*; Watkins, 1959). When H becomes incorporated into the A and B determinants, the H specificity is masked but it may be exposed again by the enzymic removal of the terminal $N$-acetyl-D-galactosamine or D-galactose residues, respectively (see Watkins, 1972). Enzymic removal of the fucose from the Type 2 H-active structures exposes the Type 2 chain ending which cross reacts with anti-Type XIV pneumococcal serum, (Fig. 4) and is the determinant recognized by certain anti-I sera in partially degraded blood group substances (Feizi *et al.*, 1971*b*).

The peptide core of the blood group specific glycoproteins isolated from ovarian cyst fluids has been less thoroughly studied than the carbohydrate moiety. The major obstacle to investigations is the lack of methods for the effective removal of the complex heterosaccharide chains without damage to, or disruption of, the peptide chain. In all these glycoproteins the predominant amino acids are serine, threonine, and proline (Pusztai and Morgan, 1963; Donald, 1973), but the less soluble preparations have a significantly higher content of aspartic and glutamic acids and of cystine than those glycoproteins which are readily soluble. Donald (1973) showed that digestion of the sparingly soluble materials with pronase did not lead to loss of blood group activity or carbohydrate or cause a dramatic fall in molecular weight, but it did yield preparations with a more uniform amino acid composition. In the enzyme-digested materials, the three amino acids threonine, serine, and proline accounted for 65–70% of the total amino acids. Moreover, there was a 1:1 molar ratio of $N$-acetylgalactosamine to the sum of threonine and serine in pronase-digested B and H substances in which $N$-acetylgalactosamine is believed to occur only in the carbohydrate–peptide linkage region. It can, therefore, be assumed that in these residual glycoproteins all the serine and

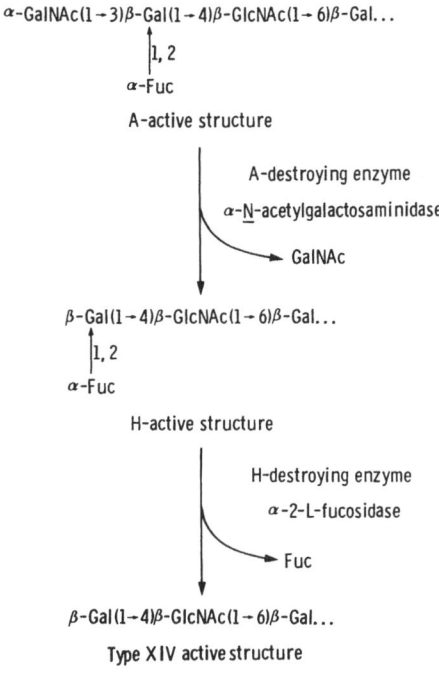

Fig. 4. Enzymic degradation of an A-active structure built on a Type 2 chain. Abbreviations as in Figs. 1 and 2.

α-GalNAc(1→3)β-Gal(1→4)β-GlcNAc(1→6)β-Gal...

|1, 2

α-Fuc

A-active structure

A-destroying enzyme

α-N-acetylgalactosaminidase

GalNAc

β-Gal(1→4)β-GlcNAc(1→6)β-Gal...

|1, 2

α-Fuc

H-active structure

H-destroying enzyme

α-2-L-fucosidase

Fuc

β-Gal(1→4)β-GlcNAc(1→6)β-Gal...

Type XIV active structure

(Determinant recognized by some anti-I sera)

threonine residues were substituted with carbohydrate chains. Isolation of a few pure peptides from the chemical degradation products of a pronase-digested glycoprotein revealed dense packing of the serine and threonine residues in the region of the peptide core carrying the carbohydrate chains (Goodwin and Watkins, 1974). No recognition signal for the initiation of glycosylation of the peptide chains is readily apparent from the amino acid sequences established, and it seems probable that for the α-N-acetylgalactosaminyltransferase adding the first sugar to a serine or threonine residue, the conformation of the peptide is more important than the precise amino acid sequence.

The peptide material removed by proteolytic digestion is believed to be covalently attached to the pronase-resistant, carbohydrate-containing region in the untreated glycoprotein molecules (Donald, 1973). The attachment of varying amounts of such peptides to the carbohydrate containing regions would give rise to products displaying a range of amino acid compositions and would explain why preparations of these substances do not have amino acids in constant ratios. The idea that the peptide moiety of the blood-group-specific glycoproteins may be built up from two kinds of structural region was previously proposed by Dunstone and Morgan (1965) and by Kristiansen and Porath (1968). Whether the varying lengths of unglycosylated peptides found in different preparations indicate polymorphism of the proteins that constitute the core of the glycoproteins, or whether they are the result of either intra- or extracellular "processing" of the protein moiety by proteolytic enzymes *in vivo*, has yet to be established. In any event, there is no apparent correlation between the amino acid composition of the peptide backbone and the A, B, or H specificity of the completed glycoprotein.

Le[a] and Le[b] blood group specificities, which are dependent upon the inheritance of an *Le* gene, are, in secretions, carried on the same glycoprotein molecules as the A, B, and H determinants. The term "secretor" refers only to the presence of A, B, and H determinants on these glycoproteins. Most "nonsecretors" have glycoproteins with Le[a] activity, and these will be discussed in more detail in the section concerned with the Lewis blood group system. About 1% of individuals are nonsecretors of ABH and also lack Lewis activity in their saliva, gastric juice, and other bodily secretions. These people have the gene combination *ABO, H, sese, lele*. The absence of ABH or Lewis blood group specificity does not, however, denote lack of glycoprotein because these individuals have macromolecules with essentially the same overall composition and properties as the blood-group-active glycoproteins (Watkins and Morgan, 1959; Vicari and Kabat, 1969, 1970). These precursor glycoproteins have a greater capacity to cross react with anti-Type XIV pneumococcal serum than do the A-, B-, and H-active glycoproteins; a reaction which is to be expected as the glycoproteins are more likely to have unsubstituted Type 2 chain endings. By the same token inhibitory action of the precursor substances with those anti-I sera that recognize the Type 2 chain ending (Feizi, 1977) is readily explicable.

## A, B, and H Antigens on Red Cell Membranes

**Glycolipids.**   Since the earliest attempts to identify the blood group A and B characters, it appeared possible that, according to the source of the blood-group-specific material, the characteristic serological properties might be associated with more than one kind of macromolecule. Blood-group-active preparations could be obtained by extraction of red cells, or red cell membranes, with ethanol or other organic solvents whereas extraction with water or salt solutions failed to yield active products (see Kabat, 1956). These results suggested a possible lipid nature for the antigens on the red cells and the term "alcohol-soluble" was used to distinguish these antigens from the "water-soluble" substances with the same specificities which occur in secretions. Many years were to elapse before the work of Yamakawa and Suzuki (1952), Koscielak (1963), and Hakomori and Strycharz (1968) showed that the "lipid" substances with A and B specificity on the red cell belonged to the class of molecules known as glycosphingolipids.

During the last fifteen years systematic investigations in the laboratories of Yamakawa in Japan, Koscielak in Poland, and Hakomori in the United States, have demonstrated that there are families of blood group A, B, and H glycosphingolipid molecules on the red cell which show considerable variation in the length and complexity of the carbohydrate chains. The qualitative composition of the carbohydrate moiety is identical in all these glycosphingolipids (Table III) except that the occurrence of N-acetylgalactosamine is confined to those that have blood group A activity (Hakomori et al., 1972; Koscielak et al., 1973; Stellner et al., 1973; Hanfland, 1975; Watanabe et al., 1975; Koscielak et al., 1976a, 1978a; Hakomori, 1978). The presence of N-acetylglucosamine and fucose differentiates these glycosphingolipids from other series of glycosphingolipids: the globosides, hematosides, gangliosides, and sulphatides, which occur in mammalian cells (see Hakomori, 1971). Irrespective of the length and complexity of the carbohydrate chains, the A, B, and H determinant structures at the nonreducing ends of the chains are identical with those established for the active fragments obtained from the degradation products of the blood-group-specific glycoproteins isolated from ovarian cyst fluids (Fig. 2). The only difference is that whereas

TABLE III. Qualitative Composition of the Glycosphingolipids with A, B, and H Specificity

| Sugar moiety | Ceramide moiety |
|---|---|
| L-Fucose | Sphingosine |
| D-Galactose | Fatty acids |
| N-Acetyl-D-glucosamine | |
| D-Glucose | |
| N-Acetyl-D-galactosamine (in A substance only) | |

in the secreted glycoproteins the active groupings are carried on both
Type 1 and Type 2 chains (see Fig. 1), in the glycosphingolipids isolated
from red cell membranes the determinants appear always to be carried
on Type 2 chain endings. The simplest H-, and A-, and B-active glycosphingolipids (Table IV) are based on the ceramide tetrasaccharide called
"lacto-$N$-neotetraosyl ceramide" [lacto-$N$-neotetraose is the trivial name
for an oligosaccharide isolated from human milk (Kuhn and Gauhe, 1962)
which has a structure identical with the carbohydrate part of this gly-
colipid] or "paragloboside." This unsubstituted ceramide tetrasaccharide
has been isolated in low yields from erythrocytes (Siddiqui and Hakomori,
1973; Ando et al., 1973). The carbohydrate chains in these glycolipids are
always attached via a glucose residue to the nitrogenous base sphingosine
in the ceramide moiety. Thus in the blood-group-active glycolipids, glucose provides the linkage between the oligosaccharide chain and the remainder of the molecule, whereas in the blood-group-active glycoproteins
from secretions, $N$-acetylgalactosamine is the sugar involved in the carbohydrate–peptide linkage. This structural difference explains why $N$-
acetylgalactosamine is always present in the secreted glycoprotein macromolecules but occurs in the blood-group-active glycosphingolipids only
if they carry group A determinants. In composition, the ceramide moieties
of the blood-group-active glycolipids are all closely similar and $C_{22}$ and
$C_{24}$ fatty acids predominate (Hakomori and Strycharz 1968; Koscielak et
al., 1973; Ando and Yamakawa, 1973).

The structures of some A, B, and H glycolipids with longer
carbohydrate chains are given in Table V. Hakomori et al. (1972) characterized four types of A-active glycolipid, $A^a$, $A^b$, $A^c$ and $A^d$. $A^a$ cor-
responds to the simplest from (Table IV) and $A^b$ (Table V) has a carbohydrate chain which is elongated by an additional β-Gal(1→4)-β-GlcNAc
unit. The third more complex type, $A^c$, has a branched structure at the
nonreducing end similar to that proposed for the A-active glycoproteins
(Fig. 3b) except that in $A^c$ both branches have the Type 2 structure. The
exact structure of $A^d$ is not yet elucidated but the authors consider it to
be similar to $A^c$ but to be even more complex with an additional branching
structure. The H-active glycolipids with larger carbohydrate moieties
(Table V) are essentially similar to the A-active glycolipids apart from the
presence of the terminal nonreducing $N$-acetylgalactosamine in the A-
active molecules. B-active glycolipids with branched structures similar
to $A^c$, except for the presence of terminal nonreducing α-galactosyl residues in place of α-$N$-acetylgalactosaminyl residues, have not yet been

**TABLE IV. Structures of the Simplest Forms of H, A, and B Glycosphingolipids Isolated from Red Cell Membranes and of Their Precursor, Lacto-N-neotetraosyl Ceramide**

| Substance | Specificity | Structure | Reference |
|---|---|---|---|
| Lacto-N-neotetraosyl ceramide (paragloboside) | Type XIV | β-Gal(1→4)β-GlcNAc(1→3)β-Gal(1→4)Glc-Ceramide | Siddiqui and Hakomori (1973); Ando et al. (1973) |
| H Glycolipid (H1) | H | β-Gal(1→4)β-GlcNAc(1→3)β-Gal(1→4)Glc-Ceramide<br>↑1,2<br>α-Fuc | Koscielak et al. (1973); Stellner et al. (1973) |
| A Glycolipid (A″) | A | α-GalNAc(1→3)β-Gal(1→4)β-GlcNAc(1→3)β-Gal(1→4)Glc-Ceramide<br>↑1,2<br>α-Fuc | Hakomori et al. (1972) |
| B Glycolipid (B1) | B | α-Gal(1→3)β-Gal(1→4)β-GlcNAc(1→3)β-Gal(1→4)Glc-Ceramide<br>↑1,2<br>α-Fuc | Koscielak et al. (1973); Hanfland (1975) |

TABLE V. Structures of More Complex H-, A- and B-Active Glycolipids Isolated from Human Red Cell Membranes

*H-active structures*

$H_2$   α-Fuc(1→2)β-Gal(1→4)β-GlcNAc(1→3)β-Gal(1→4)β-GlcNAc(1→3)β-Gal(1→4)Glc-ceramide    Koscielak *et al.* (1973); Watanabe *et al.* (1975)

$H_3$   α-Fuc(1→2)β-Gal(1→4)β-GlcNAc(1→3)⟍

                         β-Gal(1→4)β-GlcNAc(1→3)β-Gal(1→4)Glc-ceramide    Watanabe *et al.* (1975)

     α-Fuc(1→2)β-Gal(1→4)β-GlcNAc(1→6)⟋

S22   α-Fuc(1→2)β-Gal(1→4)β-GlcNAc(1→3)⟍

                         β-Gal(1→4)[β-GlcNAc(1→3)β-Gal]$_7$(1→4)Glc-ceramide    Gardas (1976*a*)

     α-Fuc(1→2)β-Gal(1→4)β-GlcNAc(1→6)⟋

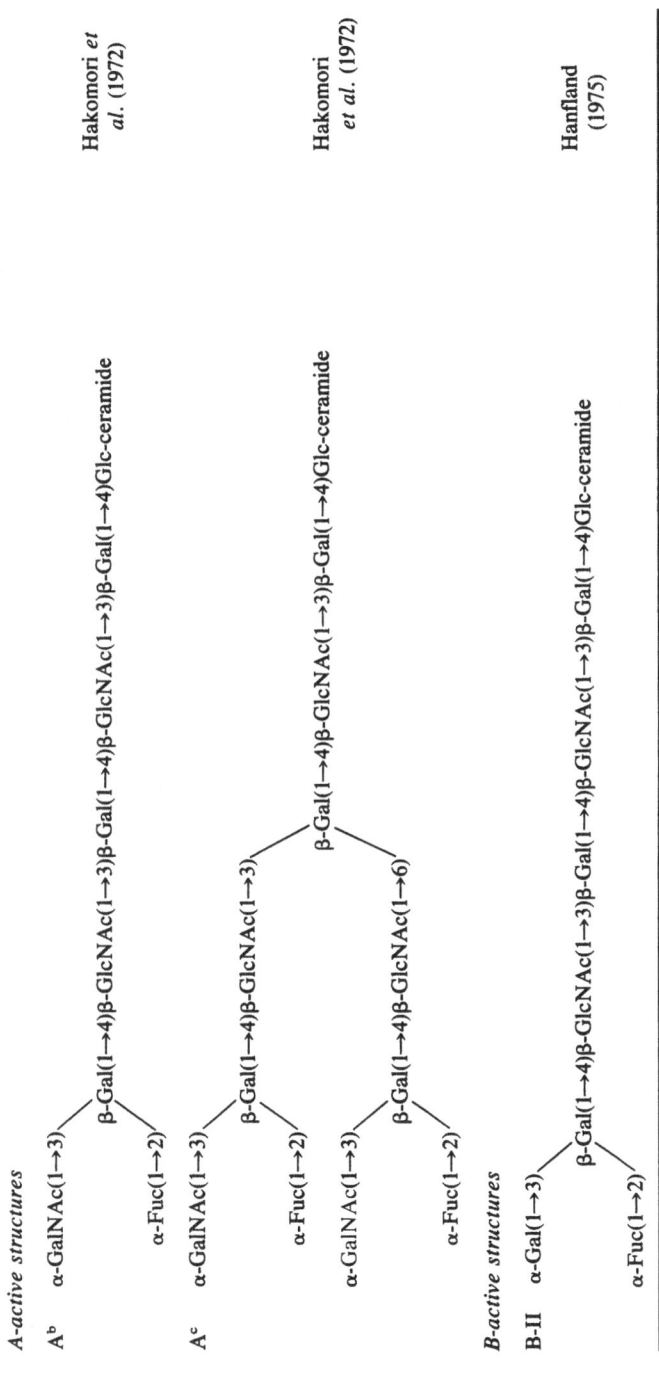

*A-active structures*

A[b]　α-GalNAc(1→3)⟍
　　　　　　　　　　β-Gal(1→4)β-GlcNAc(1→3)β-Gal(1→4)β-GlcNAc(1→3)β-Gal(1→4)Glc-ceramide　　Hakomori *et al.* (1972)
　　　α-Fuc(1→2)⟋

A[c]　α-GalNAc(1→3)⟍
　　　　　　　　　　β-Gal(1→4)β-GlcNAc(1→3)⟍
　　　α-Fuc(1→2)⟋　　　　　　　　　　　　　　β-Gal(1→4)β-GlcNAc(1→3)β-Gal(1→4)Glc-ceramide　　Hakomori *et al.* (1972)
　　α-GalNAc(1→3)⟍
　　　　　　　　　　β-Gal(1→4)β-GlcNAc(1→6)⟋
　　　α-Fuc(1→2)⟋

*B-active structures*

B-II　α-Gal(1→3)⟍
　　　　　　　　　β-Gal(1→4)β-GlcNAc(1→3)β-Gal(1→4)β-GlcNAc(1→3)β-Gal(1→4)Glc-ceramide　　Hanfland (1975)
　　　α-Fuc(1→2)⟋

characterized but there is no reason to believe that they do not occur on red cell membranes of group B individuals.

Evidence for the presence in human erythrocyte membranes of high molecular weight glycolipids with carbohydrate moieties of a size and degree of complexity hitherto unknown in glycosphingolipids was first presented by Gardas and Koscielak (1974a). These glycosphingolipids displayed A, B, H, and I blood group activity, contained 20–40 sugar residues per molecule, and were readily soluble in water because the large polar carbohydrate group masked the hydrophobic properties of the lipid component. A glycolipid with H and I activity isolated from group O red cell membranes which had 22 sugar residues was studied by Gardas (1976a) and assigned the structure S22 (Table V). Subsequently an A-active glycolipid possessing 23 sugars was assigned a structure identical with S22 except that one of the terminal β-galactosyl residues was substituted by an α(1→3) linked N-acetylgalactosamine unit (Gardas, 1978). Even more complex glycosphingolipids containing up to 60 sugar residues per molecule have been described (Koscielak et al., 1976a, 1978a). In view of their unusual complexity these compounds were designated poly(glycosyl) ceramides. Structural studies on these materials indicate that they are highly branched and may carry several blood group determinants on one molecule. In contrast to the branched structures in the ovarian cyst blood group glycoprotein (Fig. 3) these complex glycolipids have only Type 2 chains. Koscielak et al. (1976a) considered that the yields of these poly(glycosyl) ceramides were sufficiently high to suggest that they constituted the major recognition sites for A, B, and H antigens on human red cells; a view supported by the work of Dejter-Juszynski et al. (1978) who confirmed the existence of these highly glycosylated, water-soluble ABH-specific sphingolipids and, by a modified isolation procedure, succeeded in obtaining them in even higher yields.

**Glycoproteins.**   The large body of work on the ABH-active glycosphingolipids from the red cell membrane in the last few years, together with the discovery of the poly(glycosyl) ceramides with atypical solubility properties for glycolipids, seemed to be leading to the conclusion that the blood-group-active macromolecules could be neatly classified into two categories: glycoproteins in epithelial secretions and glycosphingolipids on cell surfaces. Certainly, blood-group-active glycoproteins with the composition and structure of those isolated from epithelial secretions are not integral parts of the red cell membrane, nor are they readily absorbed onto the cell surface. However, over the last fifteen years, various groups of workers have reported blood group activity in "glycoprotein" fractions isolated from red cell membranes (Pöulik and Lauf, 1965; Zahler, 1968; Whittemore *et al.*, 1969; Yatziv and Flowers, 1971; Gardas and Koscielak, 1971; Marchesi and Andrews, 1971; Liotta *et al.*, 1972; Hamaguchi and Cleve, 1972; Tanner and Boxer, 1972; Fukuda and Osawa, 1973; Fujita and Cleve, 1975). In a number of instances the inference that the active substances were glycoprotein was based on the solubility properties of the molecules and not on rigorous chemical characterization of the isolated substances; these claims, therefore, needed reinvestigation following the discovery of the poly(glycosyl) ceramides. Contamination of glycoprotein preparations with adsorbed glycolipids probably is the explanation for some of the earlier observations. Marchesi and Andrews (1971) reported that the major sialoglycoprotein component of red cell membranes had ABH activity and Fujita and Cleve (1975) found activity associated with the minor glycoproteins. Brennessel and Goldstein (1974), however, reported that, although they routinely observed H activity in glycoproteins prepared from group O red cells by the methods of Marchesi and Andrews (1971) and Hamaguchi and Cleve (1972), this activity could be dissociated from the glycoproteins by affinity chromatography. The authors concluded that the H activity was due to another class of molecule, more probably glycolipid.

The molecular features of the major sialoglycoprotein, glycophorin A, of human red cell membranes are now well established (see Marchesi *et al.*, 1977). The complete amino acid sequence and the sites of oligosaccharide attachment have been determined. The N-terminal region of the polypeptide chain has a high concentration of threonine and serine residues and it is this region which carries the carbohydrate chains. Sixteen oligosaccharide chains are attached to the peptide; one of these chains is linked through *N*-acetylglucosamine to asparagine and the remaining fifteen are *O*-glycosidically linked via *N*-acetylgalactosamine to serine or threonine. The majority of the *O*-glycosidically-linked oligosaccharides appear to be tetrasaccharides bearing two sialic acid (NeuNAc) residues (Winzler, 1972):

$$\beta\text{-Gal}(1\rightarrow 3)\alpha\text{-GalNAc-Ser or Thr}$$

$$\uparrow^{2.3} \qquad \uparrow^{2.6}$$

$$\text{NeuNAc} \quad \text{NeuNAc}$$

Hence the carbohydrate chains start off in the same way as the chains in the secreted blood-group-specific glycoproteins (Fig. 3), with the disaccharide β-Gal(1→3)α-GalNAc linked to the peptide moiety. That these chains do not normally become further elongated to form H-, A-, or B-active structures is probably attributable to the action of powerful sialyltransferases which catalyze the addition of sialic acid. The structures formed are not acceptors for the *N*-acetylglucosaminyltransferase required for further growth of the chains (see Carlson *et al.*, 1973). However, providing the appropriate glycosyltransferases are available at the site of synthesis of the glycoprotein there appears to be no *a priori* reason why a few carbohydrate chains should not escape the action of the sialyltransferases and proceed to develop into H-active structures, although too few of these chains may be synthesized for the H activity to be detectable by normal serological methods. The most compelling evidence in favor of this possibility comes from the work of Takasaki and Kobata (1976). Radioactively labeled *N*-acetylgalactosamine was transferred to group O erythrocyte membranes by means of an *A*-gene-specified α-*N*-acetylgalactosaminyltransferase purified from human milk. The specificity of the transferase is such that only H-active structures serve as acceptors for the enzyme (see section on glycosyltransferase products of *H*, *A*, and *B* genes). Repeated treatment ensured that *N*-acetylgalactosamine was transferred to all the accessible acceptors. Polyacrylamide gel electrophoresis revealed that the labeled *N*-acetylgalactosamine was incorporated into the major and minor glycoproteins of the red cell membranes. On treatment of the glycoproteins with weak alkali all the radioactivity was released. This result was taken as an indication that the radioactive sugar had been transferred to H acceptor structures in the glycoproteins and not into contaminating glycolipids since the carbohydrate chains of glycolipids are stable to mild alkaline treatment whereas carbohydrate chains in glycoproteins linked *O*-glycosidically via *N*-acetylgalactosamine to serine or threonine are labile under these conditions.

More recently Finne *et al.* (1978) reported the presence of protein-bound blood group ABH antigens in human erythrocyte membranes in which the blood-group-active carbohydrate chains are linked to peptide via relatively alkali-stable linkages. The glycopeptides carrying ABH activities were prepared by pronase digestion of red cell membranes which had previously been exhaustively extracted by methods designed to remove both the low-molecular-weight glycolipids and the poly(glycosyl) ceramides. The isolated glycopeptides contained 50–60 sugar residues per molecule and, although not structurally characterized, appeared in many ways to resemble the poly(glycosyl) ceramides except that the glycopeptides contained amino acids and were free from glucose and sphingosine. Aspartic acid was the major amino acid component, and this fact, together with the stability to mild alkali, suggests that the blood group active carbohydrate chains are linked through $N$-acetylglucosamine to asparagine. The authors have designated these compounds poly(glycosyl) peptides. Although these glycopeptides had the A or B activity appropriate to the group of the red cells used as the starting material, the activity was not compared with that of other standard blood group substances and, therefore, their total contribution to the ABH recognition sites on the cell surface cannot be assessed. Nevertheless, the yields of the blood-group-active glycopeptides (0.3 mg per liter of blood) were comparable with those found by Koscielak *et al.* (1976a) (0.6 mg/liter of blood) for poly(glycosyl) ceramides. Further investigations on the poly(glycosyl) chains of the glycoproteins (Krusius *et al.*, 1978) indicated that most, if not all, the determinants, are carried on Type 2 chains as has been found for the erythrocyte glycosphingolipids. The finding of these glycoproteins with alkali-stable carbohydrate chains carrying blood group determinants is reconcilable with the results of Takasaki and Kobata (1976) only if it is assumed that the isolation method used by the latter authors does not extract the glycoproteins carrying the poly(glycosyl) chains.

## A, B, and H Antigens in Plasma

Although the presence of A, B, and H activities in plasma has been known for many years relatively little work has been done to characterize the substances carrying these activities. Cases have been reported where there was so much A or B substance in the plasma that it interfered with the normal grouping of the red cells, but the majority of these people were suffering either from cancer or from ovarian cysts (see Race and Sanger, 1975). After removal of the ovarian cysts, the serum of the patients returned to normal, and it can be assumed that the blood-group-active substances were glycoproteins that had spilled over into the circulation. However, observations on transfused patients and those who had received grafted cells suggested that in normal persons some of the A and B activity on the red cells might be acquired from the plasma. In this respect, considerable clarification on the occurrence of A and B substances in plasma has come recently from the studies of Crookston and her colleagues in Toronto (Crookston *et al.*, 1970; Tilley *et al.*, 1975; Crookston and Tilley, 1977; Crookston, 1978).

Renton and Hancock (1962) first reported that group O cells transfused to group A or B patients became agglutinable by selected group O sera. Wherrett *et al.* (1971) confirmed that transfused O cells take up A or B antigen from a recipient's plasma and subsequently Tilley *et al.* (1975) were successful in reproducing the effect *in vitro*. Although the substances have not been rigorously characterized they are known to circulate as part of a lipoprotein complex and it is assumed that the glycosphingolipid in the complex is taken up by the red cell membrane. In a group A individual the amount of A active glycosphingolipid is affected by the A subgroup, and by the individual's endowment with respect to *secretor* genes and *Lewis* genes (Crookston and Tilley, 1977); the amount is greatest in $A_1$ secretors who are Le $(a^- b^-)$. Cells that have taken up A and B glycosphingolipid are agglutinated by a cross-reacting antibody present in most group O sera but rarely react with anti-A and anti-B formed by group B and group A donors, respectively. The presence of these acquired antigens is, therefore, not detectable with the usual blood grouping reagents which react with the A and B antigens synthesized by the red cell precursors within the hemopoietic tissue. The cellular origin of the A and B glycosphingolipids in plasma is not known.

Although the structures of the A and B glycosphingolipids in plasma have not been precisely established, because there is competition with the product of the *Le* gene (see section on Biosynthesis of $Le^a$ and $Le^b$) the determinants are assumed to be built on Type 1 chain endings and are thus derived from lacto-*N*-tetraosyl ceramide (Table X). Recent evidence (Graham *et al.*, 1977; Hirsh and Graham, 1977) indicates that the anti-H reagents in most common use, such as *Ulex europaeus*, react with the Type 2 H determinants which are synthesized as integral parts of the red cell membrane and fail to detect Type 1 H determinants acquired from the plasma. On the basis of inhibition tests with Type 1 and Type 2 H oligosaccharides, Graham *et al.* (1978) suggest that the reactions of an antibody, formerly thought to be part of the Lewis system, and called anti-$Le^d$ (Potapov, 1970), fit well with the assumption that it is detecting Type 1 H determinants taken up onto red cells from the plasma. The Type 1 H determinant in plasma is associated with glycosphingolipid (Crookston, 1978).

A sharp distinction between antibodies detecting the Type 1 and Type 2 H determinants would be in accord with the observations of Lemieux (1978) that from a stereochemical point of view the two determinants are vastly different molecular structures.

Although there is an exchange between plasma and erythrocyte pools of neutral glycosphingolipids (Dawson and Sweeley, 1970), this exchange in human blood appears to be largely restricted to glycosphingolipids with very short carbohydrate chains, namely, glucosyl ceramide and lactosyl ceramide (Koscielak et al., 1978b). Hence, although the erythrocytes can acquire blood-group-active glycosphingolipids from lipoproteins in the plasma, no exchange would be expected to occur between the plasma and the blood-group-active glycosphingolipids that are synthesized by the red cell precursors.

## Glycolipids with ABH Activity in Other Tissues

Glycolipids with A, B, and H activity have been found in parenchymatous organs and in glandular tissues (Hakomori, 1970). The quantities of blood group glycolipids in parenchymatous organs (liver, spleen, kidney) were approximately in the same range as in erythrocyte stroma but a higher quantity of blood-group-active glycolipids was generally found in glandular tissues (pancreas and stomach linings). A ceramide hexasaccharide accumulating in the pancreas of a patient with Fabry's disease, an inherited condition characterized by defective $\alpha$-galactosidase activity, was found to have blood group B serological activity. Characterization of the glycolipid (Wherrett and Hakomori, 1973) showed the following structures to be present:

$$\alpha\text{-Gal}(1\rightarrow 3)\beta\text{-Gal}(1\rightarrow 3) \text{ (and } 1\rightarrow 4)\beta\text{-GlcNAc}(1\rightarrow 3)\beta\text{-Gal}(1\rightarrow 4)\text{Glc-CER}$$
$$\uparrow {\scriptstyle 1,2}$$
$$\alpha\text{-Fuc}$$

The proportions of the two structures $\beta$-Gal($1\rightarrow 3$)GlcNAc (Type 1 chain) and $\beta$-Gal($1\rightarrow 4$)GlcNAc (Type 2 chain) was 4 : 1. Hence in the pancreas the glycolipids bearing blood group B determinants appear to be synthesized on both lacto-N-neotetraosyl ceramide (Table IV) and lacto-N-tetraosyl ceramide (Table X) precursors.

Glycolipids with A, B, and H blood group activity have also been isolated from the gastric mucosa of pigs and dogs (see McKibbin, 1978).

## Oligosaccharides with A, B, and H Activity in Milk and Urine

Naturally occurring oligosaccharides containing terminal nonreducing structures related to the A, B, and H blood group determinants occur in milk (Kobata, 1972) and urine (Lundblad, 1978). Shen *et al.* (1968) found that the trisaccharide 2'-fucosyllactose ($\alpha$-Fuc(1→2)$\beta$-Gal(1→4)Glc), earlier characterized by Kuhn *et al.*, (1955), occurred only in the milk of ABH secretors. Since this oligosaccharide has H activity (Watkins and Morgan, 1962) and the presence or absence of H had been shown to correlate with secretor status (Watkins, 1959), it appeared that the synthesis of this oligosaccharide was under the control of the *H* gene. This was the first recognition that the structures of the oligosaccharides found in human milk were regulated by genetic factors. Subsequently, Lundblad (1970) showed a correlation between the ABO blood group, secretor status, and the nature of the fucose-containing oligosaccharides in human urine.

### The A₁ and A₂ Subgroups of A

The characteristic differences between the two major inherited subgroups of A, namely $A_1$ and $A_2$, are that (1) certain sera (anti-$A_1$) react only with $A_1$ erythrocytes and (2) $A_2$ erythrocytes have more H activity than $A_1$ cells. The nature of the difference between the subgroups is still controversial. One view is that the difference is essentially quantitative and that the same A determinants are present on red cells and in the secreted substances in both $A_1$ and $A_2$ individuals, but that in $A_2$ individuals fewer H structures are changed to A determinants (Watkins and Morgan, 1957a, 1959; Mäkelä *et al.*, 1969). The second view is that a qualitative difference exists between the determinants in $A_1$ and $A_2$ phenotypes (Moreno *et al.*, 1971; Mohn *et al.*, 1977; Kisailus and Kabat, 1978).

Several groups of workers (Greenbury *et al.*, 1965; Economidou *et al.*, 1967; Williams and Voak, 1972) have established unequivocally that there are far fewer A sites on $A_2$ cells than on $A_1$ cells. More recent work has indicated that in both $A_1$ and $A_2$ phenotypes there are several different populations of red cells varying from antigen-rich to antigen-poor cells. Using a fluorescent anti-$A_1$ reagent, Rochant *et al.* (1976) observed that $A_1$ cells were a mixture of at least three populations: 20–30% of the cells gave strong fluorescence, 50–60% of the cells gave intermediate fluorescence and the remainder gave only very pale fluorescence. The $A_2$ cells showed a strikingly different pattern with the majority of the cells giving only very faint fluorescence, but even so there were rare cells which exhibited a fluorescence as strong as the strongest $A_1$ cells. Thus in group

$A_2$ individuals there is a minor cell population exhibiting $A_1$ specificity. These results therefore point to a quantitative, rather than a qualitative, difference between the two subgroups. However, Economidou *et al.* (1967) also observed differences in the equilibrium constants and rate of dissociation between anti-A antibodies and group $A_1$ and $A_2$ cells which they believed to be consistent with a difference in molecular structure between the two antigenic sites. On the basis of immunochemical studies with $A_1$ and $A_2$ glycoproteins, Moreno *et al.* (1971) and Kisailus and Kabat (1978) proposed that the qualitative difference between the $A_1$ and $A_2$ phenotypes resided in the fact that the A determinants in $A_1$ individuals are based on Type 1 chains whereas in $A_2$ individuals they are based on Type 2 chains (see Fig. 2). In competitive binding assays of $A_1$ and $A_2$ blood group substances with insolubilized anti-A serum and insolubilized A lectin from *Dolichos biflorus*, parallel inhibition lines were obtained for $A_1$ and $A_2$ substances with the insolubilized *Dolichos* reagent, but the slopes of the inhibition lines were different with the insolubilized anti-A serum. This evidence was interpreted by Kisailus and Kabat (1978) as being consistent with the proposed qualitative difference in the structure of the $A_1$ and $A_2$ determinants. That such a structural difference forms the basis of the $A_1$–$A_2$ subgroups is, however, difficult to reconcile with the observations from a number of different laboratories that only Type 2 chain determinants have been found in the A-active glycolipids and glycoproteins isolated from erythrocytes and also with the biosynthetic evidence to be discussed later.

On the basis of methylation studies on the carbohydrate moiety of the very complex poly(glycosyl) ceramides isolated from group $A_1$ and $A_2$ bloods, Koscielak *et al.* (1976a) concluded that the structures of the A determinants were identical. However, in the poly(glycosyl) ceramides isolated from group $A_1$ cells there were approximately three times as many A determinants. From a study of the smaller A-active glycolipids, Hakomori *et al.* (1977a) suggested that $A_2$ erythrocytes may be characterized by having a higher content of incomplete $A^c$ (Table V) and $A^d$ glycolipids, that is, branched structures having an A determinant on one branch and an H determinant on the other.

## Ii Specificities and Structures of Some Ii Determinants

In the ABH blood-group-specific glycoproteins from secretions, the I determinants are largely cryptic antigens revealed only after partial degradation of the carbohydrate chains (Feizi *et al.*, 1971*a*). I specificity is, however, expressed strongly on the majority of adult erythrocytes (Wiener *et al.*, 1956), and Gardas and Koscielak (1974*b*) found that on *n*-butanol extraction of human red cell membranes, I activity was associated with the antigens that also exhibit A, B, and H blood group activity. Subsequently Watanabe *et al.* (1975) showed that the branched H-active glycolipids $H_3$ (Table V) and $H_4$ exhibited I antigenic activity both by inhibition of agglutination and precipitation reactions, whereas the simpler straight chain $H_1$ and $H_2$ glycolipids (Table IV and V) were devoid of I activity. The I activity of the poly(glycosyl) ceramides examined by Koscielak *et al.* (1976*a*) increased with increasing molecular weight of the fractions and could also be correlated with the number of terminal galactose residues. These authors concluded that the terminal galactose structures were probably associated with I determinants, but removal of this galactose with β-galactosidase did not significantly affect the I activity as measured by immunodiffusion with anti-I sera. Examination of the sequential degradation products of HI-active glycolipids with ten anti-I sera and one anti-HI serum enabled the anti-I reagents to be divided into two categories (Gardas, 1976*b*). Removal of fucose destroyed the activity with anti-HI serum but left the inhibitory activity for the other anti-I sera unimpaired (Fig. 5). Removal of the terminal β-galactosyl residues destroyed the reactivity of the glycolipids with six of the anti-I reagents, but with the remaining four sera the activity was unchanged or only slightly diminished. Finally, removal of the *N*-acetylglucosamine destroyed the

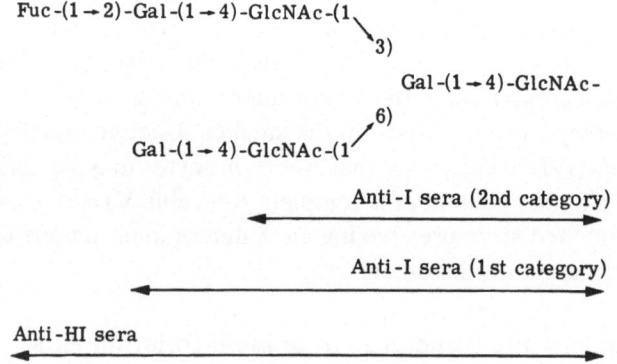

Fig. 5. Tentative structure of I-antigen complex proposed by Gardas (1976*b*). The arrows indicate the structures recognized by different anti-I sera. Abbreviations as in Figs. 1 and 2.

activity of the glycolipid with all the anti-I reagents. These experiments thus enabled the ten anti-I sera examined to be divided into a category needing a β-galactosyl end-group and a second category reacting with an internal part of the glycolipid chain of which N-acetylglucosamine is an essential constituent (Fig. 5).

Cold agglutinins with anti-I and anti-i specificity are generally monoclonal (Roelcke, 1974), and the heterogeneity of these reagents is well known to serologists (Dzierzkowa-Borodej et al., 1975). On the basis of their reaction in quantitative precipitation assays with various purified blood group substances from human ovarian cysts, anti-I sera were classified into six groups and anti-i sera into four groups (Feizi and Kabat, 1972). The combining site for one anti-I(Ma) (group 1) was shown by inhibition assays with oligosaccharides to be specific for the β-Gal(1→4)β-GlcNAc(1→6)-R structure (Feizi et al., 1971b). The presence of this sequence was recently demonstrated in I blood group active poly(glycosyl) ceramides (Zdebska and Koscielak, 1978) and a second anti-I serum (Woj) was shown to be specific for this structure. More precise definition of the combining sites of these two antibodies has been obtained from inhibition tests with chemically synthesized oligosaccharides (Feizi et al., 1978; Kabat et al., 1978). These studies confirmed that the Type 2 precursor chain in which the subterminal N-acetylglucosamine residue is linked by a (1→6) bond to the next sugar is involved in the combining site of the two anti-I sera and showed that the Type 1 precursor chain β-Gal(1→3)β-GlcNAc(1→3)Gal was inactive. Kabat et al. (1978) further delineated the relationship between the structure recognized by the group 1 anti-I sera and by anti-Type XIV pneumococcal serum. Whereas the anti-I sera require the subterminal β-N-acetylglucosaminyl residue to be linked 1→6 to the next sugar the inhibiting capacity of β-Gal(1→4)β-GlcNAc(1→6)Gal with anti-Type XIV serum was only slightly better than β-Gal(1→4)β-GlcNAc(1→3)Gal and both were only marginally more active than β-Gal(1→4)GlcNAc. The combining site of the Type XIV antiserum is therefore directed mainly towards the terminal disaccharide unit of the Type 2 precursor chain. The branched HI glycolipids examined by Gardas (1976b) failed to inhibit four autoimmune anti-i sera. Tsai et al. (1976), however, found that the agglutinins in one monoclonal anti-i serum (McC) were directed against the sequence β-Gal(1→4)β-GlcNAc(1→3)β-Gal . . . which occurs in paragloboside (Table IV). The authors found that the reactivity of adult normal I cells was increased to the same level as cord cells by mild proteolysis and suggest that short chain glycolipids behave as cryptic receptors in adult cells. A straight chain ceramide hexasaccharide that inhibited five out of six anti-i sera was described recently by Niemann *et al.* (1978). The glycolipid called "lacto-*N*-*nor*-hexaosyl ceramide" has the structure:

$$\beta\text{-Gal}(1{\to}4)\beta\text{-GlcNAc}(1{\to}3)\beta\text{-Gal}(1{\to}4)\beta\text{-GlcNAc}(1{\to}3)\beta\text{-Gal}(1{\to}4)\text{-Glc-CER}$$

This glycolipid differs from paragloboside only in the addition of an extra $\beta$-Gal$(1{\to}4)\beta$-GlcNAc disaccharide unit but paragloboside was not inhibitory in the tests carried out by Niemann *et al.* (1978). It was suggested that two repeating $\beta$-Gal$(1{\to}4)$GlcNAc residues and $\beta$-GlcNAc$(1{\to}3)$Gal residues might be essential for the full expression of activity. The glycosphingolipid was obtained by removal of sialic acid from a ganglioside isolated from bovine erythrocytes but the structure is identical with that of the $H_2$-glycolipid (Table V) isolated from human red cell membranes except for the additional fucose residue in the H-active compound. It is thus feasible to suppose that this incomplete chain occurs on the human erythrocyte surface.

## Relationship between the A, B, and H Determinant Structures and the Blood Group Genes

Toward the end of the 1950s, although knowledge of the detailed structure of the determinants was still fragmentary, sufficient genetic, serological, and biochemical information was available for profitable speculation on the relationship between the blood group genes and the serologically active structures (Watkins and Morgan, 1959; Watkins, 1959; Ceppellini, 1959). The molecular theory of inheritance had at that time recently highlighted the fact that the DNA of the structural gene loci coded for the primary amino acid sequence of the polypeptide chains of specific proteins (see Brenner, 1959). It was therefore evident that the carbohydrate structures of the determinants were not the primary products of the blood group genes, despite the clear cut manner of the inheritance of the blood group characters which render them so valuable as genetic markers in family studies. Essentially, the biosynthetic schemes proposed that the determinants are built up by the sequential addition of sugar units to a carbohydrate chain in a precursor molecule and that the blood group genes control the formation or functioning of the enzymes required for the attachment of those sugar residues that constitute the "immunodominant" sugars in each determinant structure. A new structure formed becomes the substrate for the next enzyme and the addition of another sugar residue masks the serological specificity of the preceding structure (Watkins, 1966). Thus a new phase in the biochemical genetics of the blood groups was launched in which the possibility arose of investigations on the enzymes concerned in the biosynthesis of the carbohydrate structures constituting the determinants. Guidelines for this research were available from the pioneering studies of Leloir and his co-workers (for review, see Leloir, 1964) which revealed the central role played by nucleotide-bound sugars in the biosynthesis of oligo- and polysaccharides, and the existence of glycosyltransferase enzymes whose function is to convey sugars from a nucleotide-sugar donor to an appropriate acceptor substrate. The blood group gene-specified enzymes were therefore assumed to be glycosyltransferases that catalyzed the transfer of sugars from a nucleotide sugar to the requisite acceptor structure in the carbohydrate chain of a glycoprotein or glycolipid molecule (Watkins, 1967). Experimental verification of these ideas has been obtained in many different laboratories and it is now established that the functional alleles at the *ABO* and *Hh* loci each code for, or control the functioning of, highly specific glycosyltransferase enzymes. Much of this evidence has been reviewed (Ginsburg, 1972; Watkins, 1974; Hakomori and Kobata, 1974; Schachter and Tilley, 1978; Cartron, 1978).

## *Glycosyltransferase Products of the H, A, and B Genes*

The *H*-gene-specified enzyme is a guanosine diphosphate L-fucose: β-D-galactosyl α-2-L-fucosyltransferase (E.C. 2.4.1.69) which catalyzes the reaction

$$\text{GDP-Fuc} + \beta\text{-Gal-R} \rightarrow \alpha\text{-Fuc}(1\rightarrow2)\beta\text{-Gal-R} + \text{GDP}$$

H-active structure

where R represents the remainder of a glycoprotein, a glycolipid, or an oligosaccharide. The rare alternative allele at this locus, *h*, either does not give an enzymically active product or gives one of such diminished activity that it cannot be detected by the methods available at present.

The H-active structures formed by the action of the *H* transferase are the substrates for the enzymic products of the *A* and *B* genes. The transferase controlled by the blood group *A* gene is a uridine diphosphate $N$-acetylgalactosamine: $O$-$\alpha$-L-fucosyl(1→2)D-galactose $\alpha$-3-$N$-acetyl-D-galactosaminyltransferase (E.C. 2.4.1.40) which catalyzes the reaction:

$$\text{UDP-GalNAc} + \beta\text{-Gal-R} \xrightarrow{\text{Mn}^{2+} \text{ ions}} \alpha\text{-GalNAc}(1\to3)\,\beta\text{-Gal-R} + \text{UDP}$$

$$\uparrow 1,2 \qquad\qquad\qquad\qquad\qquad \uparrow 1,2$$
$$\alpha\text{-Fuc} \qquad\qquad\qquad\qquad\qquad\quad \alpha\text{-Fuc}$$
$$\text{(H-active)} \qquad\qquad\qquad\qquad\qquad \text{(A-active)}$$

and the transferase controlled by the $B$ gene is a uridine diphosphate D-galactose: $O$-$\alpha$-L-fucosyl (→2) D-galactose $\alpha$-3-D-galactosyltransferase (E.C. 2.4.1.37) which catalyzes the reaction:

$$\text{UDP-Gal} + \beta\text{-Gal-R} \xrightarrow{\text{Mn}^{2+} \text{ ions}} \alpha\text{-Gal}(1\to3)\beta\text{-Gal-R} + \text{UDP}$$

$$\uparrow 1,2 \qquad\qquad\qquad\qquad\qquad \uparrow 1,2$$
$$\alpha\text{-Fuc} \qquad\qquad\qquad\qquad\qquad\quad \alpha\text{-Fuc}$$
$$\text{(H-active)} \qquad\qquad\qquad\qquad\qquad \text{(B-active)}$$

These pathways are summarized in Fig. 6. The third allele at the *ABO*

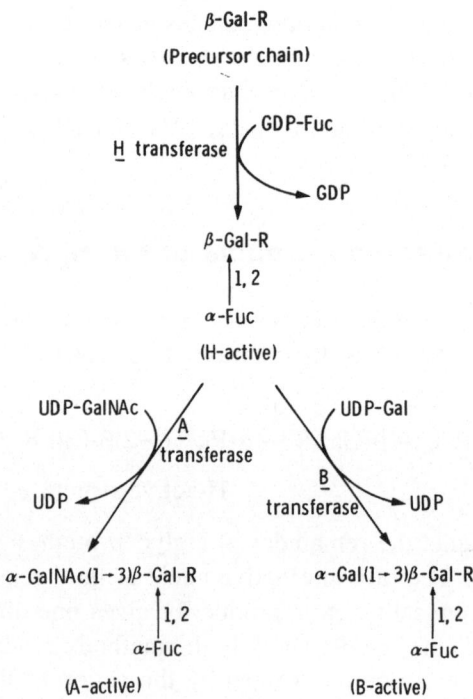

Fig. 6. Biochemical pathways for the formation of H, A, and B structures. Abbreviations as in Figs. 1 and 2.

locus, the *O* gene, is a silent allele that does not give rise to a transferase; hence in group O individuals the H-active structures do not undergo further transformation.

## The H-Gene-Specified α-2-L-Fucosyltransferase

**Methods for Detection and Assay.** Proof that an enzyme is the product of the *H* gene, ideally, should rest on the formation of H-specific structures in a precursor that lacks H serological activity. Such proof was obtained by Schenkel-Brunner *et al.* (1975), using sialidase-treated $O_h$ Bombay red cells (which owing to a genetic defect lack H activity) as the fucose acceptors, GDP-fucose as the sugar donor, and human gastric mucosa as the enzyme source; the defective cells became H-active. However, this experiment required unlabeled GDP-fucose which is not as yet commercially available and which in the hands of many workers has proved difficult to synthesize. Previously, detection of the fucosyltransferase had been achieved with radioactive GDP [$^{14}$C]fucose as the sugar donor and the inference that the enzyme was the *H* gene product was based upon the distribution of the enzyme in tissues known to be synthesizing H-specific glycoproteins or glycolipids and on the demonstration that the fucosyl residue was added in α(1→2) linkage to a terminal nonreducing β-galactosyl residue of an oligosaccharide or macromolecule (Shen *et al.*, 1968; Chester and Watkins, 1969; Schenkel-Brunner *et al.*, 1972; Munro and Schachter, 1973; Pacuszka and Koscielak, 1974).

Low-molecular-weight di- and oligosaccharides with terminal nonreducing β-galactosyl residues such as lactose (β-Gal(1→4)Glc), *N*-acetyllactosamine (β-Gal(1→4)GlcNAc), lacto-*N*-biose I (β-Gal(1→3) GlcNAc), and lacto-*N*-tetraose (β-Gal(1→3)β-GlcNAc(1→3)β-Gal(1→4)Glc) have been used by various workers as acceptors for the α-2-L-fucosyltransferase. The low-molecular-weight products have the advantage that they are separable from endogenous acceptors in the enzyme source by chromatographic procedures and can be provisionally identified by means of their $R_f$ values in various solvents. Measurement of the amount of radioactive [$^{14}$C]fucose incorporated into the product enables the activity of the enzyme to be quantitatively assayed. More rigorous characterization of the products is achieved either by treatment with linkage specific α-L-fucosidases which liberate [$^{14}$C]fucose only when it is linked α(1→2) to a β-galactosyl residue (Chester and Watkins, 1969; Schenkel-Brunner *et al.*, 1972; Pacuszka and Koscielak, 1976) or by alkaline degradation (Shen *et al.*, 1968; Munro and Schachter, 1973; Pacuszka and Koscielak, 1974). An $\alpha(1\rightarrow2)$ glycosidic linkage between fucose and the subterminal $\beta$-galactosyl residue of an oligosaccharide is stable to alkali yielding $\alpha$-2-L-fucosylgalactose and $\alpha$-2-L-fucosyltalose as the products of alkaline degradation whereas free fucose is the product when the sugar is bound in other positional linkages to galactose (Kuhn *et al.*, 1958).

Macromolecular substances, such as human blood group precursor glycoprotein (Schenkel-Brunner *et al.*, 1972), $\alpha_1$-acid glycoprotein treated with sialidase to expose terminal $\beta$-galactosyl residues (Munro and Schachter, 1973), the glycosphingolipid lacto-*N*-neotetraosyl ceramide (Pacuszka and Koscielak, 1976), and porcine submaxillary mucin (Bosmann *et al.*, 1968) have also been used as acceptor substrates for the detection of the $\alpha$-2-L-fucosyltransferase. In general, when radioactive GDP-L-fucose is used as the sugar donor, determination of the positional linkage of the added L-[$^{14}$C]fucose is more difficult to ascertain with macromolecular substrates than when low-molecular-weight acceptors are employed. The tissue homogenates or body fluids being analyzed for the $\alpha$-2-fucosyltransferase may contain at least three other fucosyltransferases; one is the Lewis *Le* gene specified $\alpha$-4-L-fucosyltransferases which catalyzes the addition of L-fucose to the C-4 position of subterminal *N*-acetyl-D-glucosaminyl residues (Chester and Watkins, 1969; Grollman *et al.*, 1969); a second is the $\alpha$-3-L-fucosyltransferase which catalyses the transfer of L-fucose into the C-3 position of subterminal *N*-acetyl-D glucosaminyl or D-glucosyl residues (Shen *et al.*, 1968; Chester and Watkins, 1969; Schenkel-Brunner *et al.*, 1972); the third is an L-fucosyltransferase that catalyzes the addition of fucose to *N*-acetylglucosamine residues which are linked to asparagine in the peptide backbone of a glycoprotein (Wilson *et al.*, 1976). It is therefore very important to use methods that distinguish the product of action of the $\alpha$-2-L-fucosyltransferase from the products given by the other fucosyltransferases. In the search for a more specific acceptor, and a more rapid assay procedure, phenyl-$\beta$-D-galactoside was found to be an efficient substrate for the $\alpha$-2-L-fucosyltransferases (Chester *et al.*, 1976). The results of chemical and enzymic degradation of the product were consistent with the interpretation that the L-fucosyl residue is transferred from GDP-fucose to phenyl-$\beta$-D-galactopryanoside in $\alpha$-anomeric linkage to the C-2 position of the $\beta$-galactosyl moiety to give the compound phenyl 2-*O*-($\alpha$-L-fucopyranosyl)-$\beta$-*D*-galactopyranoside. The mobility of this product is such that it can be clearly separated from the other radioactive components in the reaction mixture by chromatography for only four hours. In the author's laboratory this substrate is now used for all routine measurements of the α-2-fucosyl-transferase.

**Role of the Secretor Gene *Se*.** As mentioned previously, *A*, *B*, and *H* genes, are, with very rare exceptions, expressed on the red cells whenever they are part of the genome, but their expression in the secreted glycoproteins depends upon the inheritance of another gene *Se*, which segregates independently of *ABO* and *Hh*. The *Se* gene may be considered a type of regulator, or "switch" gene, which in secretory cells allows the expression of the *H*-gene-dependent α-2-fucosyltransferase. The mechanism by which the control is effected is unknown and it could be equally suggested that in these same cells a double dose of the allele *se* suppresses the formation of the α-2-fucosyltransferase. Ganshow and Paigen (1967) described a Mendelian factor in mice, distinct from the glucuronidase structural gene, which is required for the incorporation of β-glucuronidase into the microsomal membranes of liver cells. This second gene functions only in certain tissues and the authors suggest that perhaps many proteins are under the control of a special class of genetic elements which determine whether a protein can exist in functional state at a particular genetic location. The possible relationship between this finding and the mode of operation of the *Se* gene was pointed out by Ginsburg *et al.* (1971).

**Distribution of the α-2-L-Fucosyltransferase in Different Tissues.** α-2-L-Fucosyltransferases have been characterized in human milk (Shen *et al.*, 1968), submaxillary gland and stomach mucosal tissue (Chester and Watkins, 1969), serum (Schenkel-Brunner *et al.*, 1972) and bone marrow (Pacuszka and Koscielak, 1974). In agreement with the theory that in tissues producing the secreted blood group substances the gene *Se* controls the expression of the *H* gene, the α-2-L-fucosyltransferase is found in milk and submaxillary glands when the specimens come from ABH secretors and is absent in these tissues from nonsecretors. The secretor gene is not expressed uniformly throughout the body even in mucus-producing tissues. Hartmann (1941) demonstrated the persistence of small amounts of A and B substances in stomach and other organs from nonsecretors and Szulman (1966) confirmed by the immunofluorescence technique that in the deeper reaches of gastric mucus-secreting membranes synthesis of ABH substances goes to completion irrespective of secretor status. In accordance with these observations, when stomach mucosal preparations are used as an enzyme source small amounts of α-2-L-fucosyltransferase activity are found even in tissues obtained from donors grouped as nonsecretors on the basis of saliva-inhibition tests (Chester, 1971). In human bone marrow (Pucuszka and Koscielak, 1974) the transferase is detectable irrespective of the ABH secretor status of the donors, a finding to be expected since in the hemopoietic tissue the *H* gene is not under the control of the secretor gene. The α-2-L-fucosyltransferase is also present in the serum of both secretors and nonsecretors (Schenkel-Brunner *et al.*, 1972; Munro and Schachter, 1973) and the levels do not appear to be related to secretor–nonsecretor status (Chester *et al.*, 1976). Evidence derived from measurements of α-2-L-fucosyltransferase activity in the sera from individuals of the para-Bombay phenotype (see section on rare ABO variants) indicates that the α-2-L-fucosyltransferase in plasma originates largely, if not exclusively, from the hemopoietic tissue (Mulet *et al.*, 1977; Watkins, 1978).

**Purification of the α-2-Fucosyltransferase.** Prieels *et al.* (1977) reported an 18,000-fold purification of the α-2-fucosyltransferase in human milk by a two-step procedure involving ion-exchange chromatography on SP-Sephadex C-50, followed by affinity chromatography on a column of GDP--hexanolamine-agarose. The purified enzyme had a pH optimum of 5.9–6.2 and did not show a requirement for a metal ion cofactor. No evidence was given concerning the homogeneity of this enzyme.

**Acceptor Specificity.** A terminal nonreducing, unsubstituted β-D-galactopyranosyl residue appears to be the major requirement in the acceptor substrates utilized by the α-2-fucosyltransferase (Fig. 7). D-Galactose itself is a poor acceptor and D-fucose (6-deoxy-D-galactose) has

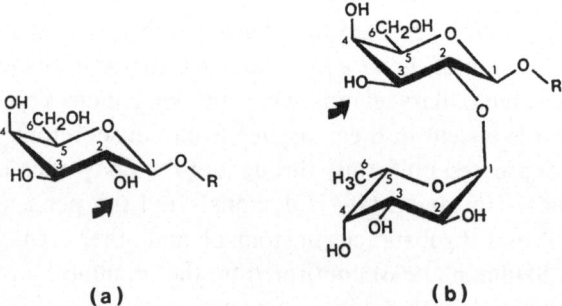

(a)                                     (b)

Fig. 7. Structures of acceptor substrates for (a) the *H*-gene-specified α-2-L-fucosyltransferase and (b) the *A*-gene-specified α-3-*N*-acetyl-D-galactosaminyltransferase and the *B*-gene-specified α-3-galactosyltransferase. The arrows indicate the positions to which the respective sugars are transferred.

about the same efficiency, indicating that the hydroxyl group at C-6 of the galactose is not necessary for binding the enzyme. That the D-configuration of the sugar is essential may be inferred from the failure of L-galactose or L-fucose to function as acceptors. Similarly, the necessity for the β-anomeric linkage of the galactose was demonstrated by tests with a series of alkyl and aryl-D-galactopyranosides. None of the α-linked galactosides accepted L-fucose but all the β-linked galactopyranosides were more efficient acceptors than galactose itself (Chester *et al.*, 1976).

In the H determinants occurring in the human-blood-group-active glycoproteins and glycolipids, the β-galactosyl residue is usually linked to *N*-acetylglucosamine by either a 1→3 (Type 1) or 1→4 (Type 2) linkage. Despite the vast difference in conformation of the Type 1 and 2 disaccharides (Lemieux, 1978), the α-2-fucosyltransferases conveys fucose to both these structures (Shen *et al.*, 1968; Chester and Watkins, 1969). Apparently, therefore, the combining site of the transferase does not include the *N*-acetylglucosamine residue. This is supported by the observation that *in vitro* both β-Gal(1→3)GalNAc and β-Gal(1→3)Fru act as acceptors for the transferase (P. H. Johnson and W. M. Watkins, unpublished observations). Although galactose linked to fructose is unlikely to occur *in vivo*, oligosaccharides have been isolated from human-H-active glycoproteins in which the β-galactosyl residue substituted with fucose is subterminal to *N*-acetylgalactosamine. Rovis *et al.* (1973) isolated, from a glycoprotein of ovarian cyst origin, an H-active oligosaccharide with the structure

$$\alpha\text{-Fuc}(1\rightarrow2)\beta\text{-Gal}(1\rightarrow3)\diagdown$$
$$\text{GalNAc}$$
$$\alpha\text{-Fuc}(1\rightarrow2)\beta\text{-Gal}(1\rightarrow4)\beta\text{-GlcNAc}(1\rightarrow6)\diagup$$

and Takasaki *et al.* (1978) characterized a trisaccharide from the glycoproteins of human erythrocyte membranes as α-Fuc(1→2)β-Gal(1→3) GalNAc.

The disaccharides α-GalNAc(1→3)Gal (A-active) and α-Gal(1→3)Gal (B-active) are not acceptors of 2-linked fucose (Chester, 1971), a finding in agreement with the concept that the fucose residue is added before the *N*-acetylgalactosamine or galactose residues in the A and B determinant structures.

**H-Gene-Specified Transferase Levels in Sera from Individuals of Different ABO Groups.** The α-2-L-fucosyltransferase occurs in the serum of all individuals with normal ABO groups. Preliminary examination of the enzyme levels in persons of different ABO groups indicated that, while there was a spread of activity for each group, the average level for donors of groups $A_1$, $A_2$, or $A_1B$ was higher than for other groups (Chester *et al.*, 1976). Subsequently, this observation was confirmed in a survey of 100 donors of each of the groups A, B, AB, and O when phenyl-β-D-galactoside was used as the acceptor for the α-2-linked fucose (Fig. 8). Mulet *et al.* (1977) reported similar findings using lacto-*N*-biose I as the acceptor substrate.

There is no explanation at present for the association between the *H* transferase level and ABO group but the possibility that the level of α-2-L-fucosyltransferase in the serum may be higher in an individual carrying an *A* gene has to be borne in mind in any attempts to assess dosage effects for the *H* transferase.

In the 400 serum samples from individuals of different ABO groups, there was no apparent correlation between the level of the *H*-gene-specified transferase activity and the age or sex of the donor (P. Greenwell and W. M. Watkins, unpublished results).

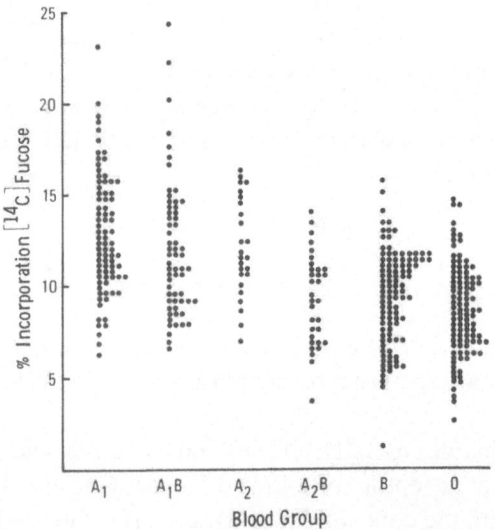

Fig. 8. *H*-gene-specified α-2-L-fucosyltransferase levels in sera from donors of different ABO blood groups (Chester *et al.*, 1977, cited in Watkins, 1978). Transferase activity was measured by the incorporation of [$^{14}$C]fucose into phenyl-β-D-galactoside as described by Chester *et al.* (1976). Each dot on the figure depicts the result of one assay. The mean incorporation for each group was $A_1$ 12.9% S.D. 2.5; $A_1B$ 11.9% S.D. 3.6; $A_2$ 12.1% S.D. 2.7; $A_2B$ 9.0%, S.D. 2.4; B 9.4% S.D. 2.5; O 8.6% S.D. 2.5.

## The *B*-Gene-Specified α-3-D-Galactosyltransferase

**Methods of Detection and Assay.** The *B*-gene-specified transferase may be detected and assayed by the transfer of radioactively labeled galactose from UDP-[$^{14}$C]galactose to low- or high-molecular-weight acceptors containing H-active structures (Race *et al.*, 1968; Kobata *et al.*, 1968*a*; Poretz and Watkins, 1972) or by its capacity to convert group O and A red cells into B- or AB-active cells, respectively, when unlabeled UDP-galactose is used as the sugar donor (Schenkel-Brunner and Tuppy, 1970; Race and Watkins, 1972*a*; Pacuszka and Koscielak, 1972).

The trisaccharide 2'-fucosyllactose (α-Fuc(1→2)β-Gal(1→4)Glc) which occurs in human milk (Kuhn *et al.*, 1955), and has H-serological activity (Watkins and Morgan, 1962), is a convenient low-molecular-weight acceptor substrate for the *B*-gene-dependent enzyme. The tetrasaccharide product is separated from the charged compounds in the reaction mixture by paper electrophoresis (Ziderman *et al.*, 1967; Race *et al.*, 1968) or by passage through an ion-exchange column (Kobata *et al.*, 1968*a*) and then separated from other neutral sugars by paper chromatography. The anomeric linkage of the radioactive product is established as α by treatment with α- and β-galactosidases of established specificity. This step is especially necessary when tests are being made for products of the *B* transferase because the sources of this enzyme usually contain β-galactosyltransferases in addition to the α-3-galactosyltransferase. Unequivocal proof of the positional linkage of the added galactose was obtained by the synthesis of the tetrasaccharide on a sufficiently large scale for methylation analysis (Race and Watkins, 1970). Confirmation that the α-linked galactose was transferred to the C-3 position of the acceptor β-galactosyl residue, together with the demonstration that the tetrasaccharide had B-serological activity, established that the enzyme associated with the blood group B character is a uridine diphosphate D-galactose: [α-1,2-L-fucosyl]-β-D-galactosylsaccharide α-3-galactosyltransferase.

The use of low-molecular-weight oligosaccharides as acceptors for the *B*-gene-specified transferase has made easier the task of determining the positional linkage of the transferred sugar and the nature of the acceptor. However the transferase has also been shown to work with macromolecular acceptors. The transfer of D-galactose in α-linkage to human H-active glycoproteins was achieved with submaxillary gland and stomach mucosal preparations from group B and AB individuals and not with similar preparations from group A or O individuals (Poretz and Watkins, 1972). A *B* transferase prepared from human milk also catalyzed the transfer of $\alpha$-linked galactosyl residues to H substance isolated from human erythrocytes (Pacuszka and Koscielak, 1972). More recently, net conversion of H-active glycoprotein into a B-active glycoprotein which inhibited the hemagglutination of B cells by anti-B serum, was obtained with a highly purified B transferase isolated from human serum (Carne and Watkins, 1977).

The transformation of group O red cells into B-active red cells was first demonstrated by Schenkel-Brunner and Tuppy (1970) by means of a *B* transferase extracted from human gastric mucosal microsomes. A similar conversion was achieved with the enzymes in group B milk (Pacuszka and Koscielek, 1972), group B serum (Race and Watkins 1972a), and group B saliva (Kogure and Furukawa, 1976). The failure of the $\alpha$-galactosyltransferase in human serum to transform cells of the Bombay $O_h$ phenotype was taken as support for the concept that H-active structures are the acceptors of the transferred galactosyl residues (Race and Watkins, 1972a). The activity of the *B* transferase can be assessed by titration of the converted cells against serial dilutions of anti-B serum.

**Distribution of the $\alpha$-3-D-Galactosyltransferase in Different Tissues.** An $\alpha$-galactosyltransferase found only in group B and AB subjects occurs in human stomach mucosa and submaxillary glands (Ziderman *et al.*, 1967; Race *et al.*, 1968), milk (Kobata *et al.*, 1968a), plasma (Sawicka, 1971), saliva (Kogure and Furukawa, 1976), red cell membranes (Koscielak *et al.*, 1976b) and ovarian cyst linings and fluids (Hearn *et al.*, 1972). In contrast to the *H*-gene-specified fucosyltransferase the B-gene-specified enzyme is found in submaxillary gland tissue, saliva, and milk from both secretors and nonsecretors; thus support is given for the hypothesis that failure to secrete B substance arises from the absence of the requisite H-acceptor substance and not from failure of expression of the *B* gene. The *B* transferase has also been found in particle-bound form in sublingual and palatine glands, lung, kidney, and bone marrow (C. Race, P. Greenwell, and W. M. Watkins, unpublished observations). The activity was particularly strong in the microsomal fraction from the kidney. No significant levels of $\alpha$-3-galactosyltransferase activity were detected in similar fractions from parotid glands, heart, liver, or spleen.

**Purification.** Two groups of workers have attempted to purify the blood group *B*-gene-dependent $\alpha$-3-galactosyltransferase in human plasma. A one-step affinity procedure which involved specific adsorption onto the

H determinants on group O erythrocyte membranes, followed by elution with the H-specific trisaccharide, 2'-fucosyllactose, yielded over 100,000-fold purification of the transferase (Carne and Watkins, 1977). There was evidence, however, that the enzyme had not been purified to homogeneity. Procedures based on conventional, multistep, chromatography were reported by Nagai *et al.* (1978*b*) to yield a product which was 400,000-fold purified and gave a single protein band on polyacrylamide gel electrophoresis at two different pH values. These authors started with four liters of plasma and estimated the final yield of purified enzyme to be about 40 µg. Hence plasma, although a convenient source of the *B* transferase, appears to contain very small amounts of the enzyme.

**Acceptor Specificity.** The *B* transferase has a high degree of specificity for the acceptor substrate (Kobata *et al.*, 1968*a*; Race *et al.*, 1968; Race and Watkins, 1969). All the low-molecular-weight oligosaccharides so far tested that function as acceptors of α-linked galactose (Table VI) contain a terminal β-galactosyl residue substituted at the C-2 position with L-fucose (Fig. 7). Whether the sugar next to the β-galactosyl residue is *N*-acetylglucosamine or glucose does not influence the capacity of the oligosaccharides to serve as acceptors. However, a fucosyl substituent on this subterminal sugar either alters the conformation of the molecules, or in some way sterically hinders the enzyme, so that transfer of the galactose unit is prevented (Table VI). The B transferase purified from plasma (Carne and Watkins, 1977) has the same acceptor specificity as the unpurified enzymes in milk (Kobata *et al.*, 1968*a*), stomach mucosa, and submaxillary glands (Race and Watkins, 1969).

**Metal Ion Requirements.** The *B* transferase has a requirement for $Mn^{2+}$ ions which cannot be replaced by other divalent metal ions (Carne and Watkins, 1977; Nagai *et al.*, 1978*b*).

**pH Optimum and Isoelectric Point.** The pH optimum of the α-3-galactosyltransferase in crude plasma has been reported as pH 6.5 (Topping and Watkins, 1975) and as pH 7.0 (Nagai *et al.*, 1978*b*). Differing values have also been reported for the purified enzyme: pH 6.5 (Carne and Watkins, 1977) and pH 7.5 (Nagai *et al.*, 1978*b*).

The isoelectric points of the *B* transferases in serum and ovarian cyst fluids from group B and AB individuals were determined by isoelectric focusing (Topping and Watkins, 1975). The major peaks of activity from both sources focused within the pH range 9–10. Kishi *et al.* (1977) also found that the major peak of α-3-galactosyltransferase activity in serum from group B and AB donors focused at about pH 9 and reported an

**TABLE VI.** Low-Molecular-Weight Acceptor Substrates for the Blood Group *A*- and *B*-
Gene-Specified Glycosyltransferases

| Name | Structure |
|---|---|
| Acceptor substrates | |
| 2-Fucosylgalactose[a] | α-Fuc(1→2)Gal |
| 2'-Fucosyllactose[b] | α-Fuc(1→2)β-Gal(1→4)Glc |
| 2'-Fucosyllactosamine[c] | α-Fuc(1→2)β-Gal(1→4)GlcNAc |
| Lacto-N-fucopentaose I[b] | α-Fuc(1→2)β-Gal(1→3)β-GlcNAc(1→3)β-Gal(1→4)Glc |
| Nonacceptors | |

3-Fucosyllactose[b]          β-Gal(1→4)
                                       \
                                         Glc
                                       /
                             α-Fuc(1→3)

Lacto-N-fucopentaose II[b]   β-Gal(1→3)
                                         \
                                           β-GlcNAc(1→3)β-Gal(1→4)Glc
                                         /
                             α-Fuc(1→4)

Lacto-N-difucohexaose I[b]   α-Fuc(1→2)β-Gal(1→3)
                                                   \
                                                     β-GlcNAc(1→3)β-Gal(1→4)Glc
                                                   /
                               α-Fuc(1→4)

Lactodifucotetraose[b]       α-Fuc(1→2)β-Gal(1→4)
                                                   \
                                                     Glc
                                                   /
                                         α-Fuc(1→3)

[a] Alkaline degradation product of Lacto-N-fucopentaose I (Kuhn *et al.*, 1958).
[b] Oligosaccharides isolated from human milk (see Kobata, 1972).
[c] Trisaccharide isolated from human H-substance (Rege *et al.*, 1964a) and prepared by chemical synthesis (Jacquinet and Sinäy, 1976).

additional minor peak which focused within the range 4.4–5.6. On the other hand saliva from the same donors gave only a single peak of α-3-galactosyltransferase activity which focused at about pH 8.

**Inhibition.** In contrast to the *A* transferase which is strongly inhibited by UDP-galactose the *B* transferase in crude serum appeared not to be inhibited by UDP-*N*-acetylgalactosamine (Race and Watkins, 1974). It was postulated that the difference in the combining sites of the *A* and

$B$ transferases may be such that the $A$-gene-specified enzyme can accommodate the smaller D-galactosyl residue in UDP-galactose whereas $N$-acetylgalactosamine, with the bulkier $N$-acetyl amino group at carbon-2 of the hexose ring, may not fit into the combining site of the $B$-gene-specified α-3-galactosyltransferase. Investigations with the purified $B$ transferase from serum showed that UDP-$N$-acetylgalactosamine is in fact a weak inhibitor of the enzyme but the apparent $K_i$ ($1 \times 10^{-4}$ M) is an order higher than the apparent $K_m$ for UDP-galactose ($1 \times 10^{-5}$ M) (Carne and Watkins, 1977). UDP is a strong competitive inhibitor of the $B$ transferase.

**Molecular Weight.** Gel filtration of crude plasma on a calibrated Sephadex G-200 column gave two peaks of α-3-galactosyltransferase activity (Nagai *et al.*, 1978*b*) One had a molecular weight of 200,000 and the other about 100,000. In the presence of 0.2 M NaCl only one active peak was eluted with a molecular weight of 80,000. Electrophoresis on SDS polyacrylamide gel indicated a subunit size of 40,000 and Nagai *et al.* (1978*b*) concluded that the active enzyme in 0.2 M NaCl is in dimeric form and that the transferase may assume an aggregated form at lower ionic strengths.

**Stability.** In crude serum the α-3-galactosyltransferase is stable to heat for 20 minutes at 55°C (Cartron *et al.*, 1978) but this property is lost on purification; the purified enzyme loses 60% of its activity after 20 minutes at this temperature (Carne and Watkins, 1977). Both the enzyme in whole serum and the purified transferase are labile if stored at $+4°$ but retain activity largely unchanged on storage at $-40°$ for several months (Carne and Watkins, 1979).

**Levels of Activity in the Sera of Individuals with a Normal Group B Red Cell Phenotype.** Badet *et al.* (1974) noted a bimodal distribution when they studied the α-3-galactosyltransferase levels in the Caucasian population of blood donors in Paris with a normal group B red cell phenotype. The major group, representing 85% of the whole, had an average level of transferase activity approximately one third to one half of the average found in the remaining 15%. The two groups were not related to the secretor status or to the genotype, *BB* or *BO,* of the individuals studied. However, the groups were clearly related to the agglutinability of the red cells by anti-B serum. In an African population comprising individuals of various ethnic groups, a third category was found in which the $B$ transferase levels were higher than any of those observed in the Caucasian population. In both populations the agglutinability of the B red cells by anti-H (*Ulex europaeus*) varied inversely with the level of *B* transferase activity, that is, the stronger the transferase the smaller the amount of H antigen detectable on the red cells. The two populations differed, however, in that for the African population there was no relationship between the agglutinability of the red cells by anti-B serum and the *B* transferase level (Badet *et al.*, 1976; Badet, 1976). The authors concluded that the strength of the B antigen on the erythrocyte depends upon both the strength of the H antigen and the strength of the α-3-galactosyltransferase and that the different results found for the two populations could probably be explained on the basis of the greater variability in the strength of the H antigen in the African population than in the Caucasian population.

## The *A*-Gene-Specified α-3-*N*-Acetylgalactosaminyltransferase

**Methods of Detection and Assay.**    The *A* transferase may be assayed in essentially the same way as the *B* transferase. The method most frequently employed is the transfer of [$^{14}$C]-*N*-acetylgalactosamine from the nucleotide donor UDP-[$^{14}$C]-*N*-acetylgalactosamine to the low-molecular-weight acceptor 2′-fucosyllactose. The labeled tetrasaccharide reaction product, α-[$^{14}$C]-GalNAc(1→3)[α-Fuc(1→2)]β-Gal(1→4)Glc, is separated from the charged components of the reaction mixture by paper electrophoresis (Hearn *et al.*, 1968), passage through ion exchange resin (Kobata *et al.*, 1968b), or ion exchange paper (Race and Watkins, 1974) and the neutral sugars are then separated by paper chromatography in an appropriate solvent. The tetrasaccharide is tentatively identified by its R$_f$ value but more rigorous characterization is achieved by testing with purified α-*N*-acetylgalactosaminidase and by comparison of the partial hydrolysis products with compounds of known structure (Hearn *et al.*, 1968; Kobata and Ginsburg, 1970). Synthesis of the tetrasaccharide on a larger scale enabled Kobata and Ginsburg (1970) to establish by periodate oxidation experiments that the *N*-acetylgalactosamine had been added to the C-3 position of the galactosyl residue of 2′-fucosyllactose and also to demonstrate that the product had blood group A serological specificity. The transferase may also be assayed by transfer of $^{14}$C-labeled *N*-acetylgalactosamine to the disaccharide 2-fucosylgalactose, to the Type 1 H chain analogue, lacto-*N*-fucopentaose I (Hearn *et al.*, 1968; Kobata and Ginsburg, 1970), and to macromolecular H-active glycoprotein (Tuppy and Schenkel-Brunner, 1969).

Conversion of group O red cells into A-active cells was first achieved by Schenkel-Brunner and Tuppy (1970) by means of an *A* transferase extracted from human gastric mucosa. The enzyme was incubated with group O cells in the presence of UDP-*N*-acetylgalactosamine and manganese ions. This method may be used to assay the *A* transferase but when serum is the enzyme source under test it has to be borne in mind that the transferase in the sera of group $A_2$ individuals confer only very weak A agglutinability on the red cells (Race and Watkins 1972*b*; Cartron *et al.*, 1975). That the degree of conversion of O cells into A-active cells cannot be directly related to the activity measured by the transfer of [$^{14}$C] *N*-acetylgalactosamine to an H-active glycoprotein was noted by Schenkel-Brunner and Tuppy (1973). With an enzyme extracted from the gastric mucosa of an $A_1$ individual the O cells first acquired $A_2$ specificity and only after prolonged incubation did the cells become agglutinable by anti-$A_1$ reagents. The H specificity of the cells gradually decreased as the A activity increased. With an enzyme extracted from the gastric mucosa of an $A_2$ individual the speed of conversion of O cells into A-active cells was much slower and when the $A^1$ transferase was diluted so as to have the same activity towards H-active glycoprotein as the $A^2$ transferase there was still a marked difference in the speed with which the two enzymes converted O red cells into A-active cells. A most interesting observation (Salmon and Cartron, 1976) is that when an $A^2$ gene is inherited together with a *B* gene in a group $A_2B$ individual, the α-*N*-acetylgalactosaminyltransferase in the serum has an increased capacity to confer A activity on group O cells. This phenomenon has been taken as an expression of allelic enhancement.

**Distribution of the α-3-*N*-Acetylgalactosaminyltransferase in Different Tissues.** The distribution of the *A*-gene-specified transferase in human tissues parallels the distribution of the *B*-gene-specified enzyme. An α-3-*N*-acetylgalactosaminyltransferase found only in group A and AB individuals occurs in milk (Kobata *et al.*, 1968*b*), human submaxillary glands (Hearn *et al.*, 1968), human gastric mucosa (Tuppy and Schenkel-Brunner, 1969*a*), plasma (Sawicka, 1971; Schachter *et al.*, 1971; Kim *et al.*, 1971*a*), saliva (P. Greenwell, unpublished observations), red cell membranes (Kim *et al.*, 1971*a*), and ovarian cyst linings and fluids (Hearn *et al.*, 1972). The *A* transferase resembles the *B* transferase in that it occurs in normal amounts in submaxillary glands and milk from both secretors and nonsecretors, although A serological activity is found in saliva and milk only of secretors. The *A* transferase has also been detected in particle-bound form in sublingual and palatine glands, lung, kidney, and bone marrow, although no significant levels of the enzyme were found in similar preparations from parotid glands, heart, liver, or spleen tissue (C. Race, P. Greenwell, and W. M. Watkins, unpublished observations).

α-$N$-Acetylgalactosaminyltransferases which catalyze the formation of structures with blood group A serological properties have been described in tissues from pigs (Tuppy and Schenkel-Brunner, 1969b; McGuire, 1970; Schwyzer and Hill, 1977a), dogs (Baker et al., 1973) and rats (Kim et al., 1971b).

**Purification.** The α-3-$N$-acetylgalactosaminyltransferase in human milk from a group $A_2$ woman was purified 55-fold by a procedure involving ammonium sulfate fractionation, Sephadex G-200 chromatography, and fractionation with $MnCl_2$ (Kobata and Ginsburg, 1970). In the light of subsequent observations on the very low concentration of the A and B transferases in serum and milk, this preparation was probably far from homogeneous. The same can be said of the $A^2$ transferase purified 500-fold from ovarian cyst fluid by isoelectric focusing (Topping and Watkins, 1975). Indeed, attempts to induce antibodies in rabbits to this enzyme preparation gave rise to strong precipitins for human γ-globulin, indicating that the latter protein was a major contaminant in the partially purified transferase preparation (Topping, 1976). Nevertheless, isoelectric focusing enables the A transferase in serum from $A_1$ individuals to be separated from β-galactosyltranferase and from the α-$N$-acetylgalactosaminyltransferase that catalyzes the addition of the first $N$-acetylgalactosamine residue to peptide chains in glycoproteins (Topping and Watkins, 1975). A one-step purification procedure involving binding of the A transferase to agarose gel beads followed by elution with UDP was described by Whitehead et al. (1974a). This purification scheme resulted in an increase in specific activity of over 1000-fold when pooled plasma from group A donors was used as the starting material. Other glycosyltransferases tested under the same conditions, including the B-gene-specified α-galactosyltransferase, failed to adsorb to the agarose. Agarose is primarily a linear polymer of alternating β-D-galactose and 3,6-anhydro-α-L-galactose residues and the reason why the α-3-$N$-acetylgalactosaminyltransferase has an affinity for this adsorbent is unknown. The authors suggest that other sugars present as minor constituents of the agarose may constitute inhibitors for the A transferase. Whitehead et al. (1974a) used a commercially available agarose preparation, Sepharose 4B, and the capacity of this material to function as an adsorbent of the A transferase has been confirmed in many laboratories. However, some investigators have experienced difficulties in obtaining adequate adsorption and elution of the A transferase. Nagai *et al.* (1978*a*) found that the adsorption capacity varied with different batches of Sepharose 4B; some batches cannot be used because of irreversible adsorption and others are unsuitable because of lack of affinity for the transferase. By careful selection of the batch of Sepharose 4B, and reexamination of the optimum conditions for adsorption and elution, Nagai *et al.* (1978*a*) achieved an increase in specific activity of 70,000- to 100,000-fold, with recovery of 80% of the $\alpha$-$N$-acetyl-galactosaminyltransferase activity from plasma. This preparation was further purified by chromatography on Bio-Gel P and the recovered enzyme was apparently homogeneous, although the overall yield after this step was reduced to 10%.

A membrane-bound $N$-acetylgalactosaminyltransferase from porcine submaxillary glands which confers A blood group specificity on submaxillary mucin has been purified 38,000-fold by affinity chromatography on UDP-hexanolamine-agarose in aqueous Triton X-100. The purified enzyme is a glycoprotein with an apparent molecular weight of 100,000 and is thought to contain two subunits (Schwyzer and Hill, 1977*a,b*). It has a specific activity of 30 $\mu$mol/min/mg of enzyme which is 55,000 times that recorded by Whitehead *et al.* (1974*a*) for the enzyme isolated from human serum. If the soluble $\alpha$-$N$-acetylgalactosaminyltransferase in human serum has the same specific activity as the membrane-bound porcine enzyme this result may indicate that even the preparation isolated by Nagai *et al.* (1978*a*) is not yet homogeneous.

**Acceptor Specificity.** The A transferase in human milk (Kobata and Ginsburg, 1970), submaxillary glands, stomach mucosa (Hearn *et al.*, 1968; Watkins, 1974), and serum (Whitehead *et al.*, 1974*b*; Schachter *et al.*, 1973) from group $A_1$ and $A_2$ individuals exhibits the same acceptor specificity toward low-molecular-weight substrates as does the B transferase (Table VI). All the acceptor substrates contain the H-active structure, $\alpha$-Fuc(1$\rightarrow$2)$\beta$-Gal-R (Fig. 7), as the terminal nonreducing group. A second fucose residue on the sugar subterminal to the $\beta$-galactosyl residue destroys the capacity of the molecule to function as an acceptor. Despite the ideas advanced that $A_1$ specificity in macromolecular A substances is determined by the Type 1 chain and $A_2$ specificity by the Type 2 chain (Moreno, *et al.*, 1971; Kisailus and Kabat, 1978) both the low-molecular-weight Type 1 chain analogue, lacto-$N$-fucopentaose I, and the Type 2 chain analogue, 2'-fucosyllactose, are acceptors of $N$-acetylgalactosamine irrespective of the A subgroup of the person from whom the transferase is derived. The $A^2$ transferase is, however, a less effective enzyme and has an appreciably higher $K_m$ value than the $A^1$ transferase with either of these substrates (Schachter *et al.*, 1973). Both the $A^1$ and the $A^2$ transferases appear to have a higher affinity for 2'-fucosyllactose than for lacto-*N*-fucopentaose I. The enzyme purified by Whitehead *et al.* (1974*b*) from pooled group A plasma had the same acceptor specificity as the crude serum. As already indicated, however, there is a more marked difference between the effectiveness of the $A^1$ and $A^2$ transferases when red cells are the carriers of the acceptor H-active structures than when low-molecular-weight acceptors are used. This difference is also observed when H-active glycoprotein functions as the acceptor (Table VII). The reason for these discrepancies is not understood but they may be related to the accessibility of the H-structures in the H-active glycoproteins and on group O red cells in comparison to their ready accessibility in the low-

TABLE VII. Activities of $A^1$- and $A^2$-Gene-Specified $\alpha$-$N$-Acetylgalactosaminyltransferases in Serum Assayed with Low-Molecular-Weight, Macromolecular, and Cellular Acceptor Substrates[a]

| Serum | | | % Incorporation of [b] [$^{14}$C]-GalNAc into acceptor | | Red cell conversion[c]: |
|---|---|---|---|---|---|
| Donor | Blood group | pH of assay | 2'-Fucosyl lactose | H-Active glycoprotein | agglutination titer with anti-A serum |
| C.R. | A₁ | 6.0 | 25 | 12 | — |
|      |    | 8.0 | 14 | 8  | — |
|      |    | 7.0 | —  | —  | 256 |
| S.B. | A₂ | 6.0 | 9  | 0.7 | — |
|      |    | 8.0 | 20 | 1.6 | — |
|      |    | 7.0 | —  | —  | 2 |

[a] From C. Race (unpublished observations).
[b] With 2'-fucosyllactose as acceptor the assays were carried out as described by Sabo *et al.* (1978) and with H-active glycoprotein as acceptor the assays were carried out as described for the *B* transferase by Carne and Watkins (1977) except that UDP-[$^{14}$C]-GalNAc was used as the sugar donor. The results are expressed as the percentage of the total radioactivity incorporated into the acceptor substrates under standard conditions of time and enzyme concentration.
[c] Red cell conversion assays were performed as described by Race and Watkins (1972*a*).

molecular-weight oligosaccharides. Schachter (1974*a*) and Hakomori *et al.* (1977) have suggested models for the structures of the $A_1$ and $A_2$ antigens in which both branches of a branched carbohydrate chain (Fig. 3 and Table 5) are substituted with *N*-acetylgalactosamine in the $A_1$ determinant and only one of the branches in an $A_2$ determinant.

**Metal Ion Requirements.** The $A^1$ and $A^2$ transferases in all tissues examined have a requirement for divalent cations and $Mn^{2+}$ ions are the most effective (Kobata *et al.,* 1968*b*; Hearn *et al.,* 1968, 1972; Schachter *et al.,* 1971). In serum, $Mg^{2+}$ ions can replace $Mn^{2+}$ ions in assays for the $A^1$ transferase but not for the $A^2$ transferase (Schachter *et al.,* 1973). With $Mg^{2+}$ ions as cofactors the pH optimum of the $A^1$ transferase shifts to pH 7.0 but the optimum of the $A^2$ transferase does not change (Cartron, 1976).

**pH Optima and Isoelectric Points.** In serum the $A^1$ transferase has a pH optimum of about 6 whereas the $A^2$ transferase has a broad pH optimum between 7 and 8 (Schachter *et al.,* 1973; Topping and Watkins, 1975; Cartron *et al.,* 1975). Previously, the $A^1A^2$ genotype could not be distinguished from $A^1A^1$ and $A^1O$ because at the antigenic level the expression of $A_2$ appears to be recessive to the $A_1$ character. The difference in pH optima of the two transferases, however, enables the $A_1A_2$ phenotype to be differentiated because the ratio of activities at pH 6 and pH 8 is very different in the serum from an $A^1A^2$ individual from that in the serum of an $A^1A^1$ or $A^1O$ individual (Topping and Watkins, 1975; Cartron *et al.,* 1976*b*). Typical pH curves obtained in the author's laboratory for the α-3-*N*-acetylgalactosaminyltransferase activities in the serum of an $A_1$, an $A_2$, and an individual of authentic $A^1A^2$ genotype, are given in Fig. 9. The $A^1$ and $A^2$ transferases in serum are dissimilar in their isoelectric points as well as in their pH optima. Isoelectric focusing of $A_2$ sera on a pH 3–10 gradient gave major peaks of α-*N*-acetylgalactos-aminyltransferase activity in the pH range 6–7 whereas $A_1$ sera gave major peaks in the range pH 9–10. This difference in the pI values enabled two α-*N*-acetylgalactosaminyltransferases to be preparatively separated from the serum of a donor of the genotype $A^1A^2$. Two peaks of transferase activity were found, one with a pI of 6.9 and the other a pI of 9.9. After separation the enzyme with the pI of 6.9 was found to have pH optimum of 7.5–8.0, characteristic of an $A^2$ transferase, whereas the enzyme with a pI of 9.9 had a pH optimum of 6.5 characteristic of the $A_1$ transferase (Topping and Watkins, 1975). These results indicate that two distinct and separable enzyme species are produced by persons of the genotype $A^1A^2$.

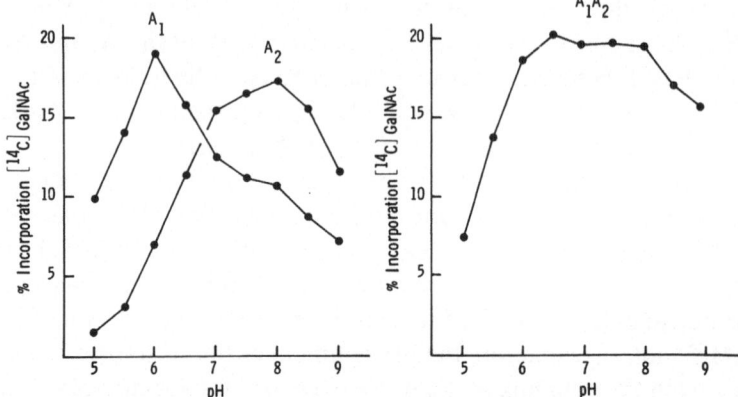

Fig. 9. Typical pH curves for the α-3-*N*-acetyl-D-galactosaminyltransferases in serum of $A_1$, $A_2$, and $A_1A_2$ individuals. Enzyme activity was assayed by the transfer of $[^{14}C]$-GalNAc to 2'-fucosyllactose as described by Sabo *et al.* (1978).

Two ovarian cyst fluids, one from a group $A_2$ and the other from a group $A_2B$ patient, had α-*N*-acetylgalactosaminyltransferase activities that focused at pH 10.0 and 9.5, respectively, although the corresponding transferase in these patients' sera focused at pH 6.8 and 6.2, respectively. The *A* transferase in ovarian cyst fluids from group $A_1$ patients focused in the pH range 9.5–10 in agreement with values found for the major peaks of activity in group $A_1$ sera. The isoelectric point of the $A^2$ transferase in different tissues thus appears to arise from secondary modifications of the enzyme protein and cannot be a direct result of the coded amino acid sequence of the protein. Nevertheless it must be assumed that there is a difference in the primary structures of the $A^1$ and $A^2$ transferases which enables the secondary modification to occur in one and not the other.

The techniques used for these isoelectric focusing experiments involved focusing by a column procedure for 72 hours, and the recoveries of enzyme were very low. The transferase measured at the end of the experiments therefore represented those enzyme molecules which were most stable under the prevailing conditions of temperature and pH. Recently, the isoelectric points have been redetermined by a flat-bed focusing technique in which the various molecular species reach their isoelectric points within 16 hours. This has resulted in a greater recovery of enzyme although losses of activity still occur. The earlier results have been essentially confirmed but a second minor, although definite, peak of α-*N*-acetylgalactosaminyltransferase activity is found at pH 5.5–6.5 in sera from group $A_1$ individuals in addition to the major peak at pH 8.5–9.5 (P. Greenwell and W. M. Watkins, unpublished results).

**Inhibition.**   The α-*N*-acetylgalactosaminyltransferases in sera from group $A_1$, $A_2$, and $A_1B$ individuals are competitively inhibited by UDP-galactose (Race and Watkins, 1974). The apparent Km of the enzymes for UDP-*N*-acetylgalactosamine and the apparent $K_i$ for UDP-galactose are closely similar indicating that both nucleotide sugars bind to the active site of the enzymes although they catalyze the transfer only of *N*-acetylgalactosamine.

**Molecular Weight.**   On the basis of sucrose density gradient and gel filtration methods (Whitehead *et al.*, 1974*b*; Nagai *et al.*, 1978*a*) a molecular weight between 80,000 and 100,000 has been reported for the *A* transferase. SDS polyacrylamide gel electrophoresis of the S-carboxymethylmaleyl derivative of the $A^1$ transferase gave an estimated molecular weight of 52,000 (Nagai *et al.*, 1978*a*); hence the enzyme was considered to be in dimeric form. Indeed, Nagai and Yoshida (1978) postulated the existence in heterozygous $A_1B$ subjects of a hybrid enzyme (ab) made up of a subunit of A enzyme (aa) and a subunit of B enzyme (bb). Some evidence, based on adsorption on to Sepharose 4B, was presented in support of this concept.

**Stability.**   The transferase in crude plasma rapidly loses activity when stored at $+4°$ but retains activity for several years on storage at $-40°$. The highly purified enzyme from plasma was found to be even more labile at $+4°$ than the enzyme in whole plasma but was stable at $-60°$ for up to 30 days in the presence of manganese chloride, EDTA, and UDP (Nagai *et al.*, 1978*a*).

**Levels of Activity.**   The *A* transferase level in the serum of adults is generally higher in those of group $A_1$ than $A_2$, but when measured at their respective pH optima there is some overlap between the activities in the two subgroups (Cartron, 1976). No sharp divisions into groups, as was observed for the *B* transferase (Badet, 1976), was found for the *A* transferase in the sera of those with normal $A_1$ or $A_2$ phenotypes. Tilley *et al.* (1978) observed that the level of blood group $A^1$-specified transferase in the serum of recently delivered women was appreciably lower than the level of this enzyme in the serum of nonpregnant adults and of newborn infants. A similar, but less striking, decrease was observed in the levels of the $A^2$-specified transferase. Although the red cells of newborn infants are known to have fewer A and H sites than adult cells, the serum of neonates had levels of $A^1$ and $A^2$ transferase activities as high as, if not higher than, the serum of nonpregnant adults.

## Glycosyltransferases in Weak Subgroups and Rare ABO Variants

**Bombay $O_h$ and Para-Bombay Phenotypes.** The Bombay $O_h$ phenotype, which is characterized by the absence of A, B, and H antigens from both red cells and secretions, was first reported by Bhende *et al.* (1952) in three individuals in Bombay; hence the name of the phenotype. The condition is very rare but is relatively more frequent in India than in other parts of the world. In a recent study of the Bombay population, Bhatia and Sathe (1974) found 22 with this phenotype out of 167,404 persons tested, giving an incidence of 1 : 7,600. The regional and community distribution of the $O_h$ phenotype suggested that is was more common in the Marathas from the southwest districts of Maharashtra. More $O_h$ persons were revealed in family studies, and consanguinity of the parents was established in 30% of the instances where such information was available. The incidence of the $O_h$ phenotype is thought to be much lower in the European population, but examples have now been described in English, French, and Italian families and in American and Canadian families of European extraction (see Race and Sanger, 1975).

Various explanations have been advanced to explain the Bombay $O_h$ phenotype. A new allele at the *ABO* locus was suggested in the original paper (Bhende *et al.*, 1952) but Ceppellini *et al.* (1952) considered that an inhibitor gene at an independent locus might be involved. As the role of H as a precursor of A and B was elucidated, it became clear that H was the product of a locus independent of *ABO* and, since individuals with the Bombay phenotype are devoid of the H character, Watkins and Morgan (1955*a*) suggested that such persons could be homozygous for a rare silent allele of *H*, that is, their genotype is *hh*. That some form of suppression was involved and not a new allele at the *ABO* locus was revealed by the classical family study of Levine *et al.* (1955). The ABO blood groups of this family made it clear that the proposita with the Bombay phenotype had an unexpressed *B* gene which she had inherited from her mother and transmitted to her daughter. The family study also showed her to be carrying an unexpressed secretor gene *Se*. Subsequently, other family studies revealed instances where persons with the Bombay $O_h$ phenotype were carrying unexpressed $A^1$ and $A^2$ genes (see Race and Sanger, 1975).

The discovery of the enzymic products of the *H*, *A*, and *B* genes enabled a fresh approach to be made to an understanding of this rare phenotype. Examination of the serum of $O_h$ donors by several groups of workers has demonstrated that they are completely deficient in the *H*-gene-specified α-2-L-fucosyltransferase which is present in all individuals with normal ABO groups (Schenkel-Brunner *et al.*, 1972; Munro and Schachter, 1973; Chester *et al.*, 1976; Pacuszka and Koscielak, 1976). Mulet *et al.* (1977) also demonstrated that the *H* transferase was deficient in the red cell stroma of Bombay $O_h$ individuals. In contrast, the *A* and *B* transferases appropriate to their true *ABO* genotype are readily detectable in serum and red cell stroma of $O_h$ individuals (Race and Watkins, 1972*b*; Mulet *et al.*, 1977), thus supporting the view that the absence of A and B activity results from lack of the H acceptor substrate and not from failure of expression of the *A* and *B* genes. Further confirmation came from the work of Schenkel-Brunner *et al.* (1975) who demonstrated that neuraminidase-treated $O_h$ cells could be converted to H-active cells by incubation with GDP-fucose and an α-2-fucosyltransferase from human gastric mucosa; the converted cells were then suitable acceptors for an *A* transferase. The necessity to treat the $O_h$ cells with neuraminidase before H-active structures can be synthesized is probably due to the fact that paragloboside (Table IV) and other longer-chain glycolipid precursors of H are also acceptors for sialyltransferases (Koscielak *et al.*, 1973). In the absence of the *H* transferase, the precursor structures are probably substituted with sialic acid, and until this sugar has been removed the addition of fucose cannot take place.

Part of the pedigree of a family with the Bombay $O_h$ phenotype, studied by Phyllis P. Moores and D. Naidoo, The Natal Blood Transfusion Service, Durban, South Africa, is shown in Fig. 10. The family, although living in South Africa, was of Indian extraction. Three members in generation II had the Bombay $O_h$ phenotype. From the ABO groups of his children, the genotype of the father in generation I can be inferred to have been *BO*. Similarly, the genotype of I 1 must be *A¹O*. The true ABO groups of the $O_h$ family members could therefore have been group $A_1$, B, $A_1B$, or O. The only one for whom a partial deduction could be made was II 20 who could be inferred to be carrying an *A¹* gene since he must have passed this gene on to his group AB child III 26. However, on the blood group evidence available from the other family members his genotype could have been either *A¹O* or *A¹B*.

Ms. Moores kindly sent serum from six members of this family to

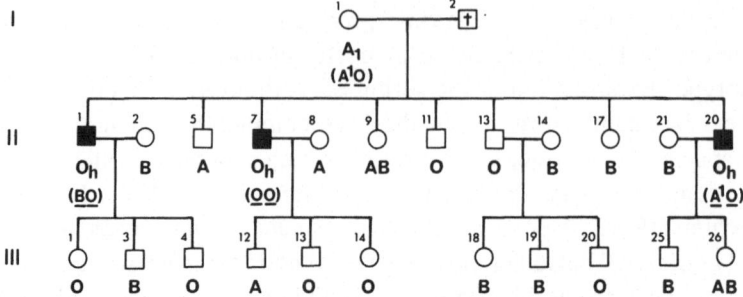

Fig. 10. Pedigree and ABO blood groups of Durban family Nar. (P. P. Moores and D. Naidoo, unpublished observations). The notations inside the parentheses represent the genotypes.

the author's laboratory for transferase investigations. As expected, the $H$-gene-specified α-2-fucosyltransferase was missing from the serum of the three $O_h$ members, II 1, II 7 and II 20, but was present in the serum of the group $A_1$ mother I 1 and the normal group O sibs II 11 and II 13 (Table VIII). Assays for the $A$ and $B$ transferases clearly demonstrated that the II 1 was carrying an unexpressed $B$ gene, II 7 was carrying neither $A$ nor $B$ genes, and II 20 was carrying an unexpressed $A$ gene with a higher activity at pH 6 than at 8, which distinguished it as an $A^1$ gene. If, as proposed, the Bombay $O_h$ phenotype arises from the inheritance of two $h$ genes, then I 1 and I 2 in this Durban family must be heterozygous $Hh$. Since I 1 had passed on an $O$ and an $h$ gene to two of her $O_h$ children and an $A^1$ gene and an $h$ gene to the third, and I 2 had similarly passed on an $O$ gene and an $h$ gene to two of his offspring and a $B$ gene and an $h$ gene to a third, the genes at the $ABO$ locus and the $Hh$ locus appear to be segregating independently. Dr. Peter Cook of the MRC Human Biochemical Genetics Unit, London, calculated the lod scores (log to base 10 of odds on linkage) for this family and suggested that the values found effectively rule out very close linkage between the two markers $ABO$ and $Hh$. Thus one locus is unlikely to have evolved from the other by tandem duplication. Obviously, on the basis of one family, only tentative conclusions can be reached with regard to linkage but the results serve to illustrate the genetic information contributed by transferase studies over and above that which is obtainable by serological investigations of the blood group characters on the red cells.

All the manifestations of the $O_h$ phenotype are explicable on the assumption that the individuals lack a functional $H$ gene. In the absence of an $H$ gene, the $Se$ gene has no regulatory role to exert and thus $Se$ would of necessity be unexpressed in persons with the $O_h$ phenotype. A child who inherited an *h* and an *Se* gene from his $O_h$ parent, and an *H* and an *Se* gene from his other parent, could reexpress the *Se* gene, as indeed happened in the family studied by Levine *et al.* (1955). Red cells of the $O_h$ phenotype frequently give stronger reactions with anti-I and anti-i sera than control adult or cord group O cells (Bhatia, 1977). Since the Ii reagents are detecting precursor carbohydrate chains which are normally masked by the H, A, and B determinants, such increased reactivity is not unexpected. The Lewis $Le^b$ phenotype is never found in $O_h$ individuals; the Lewis groups are always either Le $(a^+b^-)$ or, more rarely, Le $(a^-b^-)$ (see Race and Sanger 1975; Bhatia, 1977). The presence of a functional *H* gene, as well as an *Le* and an *Se* gene, is an essential prerequisite for the formation of the $Le^b$ specific determinant (Marr *et al.*, 1967); hence the absence of this specificity in persons with the $O_h$ phenotype is to be anticipated. The simplest explanation for the deficit of H activity in the Bombay phenotype is that the individuals are homozygous for a silent

**TABLE VIII. Glycosyltransferase Assays on Durban Bombay $O_h$ Family**[a]

| Family member | ABO group | A transferase[b] | | B transferase[b] | H transferase[c] | Latent ABO group |
|---|---|---|---|---|---|---|
| | | pH 6 | pH 8 | | | |
| I  1 | $A_1$ | 18 | 13 | 0 | 4 | |
| II  1 | $O_h$ | 0 | 0 | 18 | 0 | B |
| II  7 | $O_h$ | 0 | 0 | 0 | 0 | O |
| II  11 | O | 0 | 0 | 0 | 4 | |
| II  13 | O | 0 | 0 | 0 | 6 | |
| II  20 | $O_h$ | 31 | 19 | 0 | 0 | $A_1$ |
| Controls | $A_1$ | 20 | 13 | 0 | 7 | |
| | B | 0 | 0 | 21 | 5 | |
| | O | 0 | 0 | 0 | 5 | |

[a] From P. P. Moores, A. D. Yates, and P. Greenwell (unpublished observations).
[b] Assayed by the transfer of [$^{14}$C]-GalNAc (*A* transferase) or [$^{14}$C]-Gal (*B* transferase) to 2'-fucosyllactose as described by Sabo *et al.* (1978). Results expressed as the percentage of the total radioactivity incorporated into the acceptor under standard conditions.
[c] Assayed by the transfer of [$^{14}$C]fucose to β-phenyl-D-galactoside as described by Chester *et al.* (1976). Results expressed as the percentage of the total [$^{14}$C]fucose transferred to the acceptor under standard conditions.

allele *h*, but the evidence so far available does not allow the possibility to be ruled out that suppressor genes situated at an independent genetic locus, when inherited in double dose, modify the expression of the α-2-L-fucosyltransferase at the site of synthesis of both the membrane-bound H antigens and the secreted H-active glycoproteins. If such a suppressor mechanism were the correct explanation, then the arguments concerning the lack of close linkage between the *ABO* and *Hh* loci would lose their validity. Cell hybrid studies, combined with measurement of *H* transferase activity, might enable both the *H* gene to be mapped and an answer found to the question of whether *h* or suppressor genes are the basis of the $O_h$ phenotype.

Hesitation to accept that the Bombay $O_h$ phenotype results from the *hh* genotype arises in part from the discovery of other classes of ABO variants called "para-Bombay" phenotypes (see Race and Sanger, 1975; Bhatia, 1977). One class closely resembles the Bombay phenotype except that the red cells exhibit very weak A or B activity although they are negative for H. Anti-H occurs in the serum; A, B, and H antigens are missing from the saliva. The usual notation for this class of para-Bombays is $A_h$ or $B_h$. Tests for *H*, *A*, and *B* glycosyltransferases in the blood of individuals with $A_h$ and $B_h$ phenotypes give results which are indistinguishable from those obtained for Bombay $O_h$ phenotype. No *H* transferase activity is detectable in serum or red cell membranes, but the *A* and *B* transferases appropriate to the inherited *ABO* genes are expressed in normal amounts (Schenkel-Brunner *et al.*, 1972; Mulet *et al.*, 1977). The occurrence of these phenotypes with weak A or B activity, but no detectable H, has led some serologists to question the place of H in the pathway to A and B (Solomon *et al.*, 1965; Voak and Lodge, 1968). The biochemical view that a limited amount of H is completely converted to A or B structures has recently been vindicated by some elegant experiments of Mulet *et al.* (1978*a*). Red cells from a person with the $B_h$ phenotype were treated with a purified B-degrading α-galactosidase from *Trichomonas foetus*. The cells lost B activity, and H determinants, which were uncovered, then became substrates for an *A*-gene-specified α-*N*-acetylgalactosaminyltransferase from human group A serum. The cells developed A activity and lost H activity and hence had been converted to $A_h$ cells. If the B-negative, H-positive cells were treated with an α-2-L-fucosidase from *T. foetus*, the H activity was lost and conversion into A-active cells could not be achieved with the *A* transferase. These results demonstrate that the A and B antigens on $A_h$ and $B_h$ cells are built upon an H precursor in the normal way and also provide evidence that $H$ is not a completely silent allele in these para-Bombay phenotypes. The failure to demonstrate the $H$-gene-specified transferase in the serum of these individuals probably results from the levels being too low to be detected by the techniques at present in use for the assay of the $\alpha$-2-L-fucosyl-transferase. Bhatia (1977) and Cartron (1978) suggest a series of mutant alleles at the $H$ locus, some of which are completely silent while others allow the production of a limited quantity of H substance. Equally, a series of suppressor genes of varying effectiveness could be postulated.

The second class of para-Bombays cannot be reconciled with a mutant $H$ gene because although A, B, and H antigens are weak or absent from the red cells, these activities are expressed in normal amounts in saliva. Persons with this phenotype must, therefore, carry a normal $H$ gene in their genome. The sera of this class of para-Bombay contain antibodies reacting preferentially with O cells but several groups of workers have observed that they are not inhibited by secretor saliva and are probably anti-HI and not anti-H (see Race and Sanger, 1975). An independent genetic system $Zz$ that regulates the expression of the $H$ gene at the site of synthesis of the cellular H antigens has been postulated to explain this class of para-Bombay phenotype (Solomon $et\ al.$, 1965; Hrubisko and Mergancová, 1966); it is proposed that those lacking H antigen on the red cells are homozygous $zz$. In contrast to the Bombay $O_h$ red cells, the cells in this second class of para-Bombays frequently group as $Le(a^-b^+)$. The presence of the $Le^b$ antigen is, however, not incompatible with suppression of the $H$ gene at the level of synthesis of the red cell H structures because the Lewis antigens are taken up from the plasma and are not synthesized by the hemopoietic tissue (see section on Lewis antigens). No uniform notation for this class of para-Bombay has emerged. The earlier nomenclature of $O^h_m$, $A^h_m$, etc. was changed by Hrubisko $et\ al.$ (1970) to $O_{Hm}$, $O^A_{Hm}$, etc. in an attempt to indicate that it is the H character of the cells that is modified, but Mulet $et\ al.$ (1978$b$) suggest that $O_{Hz}$, $O^A_{Hz}$, etc. is a more appropriate notation. The A, B, and H transferase activities in four unrelated families with this phenotype were studied by Mulet $et\ al.$ (1978$b$) and in our laboratory seven Thai families, five with weakly expressed $B$ genes and two with weakly expressed $A$ genes, have been investigated (Sringarm $et\ al.$, 1979). In all these families the affected members lacked detectable $H$ transferase although the appropriate $A$ or $B$ transferases were expressed normally. Thus this second class of para-Bombays cannot be differentiated on the basis of the transferase studies from the Bombay $O_h$ or the para-Bombay $A_h$ and $B_h$ phenotypes. Race and Sanger (1975) put forward the very plausible suggestion that the two classes of para-Bombays may have the same genetic background $zz$, which allows H in saliva but not on the red cells, and that the first class is $zz$, $sese$, and hence nonsecretors, whereas the second class is $zz$, $Se$, and hence secretors.

The Bombay and para-Bombay phenotypes described above are inherited as recessive characters. Hrubisko (1976) has, however, described three Czechoslovakian families in which modified H phenotypes are inherited as a dominant trait. The H antigen on the red cells of the affected members of these families is diminished in comparison with normal cells but the activity is not nearly as weak as in the classical Bombay and para-Bombay families. Examination of the glycosyltransferase levels in one of these families by Mulet et al. (1978b) failed to reveal any deficiency of $H$ transferase and it must be assumed that the biochemical block in the synthesis of the blood group antigens lies in the glycosyltransferases synthesizing the precursor oligosaccharide chains or in enzymes making the GDP-fucose donor substrate for the $H$-gene-specified fucosyltransferase.

**Weak Subgroups of A and B.**   In addition to the major $A_1$ and $A_2$ subgroups, there are numerous variants in which the expression of A is reduced (see Race and Sanger, 1975). These rare variants are characterized by a continuous spectrum of A antigen site density directly related to red cell agglutination as measured with anti-A sera under carefully standardized conditions (Cartron et al., 1974).

The $A_3$ phenotype, first recognized by Friedenreich (1936), gives a characteristic red cell agglutination pattern in which small agglutinated clumps are vastly outnumbered by unagglutinated cells. However, the red cells are not a mosaic of A and O cells because the cells which fail to agglutinate with anti-A nevertheless combine with the antibody. The $A_3$ character is inherited and the responsible gene is considered to be an allele at the $ABO$ locus (see Race and Sanger, 1975). Examination of the $A$-gene-specified $\alpha$-$N$-acetylgalactosaminyltransferase activity in serum has indicated that $A_3$ does not constitute a homogeneous group (Cartron, 1976; Cartron et al., 1978; Greenwell and Watkins, 1978). Three categories can be distinguished. In the first the enzyme activity is about a third to a half of that found in normal group $A_1$ sera and the enzyme has a pH optimum at 6.0, thus resembling an $A^1$ gene product. In the second category the activity is much lower and the pH optimum of the enzyme is at 7–8, that is, it behaves like a weakened form of an $A^2$ gene product. The third category consists of individuals clearly grouped as $A_3$ but completely lacking detectable $A$ transferase in their sera. Only serum from the first category of $A_3$ individuals converts O red cells into A-active cells in the presence of the appropriate additives; the agglutination is stronger than that achieved by incubation of the O cells with $A_2$ sera (Cartron, 1976; Greenwell and Watkins, 1978) and the agglutination pattern is normal and not characteristic of that given by $A_3$ cells. Cartron *et al.* (1978) examined red cell membranes from $A_3$ individuals belonging to the second and third categories and failed to detect any $A$-transferase activity but membranes from an $A_3$ donor belonging to the first category gave weak but definite activity with a pH optimum at 6 (P. Greenwell, unpublished observations). Isoelectric focusing of the serum of this same $A_3$ donor gave a major peak of $\alpha$-$N$-acetylgalactosaminyltransferase activity with a pI of 9.6 and a smaller peak with a pI of 5.4 (Topping, 1976). The physical properties of the $\alpha$-$N$-acetylgalactosaminyltransferase in this $A_3$ sample thus resembled the enzyme in $A_1$ serum both with regard to the pH optimum and the isoelectric point of the major part of the enzymically active protein. The H-gene-specified $\alpha$-2-fucosyltransferase was readily detected in the $A_3$ serum samples but the levels were on average considerably lower than those observed for group $A_1$ or $A_2$ sera (Greenwell and Watkins, 1978). The transferase studies suggest that if the $A^3$ gene is an allele at the ABO locus it may be a mutant form of either an $A^1$ or an $A^2$ gene. The variable density of A-active sites on the red cells, and hence, the mixed field agglutination pattern which is so characteristic of this phenotype, has, however, yet to be explained.

Two other rare types of inherited A variants, in which the A character is expressed even more weakly on the red cells than in subgroup $A_3$, are designated $A_x$ and $A_m$ (see Race and Sanger, 1975). The red cells of individuals with these phenotypes are frequently first grouped as O but the presence of an A antigen is suspected because anti-A is missing from the serum. The cells are subsequently shown to have the capacity to absorb human anti-A even though they are not agglutinated by this reagent. In both types of variant the red cells react strongly with anti-H reagents, and they are thereby differentiated from the para-Bombay phenotypes. The two groups of variants differ in that $A_x$ individuals, if secretors, usually have H but no A (or very weak A) activity in saliva whereas most $A_m$ individuals have both A and H activities in saliva in normal amounts. Cartron *et al.* (1978) failed to detect any $\alpha$-$N$-acetylgalactosaminyltrans-

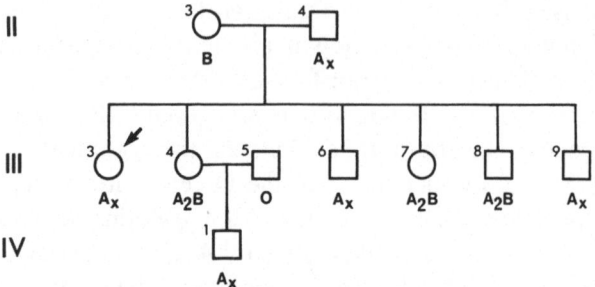

Fig. 11. Part of pedigree of family Lap. studied by Salmon and Cartron (1974) showing the transmission of an $A_x$ as $A^2$ when it is inherited together with a $B$ gene.

ferase activity in the serum or red cell membranes from $A_x$ individuals. Greenwell and Watkins (1978) similarly failed to find the $A$ transferase in serum from four $A_x$ persons but in a fifth example (V. W.) a very weak transferase with higher activity at pH 8 than at 6, was detected. This result is of considerable interest because V. W. had a child who was grouped as $A_2$ at birth but was later grouped as $A_x$ (G. W. G. Bird, personal communication). Moreover, families have been described in which a gene is expressed as $A_x$ when it is associated with an $O$ gene and as $A_2$ when it is associated with a $B$ gene in the phenotype $A_2B$ (Salmon and Cartron, 1976; Salmon, 1977; Monnet et al., 1978). In one family (Fig. 11) the number of A antigenic sites in the group $A_x$ subjects was found to be 11,000 per red cell whereas in the group $A_2B$ individuals, who had inherited the same $A$ gene, the number reached almost 100,000. Furthermore A activity was detectable in the salivary glycoproteins of the $A_2B$ person whereas it was not detectable in the $A_x$ saliva. Enzyme assays revealed weak but significant $\alpha$-$N$-acetylgalactosaminyltransferase activities in the serum of the group $A_2B$ subjects which was absent from the sera of the group $A_x$ members of the same family. Salmon (1977) suggested genetic complementation as an explanation of these facts with the corollary that if complementation can occur this implies that the $A$ and $B$ transferases are polymeric molecules.

 $H$ transferase activity was readily detectable in the sera of the $A_x$ individuals but the levels were lower than those expected for group A individuals (Greenwell and Watkins, 1978).

 Heterogeneity of the $A_m$ phenotype was established by studies of the $\alpha$-$N$-acetylgalactosaminyltransferase in the sera of 19 individuals belonging to this group (Cartron, et al., 1975; Cartron, 1976; Cartron et al.,

1978). The enzyme in the serum of fourteen individuals, who appeared to have inherited the phenotype as an allele at the *ABO* locus, had kinetic properties characteristic of an $A^1$ gene product. In one family, however, the *A* transferase in the serum of the $A_m$ member had properties characteristic of an $A^2$ gene product. On a quantitive basis the enzymic activities in these sera reached only 30–50% of the average value observed for $A_1$ and $A_2$ subjects, respectively. The authors suggest the existence of an inhibitor gene, possibly linked to the *ABO* locus which prevents either an $A^1$ or $A^2$ gene from acting at the bone marrow level although it does not affect the synthesis of A substance in mucous cells. In an interesting family study reported by Cartron *et al.* (1976*b*) two phenotypically $A_2$ children (IV 5 and IV 6) with an $A_m$ father (III 5) and $A_2$ mother (III 6) (Fig. 12) had *A* transferase in their serum with approximately equal activities at pH 6.0 and 7.0 and with a capacity to convert O cells to A-active cells which was greater than that shown by the *A* transferase in the serum of their group $A_2$ mother. These results thus enable the genotype of IV 5 and IV 6 to be recognized as $A^2A_m$. Since the $A^2$ gene is expressed normally in these children, the inhibitor gene must work only in the *cis* position; it therefore seems probable that it functions at the transcriptional level and not as a cytoplasmic modifier.

Another type of A variant, phenotypically similar to $A_m$ in that the A antigen is very depressed on the red cells but detectable in saliva, was found from family studies to result from the inheritance of modifying genes at a locus independent of *ABO* (Weiner *et al.*, 1957). The authors assumed the existence of a gene, *Y,* necessary for the development of the A antigen in red cells and postulated that these $A_m$-like individuals were homozygous for the allele *y*. One of the families studied showed that the postulated *Yy* genes cannot be closely linked to the *ABO* locus. The gene *Y* appeared to modify only the A antigenic expression and to have no

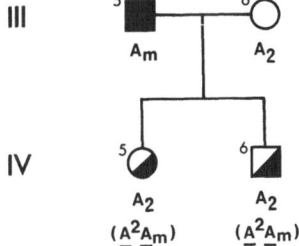

Fig. 12. Part of pedigree of $A_m$ family Min. (Cartron *et al.*, 1976*b*). The notation in parentheses indicates the probable genotype.

effect on the development of B and H antigens on the red cells or of A substance in saliva (Race and Sanger, 1975). Cartron *et al.* (1975) examined the A transferase activity in four individuals with the $A_y$ phenotype and were unable at first to detect any activity, although later, using more sensitive assays, weak but definite $\alpha$-$N$-acetylgalactosaminyltransferase activity was reported (Cartron *et al.*, 1978).

The virtual absence of the transferase in the serum of $A_y$ persons is a little puzzling in view of the presence of A activity in their saliva and the fact that the other type of $A_m$ individuals have some 30–50% of the normal level of $A$ transferase in their sera. However, in the $A_y$ individuals examined by Cartron *et al.* (1975), the amounts of secreted A substance were much weaker than in the $A_m$ individuals.

Group B antigenic expression cannot be classified into well-defined subgroups corresponding to $A_1$, $A_2$, and $A_3$, but a number of reports of weak B variants similar in general behavior to $A_x$ and $A_m$ phenotypes have appeared (see Race and Sanger, 1975). A family in which a weak B variant was characterized in four generations was studied by Simmons and Twaitt (1975). The red cells of affected members of this family showed unusually high H activity in addition to very weak B properties, but the levels of B and H substances in their saliva were normal and the authors concluded that the data represented "a $B^H_m$ family inheriting a suppressor gene which is selective on the red blood cell for the B site." Examination of the $H$ transferase levels in the sera of members of this family revealed that they fell within the ranges expected for their ABO groups, whereas the $B$-gene-specified $\alpha$-galactosyltransferase in the sera of the $B_m$ individuals was only about 50% of the normal level. Koscielak *et al.* (1976*b*) determined the $B$-gene $\alpha$-galactosyltransferase level in both serum and red cell membranes of members of a family in which the $B_m$ phenotype appeared to be inherited as a dominant character in two generations. The enzyme level in the serum of the $B_m$ (genotype $B_mO$) family member was again about 50% of the average value found for the control group B sera. In the family studied by Simmons and Twaitt and that investigated by Koscielak *et al.* (1976*b*), the family members who inherited an A gene from one parent and a $B_m$ "gene" from the other had normal expression of the $A$ gene on their red cells. Moreover, the $B$ transferase levels in the serum of these $AB_m$ individuals were approximately double those found in the $B_m$ ($B_mO$) family members. Thus these could constitute further examples of the allelic enhancement phenomenon pointed out by Salmon and Cartron (1976). In both the $B_m$ and $AB_m$ members of the family studied by Koscielak *et al.* (1976*b*), the *B* transferase activity in erythrocyte membranes was considerably reduced compared with normal B controls. This finding, together with the subsequent failure to detect *A* transferase activity in red cell membranes from individuals with the $A_m$ phenotype (Cartron *et al.*, 1978), are in agreement with the view that the weak B or A activities found in the red cells in the $B_m$ and $A_m$ phenotypes results from weakness of expression of the *B* or *A* transferases, respectively, in the hemopoietic tissues. Further support for this idea comes from the results of Kogure and Furukawa (1976), who reported that, although the α-galactosyltransferases in group $B_m$ sera were lower than those of normal group B persons, the enzyme activities in salivas from group $B_m$ individuals are comparable with those in normal group B salivas. Thus the most likely explanation of the $A_m$ and $B_m$ phenotypes is that they result from single doses of suppressor genes which act only in hemopoietic tissues and only in the *cis* position. Since these atypical expressions of A and B antigenic patterns are inherited as though they were products of alleles at the *ABO* locus, it must be inferred that the suppressor genes are very closely linked to the *A* or the *B* genes.

Another family (examined by Kogure and Furukawa, 1976) with a weak B variant, in which the B antigens on both red cells and saliva were weak, was found to have lower than normal α-galactosyltransferase activities in both serum and saliva.

**The *cis* AB Phenotype.** The term *cis* AB was introduced by Yamaguchi *et al.* (1966) to distinguish from normal "*trans*" AB phenotypes certain rare AB variants in which both the A and B characters are inherited together from one parent. Despite its rarity, the *cis* AB phenotype is of considerable interest and importance because it appears to challenge the generally accepted manner of inheritance of the ABO groups proposed by Bernstein (1924). The first ABO incompatibilities between group O mothers and their AB children were reported nearly 50 years ago (Kossovitch, 1929; Haselhorst and Lauer, 1931), but these exceptions tended to be explained away as somatic mutations or possible substitutions of the newborn infants. However, in 1964 Seyfried *et al.* produced incontrovertible evidence of an $A_2B$ phenotype that was inherited from one parent in two generations of a Polish family (Fig. 13). Family member II 3 had a group O mother (I 2) and a group O husband (II 2) but passed on her $A_2B$ phenotype to her two children, III 1 and III 2. Subsequently, O/AB and AB/O incompatibilities between a child and one of its parents have been described in a number of families in different parts of the world

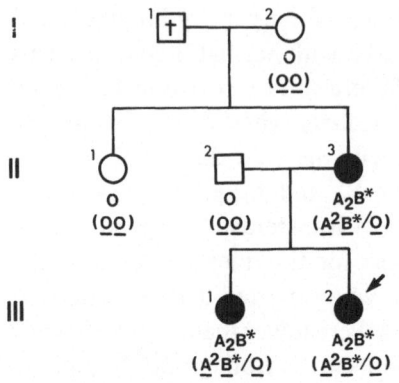

Fig. 13. Inheritance of *cis* AB in Polish family Sl. investigated by Seyfried *et al.* (1964). The notation in brackets indicates the genotype. *Weak B antigen.

(see Yamaguchi, 1973; Race and Sanger, 1975; Lopez *et al.*, 1976). The observed incidence in the European population is too low for estimates of the frequency to be made, but the condition appears to be slightly more common in the Japanese population, and Yamaguchi (1973) calculated the frequency as $1.1 \times 10^{-5}$. In nearly all instances of the *cis* AB phenotype so far recorded, the B antigen on the red cell was atypical in its behavior, and the individual's serum contained an antibody that recognized normal B cells but did not react with *cis* AB cells. The serological behavior of the A antigen on the red cells is usually more closely analogous to that of normal $A_2$ cells than of $A_1$ cells, but Reviron *et al.* (1968) described a family with the *cis* AB phenotype in which the A antigen had $A_1$ properties.

Several explanations have been advanced to explain the *cis* AB phenotype. Crossing over within the *ABO* locus has been proposed (Komai, 1950; Boettcher, 1966; Yamaguchi, 1973), resulting in a gene with dual AB properties. In biochemical terms this would probably mean a gene with the capacity to code for an enzyme protein with two active sites, one with *A* transferase activity and one with *B* transferase activity. An alternative explanation to intragenic crossing over is a mutation in or near the active site of either the *A* or *B* transferase giving rise to a rare allele that codes for an enzyme able to catalyze the transfer of either *N*-acetyl-D-galactosamine or D-galactose to H-active structures; the enzyme would thus have the capacity to synthesize both A- and B-specific groupings (Watkins, 1968; Salmon, *et al.*, 1973; Hirschfeld, 1977). Since the two sugars are structurally so similar, only a relatively small change in the active site of the transferase might be required to enable such an allele to arise. A third possibility is gene duplication followed by mutation in one of the gene copies (see Harris, 1975); this event would be expected to give rise to two separate enzymes.

Examination of the A- and B-gene-specified glycosyltransferase activities in the sera of individuals with the *cis* AB phenotype has not yet provided an answer to the question of whether one or two enzymes are involved. Pacuszka *et al.* (1975) examined three Polish families with the *cis* AB phenotype and found that all the individuals with this phenotype had strongly reduced activities of A-gene-specified α-N-acetylgalacto-saminyltransferase and only trace activities of B-gene-dependent α-gal-actosyltransferase. The authors suggested that the low activites could result from changed physicochemical properties of a mutant gene product leading to reduced solubility or stability of the enzyme. Kogure (1975), using the cell conversion technique, also failed to demonstrate B transferase activity in the sera of three individuals with the *cis* AB phenotype. On the other hand, Badet *et al.* (1978) examined the sera of thirteen *cis* AB subjects belonging to five families and found A transferase levels, which although usually weaker than the normal controls were variable and in some instances considerably stronger than the levels observed in the sera of the Polish *cis* AB families. For several of the *cis* AB sera the shape of the pH dependent curve, the effect of substitution of $Mg^{2+}$ for $Mn^{2+}$ ions and the capacity for the conversion of group O red cells into A-active cells appeared to be intermediate between that normally found for the $A^1$ and $A^2$ transferases. α-Galactosyltransferase activity was also detectable in all thirteen of the *cis* AB sera although the levels were lower than in normal B or AB persons and were sometimes at the limit of sensitivity of the techniques. One of the families (Lam.) studied by Badet *et al.* (1978) first came to the attention of serologists through a case of disputed paternity. From biostatistical evaluation of twenty-one genetic markers a high value of probability for paternity, maternity, and parentage was found between the child, the child's mother, the putative father, and his mother (Hummel *et al.*, 1977). The child, the child's father, and the father's mother all had atypical AB cells which were classified as *cis* AB (Fig. 14). This family was characterized by the presence of a much higher α-D-galactosyltransferase activity giving rise to a stronger B antigen than in any of the previously investigated *cis* AB cases. In the two family members, where only the *cis* AB gene was involved, the A transferase activities were about 20–30% of those found in the controls, although one family member, who was believed to have the genotype $A_2/cis$ AB, had

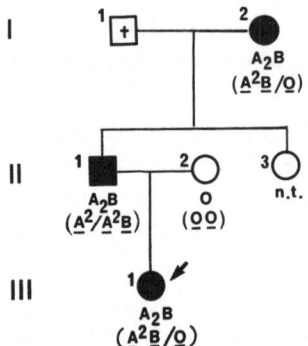

Fig. 14. Pedigree and ABO blood groups of *cis* AB family Lam. (modified from Hummel *et al.*, 1977). The notation in brackets indicates the probable genotype. n.t., Not tested.

much higher activity. Both the *A* and *B* transferases in this family could be detected by the transformation of O cells to A- or B-active cells, respectively. The data on the thirteen examples of *cis* AB examined by Badet *et al.* (1978) does not enable any definite assessment to be made as to whether one or two enzymes are responsible for the *A* and *B* transferase activities but the authors consider the results favor the interpretation of a single enzyme produced by a mutant gene.

A family (McC.) in the United States in which the *cis* AB phenotype appeared in three generations was reported by Bush and Sabo (1973). The serological behavior of the A antigen on the red cells was intermediate between that of normal $A_1$ and $A_2$ cells. The B antigen gave weak and variable reactions with naturally occurring antibodies. Examination of the transferases in the sera of the three *cis* AB family members (Fig. 15) revealed that all contained α-$N$-acetylgalactosaminyltransferase levels that were 65 to 85% of that found in a control $A_1$ serum and all had sharp optima at pH 6.0, characteristic of the $A^1$ gene product (Sabo *et al.*, 1978).

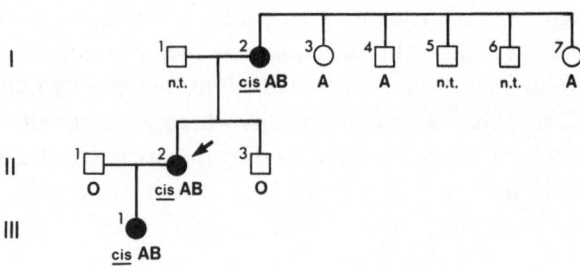

Fig. 15. Pedigree and ABO blood groups of *cis* AB family McC. investigated by Sabo *et al.* (1978). n.t., Not tested.

In cell conversion experiments the sera from the *cis* AB individuals showed a greater capacity to transform group O cells into A-active cells than did the serum from a group $A_2$ control. The *B* transferases in the *cis* AB sera of this family were very weak but both the *A* and *B* transferase levels were fairly constant when examined at intervals over a period of three years and the results were essentially similar for the three family members carrying the *cis* AB gene. This is in agreement with the view expressed by Lopez *et al.* (1976), on the basis of immunological and thermodynamic studies of the ABH antigens on *cis* AB red cells, and of Badet *et al.* (1978) on the basis of their transferase studies, that although differences occur among samples from unrelated individuals the results on samples from different members within a family are closely similar. The variations in the levels of the glycosyltransferases in the sera of unrelated individuals with the *cis* AB phenotype, together with the considerable difference in the degree of expression of the B antigen on their red cells, suggests that not only is there more than one *cis* AB gene but also that the phenotype may arise by more than one type of mechanism.

A mutant enzyme capable of transferring both *N*-acetylgalactosamine and D-galactose to H-active structures might be expected to show a greater affinity for UDP-D-galactose than that found for normal *A*-gene-specified enzymes. Earlier work had shown that UDP-galactose is in any case a strong inhibitor of normal $A^1$- and $A^2$-gene-specified transferases (Race and Watkins, 1974). However, this nucleotide sugar proved to be an even more effective inhibitor of the *A* transferase in the sera of the McC. family members with the *cis* AB phenotype (Fig. 16). The velocity of the reaction

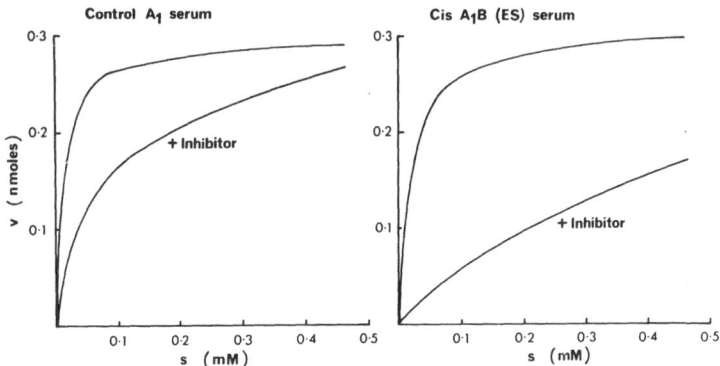

Fig. 16. Inhibition of the $\alpha$-3-*N*-acetylgalactosaminyltransferases in $A_1$ serum and in *cis* AB serum E.S. (I. 2, Fig. 15) by UDP-galactose (for details see Sabo *et al.*, 1978).

with the *cis* AB serum as the enzyme source was not very different from that of the control $A_1$ in the absence of UDP-galactose but in the presence of a constant amount of this inhibitor the velocity was decreased far more with the *cis* AB serum than with the control $A_1$ serum. Lineweaver–Burk plots derived from the substrate concentration curves showed that the inhibition was competitive. The apparent $K_m$ values for UDP-*N*-acetylgalactosamine were very similar for both the *A* transferase in the *cis* AB sera and those in normal $A_1$ and $A_1B$ sera. However, with the enzymes in the *cis* AB sera the apparent $K_i$ values for UDP-galactose were appreciably lower than the apparent $K_m$ values for UDP-*N*-acetylgalactosamine whereas with the normal $A_1$ and $A_1B$ sera the apparent $K_i$ for UDP-galactose and the apparent $K_m$ for UDP-*N*-acetylgalactosamine were approximately the same (Sabo *et al.*, 1978). These results indicate that the *A* transferases in the *cis* AB sera have a greater affinity for UDP-galactose than do the enzymes in normal A sera. The *B* transferase activity in the *cis* AB sera of the McC. family was so weak that detailed kinetic studies were not possible but inhibition experiments with two different concentrations of UDP-*N*-acetylgalactosamine revealed that the *B* transferases were more readily inhibitable by this nucleotide sugar than are the corresponding enzymes in normal B sera. Thus both the *A* and *B* transferases in the *cis* AB sera from this family behaved differently with respect to their combining power with the heterologous sugar nucleotides than do the transferases in normal A, B, or AB sera. These results still fail to answer the crucial question of whether one or two enzymes are present in the *cis* AB sera but they do imply that the phenotype does not result simply from a mixture of normal *A* transferase with a lesser amount of a normal *B* transferase.

Cytogenetic investigations of blood lymphocytes from all three *cis* AB members of the McC. family showed normal karyotypes. Specifically, the terminal bands of the long arms of the No. 9 chromosomes to which the *ABO* : *Np-1* : *AK-1* linkage group has been assigned displayed G bands similar to those in cells from normal individuals examined at the same time (Sabo *et al.*, 1978).

## Glycosyltransferases in Genetic Chimeras

Human genetic chimeras fall into two main classes, namely twin chimeras and dispermic, or tetragametic, chimeras. The twin chimeras result from placental cross circulation in dizygotic twins and the cells with different zygotic lineages are confined to hemopoietic tissue. Twin chimeras usually present as blood grouping problems, that is, they are observed to have two red cell populations carrying different antigenic determinants or they are found to lack an anti-A or anti-B agglutinin expected on the basis of their apparent ABO red cell group (see Giblett, 1969; Race and Sanger, 1975).

Measurement of the ABH glycosyltransferases in the serum and red cells contributes information on the true genetic groups of twin chimeras. A low $A$ transferase level was observed in the serum of a hemopoietic chimera who was genetically O but had 50% of grafted $A_1$ red cells (Schachter et al., 1971). This result indicated that the hemopoietic tissue made a small but significant contribution to the $A$ transferase activity detected in serum. Subsequently Wrobel et al. (1974) examined the transferases in a pair of twins, one male, one female, who each had a mixture of 99% $A_1$ red cells and 1% B cells (Fig. 17). In each twin the two populations of red cells also differed in Rhesus, MN, and Xg groups. Karyotyping of the white cells revealed them also to be mixtures of 46XY and 46XX cells in each twin, although the male twin had 80% XY and 20% XX cells and the female twin 44% XX and 56% XY cells. Examination of the $A$ and $B$ transferase activities in the serum of the parents and twins (Table IX) revealed, as expected, that the $\alpha$-$N$-acetylgalactosaminyl- and $\alpha$-galactosyltransferases were present in the serum of the group $A_1B$ mother, M. St., and absent from the serum of the group O father, H. St. Twin I, Jo. St., had a high $A$ transferase level, comparable with that in his mother's serum whereas Twin II, Ju. St., despite having 99% $A_1$ red cells in her circulation, had only 16% of the $A$ transferase activity in her mother's serum. Twin I also secreted A substance in his saliva and hence was deemed to be genetically $A^1O$ and to be the twin who had contributed

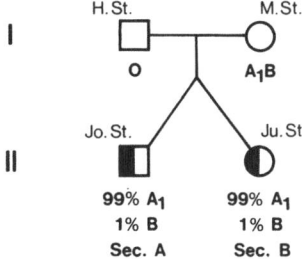

Fig. 17. Pedigree and ABO groups of twin chimera family St. investigated by Wrobel et al. (1974).

TABLE IX. Blood Group Antigens on Red Cells and Saliva and *A* and *B* Transferase
Activities in Sera of Members of St. Family[a]

| Family member | | ABO group of red cells | Blood group activity in saliva | Transferase activity[b] | | Percentage of activity of transferase in M. St.'s serum | |
|---|---|---|---|---|---|---|---|
| | | | | *A* transferase | *B* transferase | *A* | *B* |
| Father | H. St. | O | H | 0 | 0 | | |
| Mother | M. St. | A₁B | A, B, and H | 20 | 9 | | |
| Twin I | Jo. St. | 99% A₁ | A and H | 22 | 0.3 | 110 | 1 |
| | | 1% B | | | | | |
| Twin II | Ju. St. | 99% A₁ | B and H | 3 | 6.3 | 16 | 70 |
| | | 1% B | | | | | |

[a] Modified from Wrobel *et al.* (1974).
[b] Measured as percent radioactivity transferred from UDP-*N*-acetyl[$^{14}$C]galactosamine (*A* transferase) or UDP-[$^{14}$C]galactose (*B* transferase) to 2'-fucosyllactose.

A₁ red cell precursors, and XY white cell precursors, to his sister's bone marrow. The occurrence of a relatively strong *B* transferase in the serum of twin II, despite the fact that she had only 1% of circulating B cells, together with the fact that she secreted B substance, indicated that she was genetically *BO* and that the B red cells and XX white cell precursors had originated in her bone marrow. The reasons why the proportions of red cells and white cells are different is unknown but where the lymphocyte karyotypes have been determined in chimeric twins the proportion of grafted red cells and lymphocytes have been similar in some twins and dissimilar in others (see Race and Sanger, 1975). Hosoi *et al.* (1977) suggested that either the proportions of hemopoietic and lymphoid stem cells passing through a fetal anastomosis could be different or, in the early stage of embryonic development, pluripotential stem cells might reach hemopoietic sites and the antigenic expression of the hemopoietic stem cells may be modified by a mechanism which does not affect the lymphoid stem cells.

A striking example of a chimera which confirmed that the proportion of lymphocytes with the 46XX or 46XY karyotype in the circulation has no bearing on the true sex of an individual was described by Battey *et al.* (1974). A Caucasian *prima gravida* was found on routine antenatal serological investigation to have two red cell populations with differences in four blood group systems; the major population (93%) was group O and the minor population (7%) was group $A_1$. Chromosome analysis of the cultured lymphocytes showed that 96% of cells had the male karyotype 46XY. The proposita's husband was group O and she eventually gave birth to a group O child (Fig. 18). Analysis of the blood group glycosyl-transferases in the serum of the proposita showed that her A transferase level was similar to that of a normal $A_1$ control (Bird *et al.*, 1976); thus the minor group A red cell population and the minor lymphocyte population with the 46XX karyotype appeared to correspond to her true genetic make up. There was no evidence of a twin but the two genetic cell lines, as far as could be ascertained, were confined to hemopoietic tissues and it is possible that the proposita's twin may have been aborted or assimilated *in utero*.

Examination of the transferase levels in a number of other twin chimeras have shown that, provided the twins differ in their ABO groups, it is usually possible to deduce the true ABO phenotype of each twin from the enzymic analyses (P. Greenwell, A. D. Yates, L. R. Carne, and W. M. Watkins, unpublished observations). This is particularly useful then one or both of the twins are nonsecretors.

The second class of human genetic chimeras, the dispermic or tetragametic chimeras, may have two distinct genetic cell populations in many tissues. Many such chimeras have been made artifically in animals by fusion of embryos (see McClaren, 1976), but in humans they are believed to result from fertilization by two sperms of two maternal nuclei and subsequent fusion of the two zygotes so that they develop as one organism. Either the father or both the mother and the father may make two

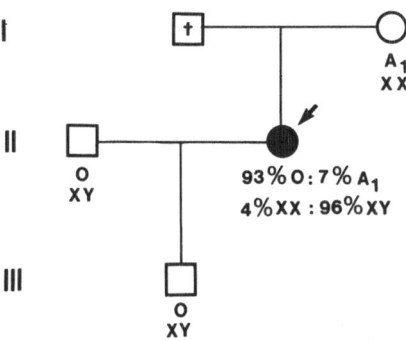

Fig. 18. Pedigree, ABO groups and karyotypes of chimera and family investigated by Battey *et al.* (1974).

genetic contributions. Dispermic chimeras usually present as gonadal abnormalities or are recognized because of an unusual external appearance such as patchy skin color or eyes of different color (Giblett, 1969; Race and Sanger, 1975). Subsequent serological and cytogenetic examination of their blood frequently reveals mixed red cell and lymphocyte populations. Recently, however, a dispermic chimera was suspected initially from the results of blood group gene-specified glycosyltransferase assays on serum and red cells (Watkins *et al.*, 1978). A normal male blood donor, at first thought to be group B was found to have no anti-A in his serum. Further investigation showed that his red cells carry a very weak A antigen detectable only by absorption and elution of anti-A. He was a nonsecretor of A, B, and H substances, and therefore little could be deduced from saliva studies. From the serological investigation he was assumed to be carrying a weak *A* gene and a normal *B* and thus to have the genotype $A^wB$. Examination of the blood of other members of his family showed that his wife was group $A_2$, one of his sons was $A_2$, and the other B. The first interpretation of the inheritance of ABO groups in this family was that shown in Fig. 19a.

Examination of the *A*-, *B*- and *H*-transferase activities in the serum of the propositus revealed that all three activities were detectable but, in contrast to the finding of a very weak A and a normal B antigen on his red cells, the *A*-transferase activity in his serum was comparatively strong and the *B*-transferase activity relatively weak. The *A* transferase on the basis of its pH optimum and capacity to convert O cells to A-active cells was characterized as the product of an $A^1$ gene. The propositus did not,

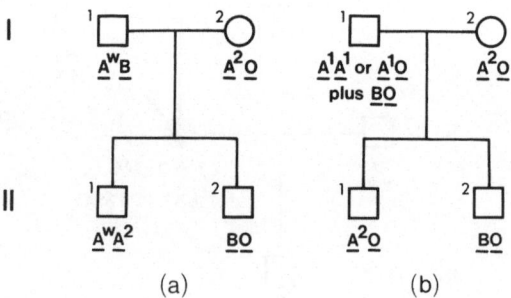

Fig. 19. Pedigree of chimera and family Sh. investigated by Watkins *et al.* (1978). (a) First interpretation of inheritance of ABO groups on the basis of serological results. (b) Final interpretation of inheritance of ABO groups based on enzymic and cytogenetic studies.

however, appear to have passed this gene on to either of his sons. The group B son must have inherited the $B$ gene from his father but the $B$ transferase level in the son's serum was three times as high as that in his father's serum. The wife and group $A_2$ son of the propositus have normal $A^2$ transferases in keeping with their $A_2$ red cell status. The $A_2$ son, therefore, appears to have inherited an $A^2$ gene from his mother but neither the $A^1$ nor the $B$ gene from his father. Examination of the red cell groups, the serum transferase levels, and the genetic characteristics of the transferases together with the unclear pattern of inheritance led to a suspicion of chimerism. Cytogenetic examination of the propositus' lymphocytes revealed them to be all of the 46XY karyotype. However, cultured skin fibroblasts were found to be a mixture of 46XX (60%) and 46XY (40%) cells and hair roots also had a mixture of male and female cells. The conclusion was reached that the propositus was probably a dispermic chimera with two genetic cell lines, one with genotype $BO$ and the other either $A^1O$ or $A^1A^1$. The $A_2$ son is assumed to have inherited an $O$ gene from his father. It is, therefore, probable that the bone marrow and reproductive organs of the propositus are predominantly group B and male whereas his skin, and the organs making the $A$ transferase that appears in his serum, are partly $A_1$ and female. A reinterpretation of the pattern of inheritance in this family is given in Fig. 19b.

## Origin of the *A*-, *B*-, and *H*-Gene-Specified Glycosyltransferases in Serum

The precise origin of the glycosyltransferases in serum is not known but some inferences may be drawn from the investigations of transferase levels in chimeras and in rare blood groups in which the expression of the *A*, *B*, or *H* genes are suppressed at the cellular level or at the site of synthesis of the secreted glycoproteins.

The *H*-gene-specified α-2-fucosyltransferase is present in the serum of both secretors and nonsecretors of ABH substances and the level of activity is not related to secretor–nonsecretor status (Schenkel-Brunner *et al.*, 1972; Chester *et al.*, 1976). The fact that in nonsecretors the *H* transferase is missing from, or only very weakly expressed in, tissues producing the secreted glycoproteins (Chester and Watkins, 1969) does not appear to influence the level of activity of this transferase in serum. These results suggest that most of the circulating enzyme originates from the blood-forming tissues and possibly other cells where the expression of H as a cell surface antigen is not under the control of the secretor gene (see Cartron, 1978). Individuals with the para-Bombay phenotype, in whom regulator or modifying genes ($zz$) suppress the expression of H on the red cells but not in secretions, have no detectable $H$ transferase in serum (Mulet et al., 1977; Watkins, 1978). These results thus lend further support to the view that the enzyme in serum originates mainly from the hemopoietic tissues.

In contrast to the $H$ transferase the major part of the $A$-gene-specified $\alpha$-$N$-acetylgalactosaminyltransferase and the $B$-gene-specified $\alpha$-galac-tosyltransferase in serum is derived from sources other than the hemo-poietic tissue. A hemopoietic chimera may receive in utero a graft of cells from a genetically group A twin which so successfully populates the bone marrow that 99% of the red cells in the circulating blood are group A. Nevertheless, if the recipient carries only $B$ or $O$ genes in other tissues, the level of $A$ transferase in the serum amounts to only 20–30% of that found in a normal group A member of the same family (Schachter et al., 1971; Wrobel et al., 1974; Cartron, 1976). Conversely a chimeric twin who is genetically group B has about 60–70% of the normal level of $B$ transferase in the serum even if only 1% of the circulating red cells are group B (Wrobel et al., 1974). Since the mucosal tissues produce the $A$ and $B$ transferases irrespective of secretor status (Hearn et al., 1968; Race et al., 1968), the enzymes in serum possibly derive from these sources, but this is not yet proved.

Cartron et al. (1975) reported that in 15 examples of the $A_m$ pheno-type, where there is failure of expression of the $A$ gene on the red cells, but normal expression in saliva, the $A$ transferase levels were 30–50% of the average values observed for $A_1$ or $A_2$ subjects, respectively. These results are consistent with the interpretation that the $\alpha$-$N$-acetylgalacto-saminyltransferase comes from other sources than the hemopoietic tissues although the values for the contributions from other tissues are lower than those suggested from the results on chimeras. On the other hand, values between 50% and 70% of those given by control sera have been reported for the activity of the $\alpha$-galactosyltransferase in examples of the $B_m$ phen-otype (Simmons and Twait, 1975; Koscielak et al., 1976b; Watkins, 1978). The considerable differences observed in the enzyme activities in unre-lated A or B persons, the possibility of interaction between the enzymic products of allelic genes (Salmon and Cartron, 1976), the likelihood that the transferases are not always tested under optimum conditions for linearity, together with the inaccuracies inherent in the rather cumbersome methods in use for the assay of the enzymes, probably account for some of the discrepancies in the results reported by different laboratories for the relative quantities of transferase contributed to the serum by the various tissues. On the other hand the mutations that give rise to the $A_m$ and $B_m$ phenotypes may affect other tissues in addition to the hemopoietic tissues and hence the contributions to the serum may be different from that in the twin chimeras.

## Are the *A*- and *B*-Gene-Specified Transferases the Products of Allelic Genes?

The blood group *ABO* locus is unique amongst the loci so far investigated in mammalian genetic systems in that the structural alleles, *A* and *B*, code for enzymes with qualitatively different specificities. The specificities of the two enzymes can in fact be considered to be very similar since each catalyzes the transfer of a sugar with a basic D-galactose configuration (Fig. 20) in $\alpha$-(1→3) linkage to the same acceptor substrate, namely an H-active structure. Nevertheless, in general, allelic genes show

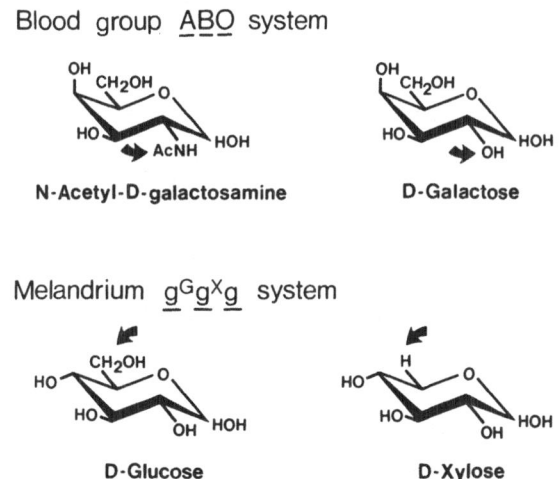

Fig. 20. Structures of the sugars transferred by the glycosyltransferase products of allelic genes in the human blood group *ABO* system and in plant *Melandrium* $g^G g^X g$ system. The arrows indicate for each pair the positions in the sugar rings where there are structural differences.

quantitative differences in biochemical action, and the finding that the $A$ and $B$ genes control the formation of transferases with qualitatively different specificities has led some geneticists (see Boettcher, 1978a) to doubt whether the genes are alleles despite the vast amount of data derived from serological studies on families which support the concept that they are alternative forms at the same locus. The report of the appearance of A antigen in cancerous tissues of groups B and O patients with gastric carcinoma (Häkkinen, 1970) has led to the suggestion that the $A$, $B$, and $O$ alleles are normally involved in the repression of ubiquitous genes and that derepression occurs in the malignant state (see Boettcher, 1978a).

However, although no other examples of mutant enzymes with altered specificity appear to have been reported for genetic loci in mammalian systems, a series of alleles has been described in the plant *Melandrium* that in many respects presents a similar picture to the *ABO* system (Brederode and Nigtevecht, 1974, 1975). In the petals of *Melandrium* the glycosylation of the 7-hydroxyl group of isovitexin is governed by a series of four alleles $g^G$, $g^X$, $g^{X'}$, and $g$. Gene $g^G$ is the structural gene for UDP-glucose:isovitexin 7-$O$-glucosyltransferase. The alleles $g^X$ and $g^{X'}$ are both structural genes for UDP-xylose:isovitexin 7-$O$-xylosyltransferase, but the two enzymes differ in their $V_{max}$ when working at saturating isovitexin concentrations. Gene $g$ is inactive and does not produce a functional glycosyltransferase. Thus the two xylosyltransferases may be considered analogous to the $\alpha$-$N$-acetylgalactosaminyltransferase products of the $A^1$ and $A^2$ genes, the glucosyltransferase analogous to the $\alpha$-galactosyltransferase product of the $B$ gene, and the silent allele $g$ analogous to the $O$ gene. The relationship between glucose and xylose is such that the structures differ only in the nature of the substituent attached to C-5 in the pyranoside ring, a $CH_2OH$ group in the hexose glucose and an H atom in the pentose xylose (Fig. 20). The enzymic products of $g^G$ and $g^X$ are analogous to those of the $A$ and $B$ genes in that, in each system, both enzymes utilize the same acceptor substrate and, although the glycosyltransferases have qualitatively different specificities the structures of the transferred sugars differ solely in the nature of the substituent at one carbon atom in the sugar ring. Brederode and Nigtevecht (1974) pointed to the possibility that a new allele with a different substrate specificity might evolve via a silent allele as the result of the accumulation of mutations affecting the active site of the enzyme protein. In a system such as the ABO system where the enzymic products of the genes are not essential for life it is possible that the silent allele may serve the same function in the evolution of a new enzyme as the duplication of genes in other genetic systems in which absence of the gene product would be lethal.

In bacteria, evidence that qualitative changes in enzyme specificity are possible has come from investigations on the stepwise evolution of enzymes in the laboratory (Wood, 1966; Wu *et al.*, 1968; Clarke 1974). Dr. Patricia Clarke and her colleagues took a single enzyme, an inducible aliphatic amidase of *Pseudomonas aeruginosa* and showed that it was possible to evolve amidases with altered substrate specificities by introducing novel substrates and selecting strains that had mutated to be able to use these substrates (Betz *et al.*, 1974). The A amidase produced by the wild-type strain hydrolyzes acetamide (1) but has no activity with *N*-phenylacetamide (2).

(1)  $NH_2COCH_3$  (2) —NHCOCH$_3$

One of the mutant enzymes (A 13) had acquired the capacity to hydrolyze *N*-phenylacetamide (acetanilide) and the change in substrate specificity to allow the enzyme to accommodate the benzene ring resulted in decreased acetamidase activity. The A 13 mutant enzyme gave complete cross reaction with an antiserum to the A amidase and the difference between the two enzymes was shown to reside in the substitution of a single amino acid residue; a threonine residue of the wild-type enzyme was replaced by an isoleucine residue in the mutant A 13 enzyme (Brown and Clarke, 1972). Although the structural differences between acetamide and *N*-phenylacetamide are not strictly analogous to the differences between D-galactose and *N*-acetyl-D-galactosamine, there is sufficient similarity to suggest that the changes required to alter the specificity of an α-D-galactosyltransferase to an α-*N*-acetyl-D-galactosaminyltransferase or vice versa might involve very few changes in the primary structure of the enzyme and could possibly result from a single amino acid substitution. The α-*N*-acetylgalactosaminyltransferases with lower activity and differing kinetic properties which give rise to the A$_2$ phenotype and weaker subgroups of A could arise from mutations which involved regions of the enzyme protein other than the active site of the transferase.

# THE LEWIS SYSTEM

The Lewis system comprises two antigens, Le$^a$ and Le$^b$, which despite their apparently antithetical relationship on red cells are not the products of allelic genes. Szulman and Marcus (1973) investigated the Le$^a$ and Le$^b$ antigens during fetal development by means of the immunofluorescence technique and found that in the salivary glands, stomachs, and intestines of human embryos there is, in general, a reciprocal relation between Le$^a$ and ABH, whereas there is a parallel relation between Le$^b$ and ABH. The Le$^a$ and Le$^b$ antigens on the red cell surface differ from the ABH antigens in that they are not synthesized in the erythrocyte precursor cells but are secondarily acquired from the plasma in which the red cells circulate (Sneath and Sneath, 1955; Mäkelä and Mäkelä, 1956). The acquired antigens are now known to be glycosphingolipids which are synthesized at an, as yet, unknown site and carried in the plasma by high- and low-density lipoproteins (Marcus and Cass, 1969). In saliva and gastric mucosa, Le$^a$ and Le$^b$ specificities are carried on the same glycoprotein molecules as those that carry A, B, and H determinants (see Watkins, 1974).

## Serology and Genetics

At the Lewis genetic locus there are two alleles: *Le*, a functional gene, and *le*, a silent gene. This locus has not yet been assigned to a chromosome (Edwards and McKusick, 1978). The *Le* gene is expressed whenever it is part of an individual's genome and is not under the control of the secretor gene. Whether the antigen on the red cells is Le$^a$ or Le$^b$, however, depends upon the genetic endowment with respect to *H* and *Se* genes. The Le$^a$ and Le$^b$ glycosphingolipids which are destined for export into the plasma, and eventual uptake onto the red cell surface are synthesized in cells where the expression of the *H* gene is controlled by the *Se* gene. In persons with an *Le* gene, an *H* gene, and an *Se* gene, the glycosphingolipid molecules carry Le$^b$ specificity, which results from the action of the enzymic products of *Le* and *H* genes on a common acceptor substrate. In those who have an *Le* gene and an *H* gene but are homozygous *se se*, the glycosphingolipid molecules have Le$^a$ specificity. About 10% of the European population is homozygous for the allele *le*; the red cells and secretions of these individuals lack both Le$^a$ and Le$^b$ antigens.

The regulation by the secretor gene *Se* of the formation of the Le[b] antigen which appears on the red cell surface and of the A, B, and H antigens that occur in secretions results in a close phenotypic linkage between the Lewis groups on the red cell and ABH secretion. As first observed by Grubb (1948), individuals who have Le[a] antigen on their red cells are nonsecretors of ABH, whereas those who have Le[b] antigens are secretors of ABH. The occurrence of Le[b] activity only on the red cells and in the tissue fluids of ABH secretors led Ceppellini (1955) to suggest that Le[b] was an interaction product of the *Le* and *Se* genes. The concept that Le[b] specificity is a gene interaction product is now well established from the structure of the Le[b] determinant (Fig. 21), but it is the gene

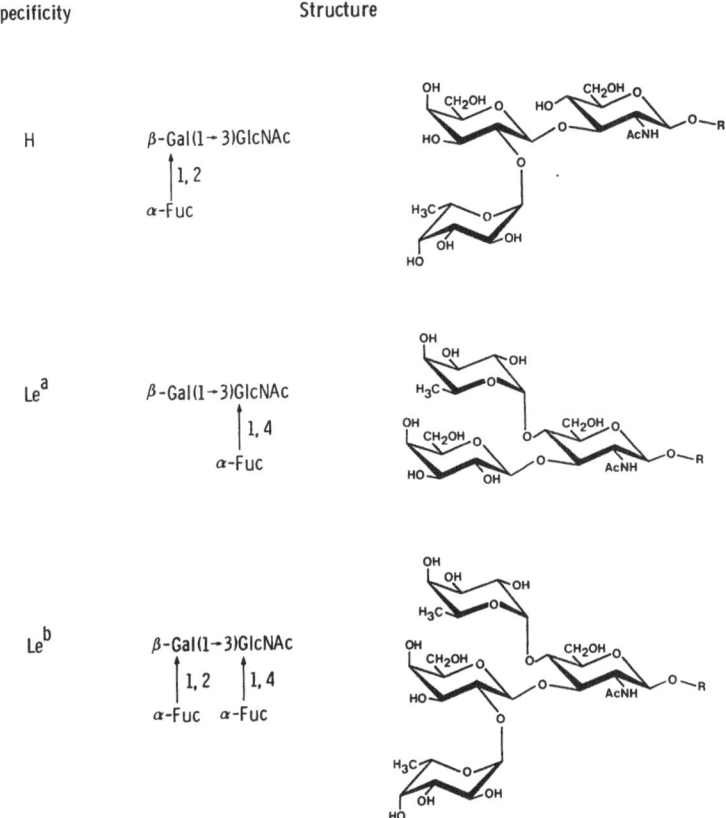

| Specificity | Structure |
|---|---|
| H | β-Gal(1→3)GlcNAc ↑1,2 α-Fuc |
| Le[a] | β-Gal(1→3)GlcNAc ↑1,4 α-Fuc |
| Le[b] | β-Gal(1→3)GlcNAc ↑1,2 ↑1,4 α-Fuc α-Fuc |

Fig. 21. Structures of Type 1 H, Le[a], and Le[b] determinants. Abbreviations as in Figs. 1 and 2.

regulated by the *Se* gene, namely *H*, that interacts with the product of the *Le* gene.


## Chemistry of Lewis Substances

### Le$^a$ and Le$^b$ Determinants

The structures of the Le$^a$ and Le$^b$ determinants (Fig. 21) were first deduced from the results of serological inhibition tests with fucose-containing oligosaccharides from human milk (Watkins and Morgan, 1957*b*, 1962) and subsequently confirmed by the isolation of oligosaccharide fragments from alkaline degradation products of Le$^a$ (Rege *et al.*, 1964*b*; Lloyd *et al.*, 1968) and HLe$^b$ (Marr *et al.*, 1967; Rovis *et al.*, 1973) blood-group-specific glycoproteins isolated from ovarian cyst fluids. Whereas two forms of H-, A-, and B-active oligosaccharides, based on the Type 1 and Type 2 chain endings (Fig. 2) were isolated from the appropriate glycoproteins, only one form of Le$^a$-active trisaccharide and one form of Le$^b$-active tetrasaccharide have been isolated. The Le$^a$ determinant contains L-fucose joined to the C-4 position of the subterminal *N*-acetylglucosamine in a Type 1 chain and since in Type 2 chains the C-4 position of *N*-acetylglucosamine is occupied by the terminal β-galactosyl residue (Fig. 1) it is not possible to form an Le$^a$-active structure on this chain. The chemical synthesis of β-Gal-(1→3)[α-Fuc(1→4)]GlcNAc (Lemieux and Driguez, 1975*b*) and the demonstration that a synthetic antigen prepared from this trisaccharide induced the formation of antibodies which agglutinated Le$^a$-positive red cells and precipitated with Le$^a$-active glycoprotein (Lemieux *et al.*, 1975*b*) has provided strong independent evidence in support of the structure assigned to the Le$^a$ determinant.

The Le$^b$ determinant, also based on the Type 1 chain has two fucosyl residues joined to adjacent sugars, one linked α-(1→4) to *N*-acetylglucosamine as in the Le$^a$ determinant and the second linked α-(1→2) to the β-galactosyl residue as in Type 1 H trisaccharide (Fig. 21). Le$^b$ is thus a hybrid antigen compounded of the H and Le$^a$ determinants but bearing a new, distinctive specificity (Marr *et al.*, 1967). This was the first example of a hybrid cell surface antigen, arising from the action of secondary gene products, to be defined both in terms of its chemical structure and the enzymes responsible for its formation. Since genes at three independent loci are required to give an Le$^b$ determinant it is possible for a child to have the antigen when it is absent from both parents. A hypothetical pedigree demonstrating such a pattern of inheritance is shown in Fig. 22.

## Glycosphingolipids with Le$^a$ and Le$^b$ Activities

Marcus and Cass (1969) demonstrated that the Le$^a$ and Le$^b$ antigens taken up onto erythrocytes are glycosphingolipids carried in the plasma by high- and low-density lipoproteins. Isolation of the Lewis antigens from red cell membranes is even more difficult than the isolation of A, B, and H antigens because the Le$^a$- and Le$^b$-active glycosphingolipids are present in relatively much smaller amounts (Hanfland and Egli, 1975). The isolation from human group O red cells of a glycolipid fraction with H and Le$^b$ activity was reported by Hakomori and Strycharz (1968) but the yield was too low for structural characterization. Lewis-active glycolipids were, however, isolated and characterized from human adenocarcinoma tissue (Hakomori and Andrews, 1970) and normal human small intestine (Smith *et al.*, 1975). Oxidation with osmium tetroxide of the Le$^a$-active, and the simplest Le$^b$-active, glycolipids isolated by Hakomori and Andrews (1970) gave the Le$^a$-active oligosaccharide lacto-*N*-fucopentaose II and the Le$^b$-active oligosaccharide, lacto-*N*-difucohexaose II (Table VI), respectively. The structure of the Le$^a$ glycolipid isolated by Smith *et al.*, (1975) was more rigorously characterized and the results confirmed that the determinant is identical with that established for the Le$^a$ active structure in the blood-group-active glycoproteins. The Le$^a$- and the Le$^b$-

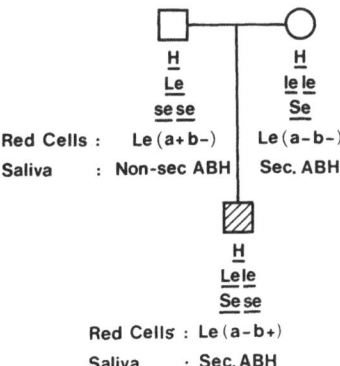

Fig. 22. Hypothetical pedigree to illustrate the inheritance of Le$^b$ character in a child whose parents lack the antigen.

active glycolipids are based on the type I chain, lacto-$N$-tetraosyl ceramide, structure (Table X). The possible existence in the tumor tissues
of families of molecules with the same determinant structure but with
different carbohydrate chain lengths was suggested by the fact that two
$Le^b$-active glycolipids were isolated (Hakomori and Andrews, 1970) one
having six and the other eight sugar residues.

More recently Hanfland (1978) examined the Lewis-active glycosphingolipids in the plasma of human $OLe^b$ individuals. Two $Le^a$-active
ceramide pentasaccharides, differing in their chromatographic properties,
and three $Le^b$-active ceramide hexasaccharides were purified. The structures of these glycolipids have yet to be established but the sugar composition and general properties indicate that the carbohydrate moieties
in the three $Le^b$-active ceramide hexasaccharides are identical. The difference in chromatographic behavior therefore probably indicates that the
glycosphingolipids differ from one another in the nature of the lipid
moiety. As little as 0.0001 $\mu$g of one of the $Le^b$-active glycolipids was
sufficient to convert $9 \times 10^7 OLe(a^- b^-)$ erythrocytes into $OLe(a^- b^+)$ cells.
This means that maximally 400 molecules per erythrocyte are sufficient
to achieve agglutinability of $Le^b$ cells. Larger quantities (0.04 $\mu$g and 0.3
$\mu$g) of the two $Le^a$-active glycosphingolipids were required to convert the
same number of $OLe(a^- b^-)$ erythrocytes into $OLe(a^+ b^-)$ cells. These
amounts are, however, still considerably less than the quantity (2.5 $\mu$g
per $9 \times 10^7$ erythrocytes) of purified blood group B-active ceramide hexasaccharide or octasaccharide required to render the same $OLe(a^- b^-)$
red cells agglutinable by normal human anti-B serum (Hanfland, 1978).

The site of synthesis of the Lewis-active glycosphingolipids that circulate in the plasma, and coat onto red cells, is unknown. Oriol $et$ $al.$
(1978$a$) reported that Lewis substances are synthesized by the kidney and
excreted into the urine. However, in patients who have received kidney
transplants the Lewis activity in the urine reflects the specificity of the
transplanted kidney but does not influence the pattern of Lewis activity
in the plasma of the recipient. The kidney is thus not the source of the
Lewis-active glycolipids circulating in the plasma. Another point with
regard to the Lewis antigens that is still not established is whether there
are specific receptor sites on the red cells for the $Le^a$ and $Le^b$ glycolipids
or whether they are nonspecifically slotted into the lipid bilayer of the red
cell membrane.

Certain antisera react only with human red cells which are both $A_1$
and $Le^b$ positive, that is, cells from individuals with $A^1$, $H$, $Se$, and $Le$

genes (Seaman *et al.,* 1968; Crookston *et al.,* 1970). The determinant recognized by anti-$A_1Le^b$ is not a mixture of A and $Le^b$ molecules but is a hybrid antigen carried by a glycosphingolipid molecule which is present in plasma and is taken up by the erythrocytes (Tilley *et al.,* 1975). Recently Karlsson (1978), by means of an improved method for the extraction of total nonacid glycosphingolipids, isolated novel fucose-containing glycolipids from human small intestine (A7, Table X) and human erythrocytes (A9, Table X) which have $ALe^b$ structures at the terminal nonreducing ends of the molecules. Most probably this is the determinant detected by the anti-$A_1Le^b$ reagents. The anti-$A_1Le^b$ sera provide useful tools for establishing the true genotype of hemopoietic chimeric twins if one of them is genetically $A^1$ and the other $B$ or $O$. All the cells in the mixed red cell population acquire the $ALe^b$ glycolipid from the plasma but, since the glycolipid is not synthesized in the hemopoietic tissue, only the twin carrying an $A^1$, *Se, H,* and *Le* gene will be capable of synthesizing the hybrid antigen (Crookston *et al.,* 1970; Wrobel *et al.,* 1974; Bird *et al.,* 1976). Certain cytotoxic sera reacting with lymphocytes appear to have anti-$ALe^b$ and anti-$BLe^b$ specificity (Jeannet *et al.,* 1973, 1974).

## Glycoproteins with $Le^a$ and $Le^b$ Activities

$Le^a$ and $Le^b$ determinants in saliva, gastric mucosa, and ovarian cyst fluids are carried on the glycoprotein macromolecules which also carry the A, B, and H determinants (see Morgan, 1960; Kabat, 1973; Watkins, 1974). In ABH nonsecretors who carry an *Le* gene, the glycoproteins have only $Le^a$ out of the five possible specificities A, B, H, $Le^a$, and $Le^b$. Because substitution with fucose to form $Le^a$ determinants can occur only on Type 1 chain endings, these glycoproteins also react with reagents that recognize unsubstituted Type 2 chain endings, such as anti-Type XIV pneumococcal serum (Morgan, 1960) and certain anti-I sera (Picard, *et al.,* 1978). In individuals with an *Se,* an *H,* and an *Le* gene, the Type 1 chains in the glycoproteins are mainly converted into $Le^b$-specific structures but the Type 2 chains will also be substituted on the terminal β-galactosyl residue with α-2-linked fucose. The molecules therefore carry both H and $Le^b$ determinants (and probably some $Le^a$ determinants) and it is not possible to isolate an $Le^b$ glycoprotein entirely free from other blood group activities.

**TABLE X. Structures of Le$^a$, Le$^b$, and ALe$^b$ Glycosphingolipids and Their Immediate Precursor Lacto-*N*-tetraosyl Ceramide**

| Glycolipid | Structure |
| --- | --- |
| Precursor (lacto-*N*-tetraosyl-ceramide)$^a$ | β-Gal(1→3)β-GlcNAc(1→3)β-Gal(1→4)Glc-CER |
| Le$^a$ | β-Gal(1→3)β-GlcNAc(1→3)β-Gal(1→4)Glc-CER<br>↑ 1,4<br>α-Fuc |
| Le$^b$ (1) | β-Gal(1→3)β-GlcNAc(1→3)β-Gal(1→4)Glc-CER<br>↑ 1,2     ↑ 1,4<br>α-Fuc     α-Fuc |

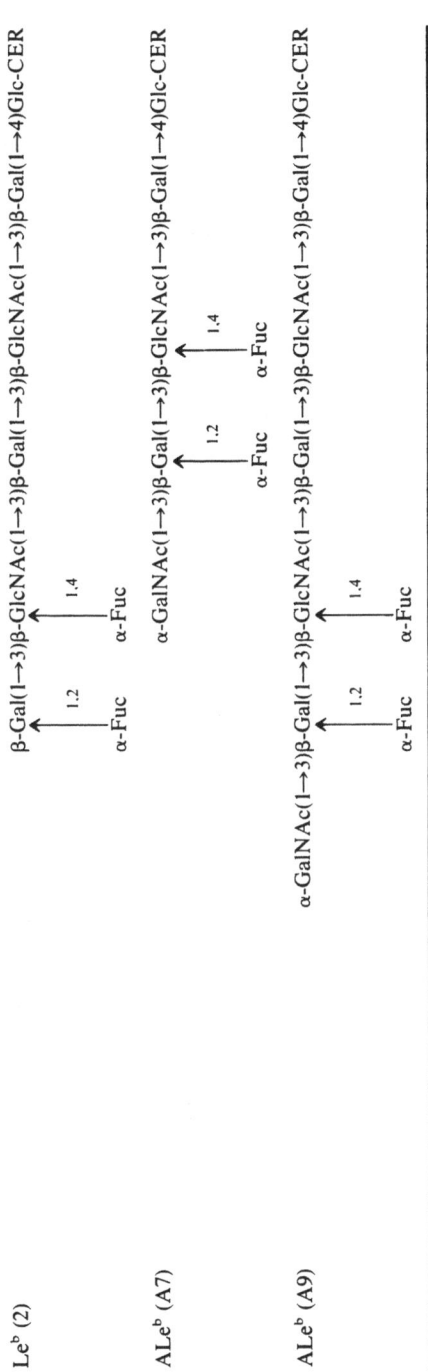

Le<sup>b</sup> (2)

$$\beta\text{-Gal}(1\rightarrow3)\beta\text{-GlcNAc}(1\rightarrow3)\beta\text{-GlcNAc}(1\rightarrow3)\beta\text{-Gal}(1\rightarrow4)\text{Glc-CER}$$

ALe<sup>b</sup> (A7)

$$\alpha\text{-GalNAc}(1\rightarrow3)\beta\text{-Gal}(1\rightarrow3)\beta\text{-GlcNAc}(1\rightarrow3)\beta\text{-Gal}(1\rightarrow4)\text{Glc-CER}$$

ALe<sup>b</sup> (A9)

$$\alpha\text{-GalNAc}(1\rightarrow3)\beta\text{-Gal}(1\rightarrow3)\beta\text{-GlcNAc}(1\rightarrow3)\beta\text{-Gal}(1\rightarrow4)\text{Glc-CER}$$

[a] The Le<sup>a</sup> glycolipid was isolated from tumor tissue (Hakomori and Andrews, 1970) and human small intestine (Smith *et al.*, 1975). The Le<sup>b</sup> glycolipids (1) and (2) were isolated from tumor tissue (Hakomori and Andrews, 1970). The ALe<sup>b</sup> glycolipids were isolated from human small intestine (A7) and human erythrocytes (A9) (Karlsson, 1978).

## Biosynthesis of Le ᵃ and Le ᵇ Determinants

The *Le* gene at the *Lewis* locus specifies an α-4-L-fucosyltransferase (E. C. 2.4.1.65) that catalyzes the formation of an Le$^a$ structure (Fig. 21) by the following reaction:

$$\text{GDP-Fuc} + \beta\text{-Gal}(1{\rightarrow}3)\beta\text{-GlcNAc-R} \rightarrow \beta\text{-Gal}(1{\rightarrow}3)\text{-GlcNAc-R} + \text{GDP}$$
$$\uparrow {\scriptstyle 1.4}$$
$$\alpha\text{-Fuc}$$

The enzyme can utilize only Type 1 chain endings in glycoproteins, gly-colipids, or oligosaccharides. The acceptor specificity of the *Le* gene spec-ified 4-fucosyltransferase is such that the enzyme does not transfer L-fucose to *N*-acetylglucosamine alone or to oligosaccharides with terminal β-*N*-acetylglucosaminyl residues (Chester, 1971). With low-molecular-weight compounds such as lacto-*N*-biose I (β-Gal(1→3)GlcNAc), or lacto-*N*-tetraose (β-Gal(1→3)β-GlcNAc(1→3)β-Gal(1→4)Glc), as acceptor substrates, this fucosyltransferase has been demonstrated in milk (Groll-man *et al.*, 1969), gastric mucosa and submaxillary glands (Chester and Watkins, 1969), ovarian cyst linings (Chester, 1971), saliva (Yazawa, 1976), and kidney (Oriol *et al.*, 1978a). In contrast to the *A*, *B*, and *H* transferases the *Le*-gene-dependent transferase has not been detected in serum or plasma (Schenkel-Brunner *et al.*, 1972) in individuals carrying the *Le* gene. Hence it seems probable that both the appropriate acceptor and the requisite enzyme for the formation of Le$^a$- and Le$^b$-active struc-tures are missing from the hemopoietic tissue.

Examination of milk from women of different Lewis groups showed the transferase to be present in milk from both Le(a$^+$) and Le(b$^+$) women but absent from milk of women whose red cell and saliva group was Le(a$^-$b$^-$) (Grollman *et al.*, 1969). These findings are in keeping with the idea that the allele *le* is silent and does not give an enzymically active product. An *Le* enzyme preparation from human milk catalyzed the trans-fer of fucose to glycoproteins devoid of blood group activity to give prod-ucts which by sensitive immunochemical techniques were found to have Le$^a$ activity (Jarkovsky *et al.*, 1970).

In tissues from individuals with an *Le* gene, an *H* gene, and an *Se* gene, both the galactosyl and *N*-acetylglucosaminyl residues in the Type 1 chain are substituted with L-fucose and an Le$^b$ structure is formed (Fig. 21). With human submaxillary glands from an Le(b$^+$) individual as the enzyme source and lacto-$N$-biose I ($\beta$-Gal($1\rightarrow3$)GlcNAc) as the acceptor molecule, a tetrasaccharide was formed which co-chromatographed with an authentic sample of Le$^b$-active tetrasaccharide isolated from a blood-group-specific glycoprotein (Chester and Watkins, 1969). More recently Prohaska *et al.* (1978) reported the isolation of a blood group Lewis precursor from the plasma of an Le(a$^-$b$^-$) individual and demonstrated that, with fucosyltransferases from human gastric mucosa of Le(a$^-$b$^+$) individuals as the enzyme source, the precursor could be converted into Le$^a$ and Le$^b$ specific glycolipids. Neither the precursor glycolipid, nor the fucosyltransferases were highly purified but the acquired Le$^a$ and Le$^b$ activities were revealed by agglutination of OLe(a$^-$b$^-$) cells with anti-Le$^a$ or Le$^b$ sera after adsorption of the converted precursor glycolipid onto the cells. Moreover Le(a$^-$b$^-$) erythrocytes were found to develop Le$^a$ and Le$^b$ activities when subjected to enzymic fucosylation, thus showing that Lewis-negative cells carry blood group Lewis precursor glycolipid on their surface.

Biochemical pathways for the formation of Le$^a$- and Le$^b$-specific structures are summarized in Fig. 23. The biosynthetic pathways proposed earlier for the formation of A, B, H, Le$^a$, and Le$^b$ structures in the secreted glycoproteins (Watkins and Morgan, 1959) assumed that the change in the precursor glycoprotein controlled by the *Le* gene occurred before the step controlled by the *H* gene. This order was inferred from the enzymic degradation experiments in which loss of A or B activity resulted in a development of H activity, and further treatment with an H-destroying enzyme then gave a product with Le$^a$ activity (Watkins, 1962). The elucidation of the structures of the A, B, H, Le$^a$, and Le$^b$ determinants has now made it clear that most of the H activity developed on loss of A and B activity probably results from removal of the terminal nonreducing sugar from Type 2 chains (Fig. 4), whereas the Le$^a$ activity developed on treatment with the H-destroying enzyme results from removal of L-fucose from Le$^b$-active structures on Type 1 chains (Fig. 24). The use of an Le$^a$-destroying $\alpha$-1,4 L-fucosidase which was free from H-destroying $\alpha$-1,2 L-fucosidase activity (Stealey and Watkins, 1971) demonstrated that either H or Le$^a$ activity may be formed from an Le$^b$ structure depending upon the order of treatment with H- or Le$^a$-destroying enzymes.

Biosynthetic experiments with low-molecular-weight acceptors have strongly indicated that the preferred pathway for the formation of an Le$^b$-active structure is (1) the formation of an H-active structure on the Type

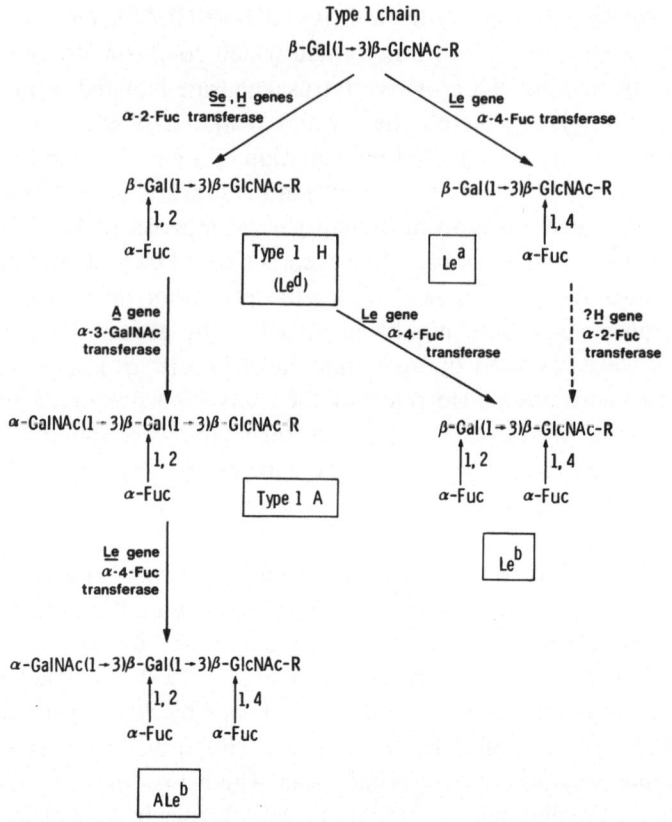

Fig. 23. Biochemical pathways for the formation of H, Le[a], Le[b], and ALe[b] structures on Type 1 chains in glycoproteins and glycolipids. Abbreviations as in Figs. 1 and 2. The pathway from Le[a] to Le[b] represented by the dotted line is uncertain.

1 chain ending catalyzed by the *H*-gene-specified enzyme and (2) the addition of a second fucose unit to *N*-acetylglucosamine catalyzed by the *Le*-gene-specified enzyme (Shen *et al.*, 1968; Chester, 1971). In their work with the Lewis precursor glycolipid, however, Prohaska *et al.* (1978) found that, on enzymic fucosylation of Le(a⁻b⁻) erythrocytes, Le[a] specificity appeared ahead of Le[b] specificity and suggested that this result supported the occurrence of 1,4-fucosylation of *N*-acetylglucosamine before 1,2-fucosylation of galactose. Further experiments are required to resolve this question.

Little published information is available on the purification of the *Le*-

gene-specified α-4-L-fucosyltransferase. In a preliminary report Prieels
*et al.* (1977) described a 56,000-fold purification of the enzyme in human
milk by ion-exchange chromatography and affinity chromatography on
GDP-hexanolamine-agarose. The purified enzyme had a pH optimum of
7.6–8 and a requirement for $Mn^{2+}$ ions.

## *"Lewis-like"* Structures and the α-3-L-Fucosyltransferase

The blood group specific glycoproteins carrying the A, B, and H
determinants have chain endings (Fig. 25) other than those already described in which L-fucose is linked α(1→3) to a subterminal *N*-acetylglu-
cosamine in a Type 2 chain (Marr *et al.*, 1968; Lloyd *et al.*, 1968). It is
evident that a third fucosyltransferase is active at the site of synthesis of

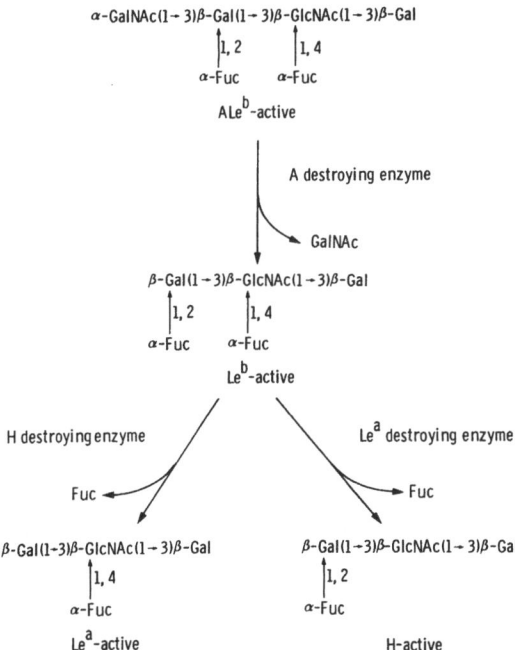

Fig. 24. Enzymic degradation of ALe[b] structure on a Type 1 chain (Stealey and Watkins,
1971; Stealey, 1973). Abbreviations as in Figs. 1 and 2.

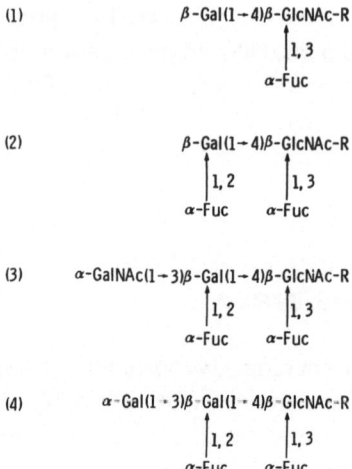

Fig. 25. Mono- and difucosyl structures based on Type 2 chains. Abbreviations as in Figs. 1 and 2.

the blood-group-specific glycoproteins which catalyzes the reaction:

GDP-Fuc + β-Gal(1→4)β-GlcNAc-R → β-Gal(1→4)β-GlcNAc-R + GDP

$$\uparrow 1.3$$

α-Fuc

The structure formed [Fig. 25 (1)] is an analogue of the Le$^a$-active tri-saccharide but it does not have Le$^a$ activity. An oligosaccharide with fucosyl residues attached (1→2) to galactose and (1→3) to N-acetylglu-cosamine on a Type 2 chain ending [Fig. 25 (2)] was isolated from an H glycoprotein (Lloyd et al., 1966). Although structurally similar to Le$^b$, this oligosaccharide does not have Le$^b$ activity. A- and B-active structures with this underlying difucosyl structure have also been isolated from al-kaline-borohydride degradation products of A and B substances (Lloyd et al., 1966). Similar oligosaccharides built upon lactose (β-Gal(1→4)Glc) in place of the β-Gal(1→4)β-GlcNAc-R structure of the Type 2 chain ending occur as free oligosaccharides in human urine (Lundblad, 1978) and in milk (Kobata 1972). From a study of three dimensional molecular models Kabat (1977) pointed out the difference in conformation of the Le$^a$ trisaccharide and the analogue on the Type 2 chain and this difference is reinforced by the conformational analyses of Lemieux (1978) based on hard sphere calculations. It is therefore not surprising that the mono- and difucosyl structures built on Type 2 chains present profiles which prevent them from interacting with anti-Le$^a$ or anti-Le$^b$ sera, respectively.

A glycolipid based on lacto-$N$-neotetraosyl ceramide (Table V) with fucose linked $\beta(1\rightarrow3)$ to $N$-acetylglucosamine was isolated from human adenocarcinoma tissue (Yang and Hakomori, 1971) and called X-hapten. Mono- and difucosyl-containing glycolipids from canine gastric mucosa, also based on Type 2 chain glycolipids, have been called Le$^a$-like and Le$^b$-like (McKibbin, 1978). Since the structures do not cross react with anti-Le$^a$ and anti-Le$^b$ sera, and the $\alpha$-3-L-fucosyltransferase is not a product of a gene at the *Lewis* locus, this nomenclature is confusing and incorrect.

The $\alpha$-3-L-fucosyltransferase has been detected in human milk (Shen *et al.*, 1968), human submaxillary glands and stomach mucosa (Chester and Watkins, 1969), and human serum (Schenkel-Brunner *et al.*, 1972; Pacuszka and Koscielak, 1976). The enzyme is not under the control of the *Se* gene and none of the serum samples examined in the author's laboratory have been found to lack this transferase, including those with the Bombay O$_h$ phenotype. If the gene locus coding for the $\alpha$-3-L-fucosyltransferase has an inactive allele it must be of much lower frequency than the *le* gene in the *Le le* system. The origin of the $\alpha$-3-L-fucosyltransferase in serum is not established. Although both glycoproteins and glycolipids bearing the structures synthesized by this enzyme occur in mucosal tissue none of the glycolipids so far isolated from erythrocytes have been found to contain $\alpha$-3-linked L-fucose (see McKibbin, 1978).

## *The Antigens "Le$^c$" and "Le$^d$"*

Potapov (1970) injected a goat with saliva from an OLe(a$^-$b$^+$) secretor person and obtained two antibodies. One was an anti-Le$^b$ and the second an antibody which failed to react with Le(a$^+$b$^-$) cells or with Le(a$^-$b$^-$) cells from ABH nonsecretors but did react with Le(a$^-$b$^-$) cells from ABH secretors. This antibody was called anti-Le$^d$, leaving anti-Le$^c$ free for the then hypothetical antibody expected to react with cells from Le(a$^-$b$^-$) nonsecretors. Subsequently an antibody (ARM) was described by Gunson and Latham (1972) which reacted only with the cells of Le(a$^-$b$^-$) non-secretor people and thus had the properties of the expected anti-Le$^c$ reagent. In tests with low-molecular-weight oligosaccharides, the trisaccharide 3-fucosyllactose ($\beta$-Gal(1$\rightarrow$4)[$\alpha$-Fuc(1$\rightarrow$3)]Glc) (Table VI) inhibited the agglutination of OLe(a⁻b⁻) cells by anti-Le$^c$ serum. A preliminary suggestion was made (Watkins, reported in Gunson and Latham, 1972) that Le$^c$ and Le$^d$ are produced by the addition of fucosyl residues to a Type 2 precursor, the monofucosyl structure Le$^c$ [Fig. 25 (1)] being formed in nonsecretors who lack a functional $H$ gene and the difucosyl structure $Le^d$ [Fig. 25 (2)] being formed in secretors who have a functional $H$ gene to catalyze the addition of α-2-linked fucose to the terminal β-galactosyl residue. Since neither of these structures would be products of genes at the $Lewis$ locus the inappropriateness of the nomenclature was pointed out. Ginsburg $et\ al.$ (1978) confirmed the inhibition of the anti-Le$^c$ serum ARM by 3-fucosyllactose and found that lacto-$N$-fucopentaitol III (β-Gal(1→4)[α-Fuc(1→3)]βGLcNAc(1→3)β-Gal(1-4)Sorbitol) was twice as effective an inhibitor on a molar basis.

More recently, further examples of anti-Le$^c$ and anti-Le$^d$ were prepared by immunization of goats with human saliva (Graham $et\ al.$, 1977). These authors reasoned that if Le$^c$ and Le$^d$ specificities result from fucosylation of Type 2 chain precursors they should be detectable in the presence of the Le$^a$ and Le$^b$ antigens built on Type 1 chains. Of the antigens, Le$^a$, Le$^b$, Le$^c$, and Le$^d$, only one of the four was found on the red cells of any one of 98 adults tested; these results suggested that Le$^c$ and Le$^d$ are formed from the same Type 1 precursor chains as the Le$^a$ and Le$^b$ determinants. Subsequently Graham $et\ al.$ (1978) demonstrated that anti-Le$^d$ was inhibited by an oligosaccharide, lacto-$N$-fucopentaose I (Table VI), containing a Type 1 H determinant and not by 2-fucosyllactosamine (Table VI) which contains a Type 2 H determinant. The additional demonstration that the widely used $Ulex\ europeaus$ anti-H lectin is specific for the Type 2 H determinant gave plausibility to the interpretation of Graham $et\ al.$ (1978) that the determinant recognized by the antisera reacting with cells from individuals with the genotype $H,\ Se,\ lele$ is an H-active structure built on a glycosphingolipid with a Type 1 carbohydrate chain ending (Fig. 23). Such a structure would be expected to occur in largest amounts in the plasma of group O individuals who lack both the $Le$ gene to compete for the Type 1 chains and $A$ or $B$ gene products to convert H structures to A or B-active determinants (Crookston, 1978). The structure of the Le$^c$ determinant remains unclear. A glycolipid with an unsubstituted Type 1 chain ending, β-Gal(1→3)β-GlcNAc, would seem the most obvious contender from the arguments advanced by Graham $et\ al.$ (1977), but evidence to support the role of this structure, or to refute the findings with the human anti-Le$^c$ serum ARM, has not yet appeared. In the absence of fucosylation by either the *H* or the *Le* gene product it is possible that addition of sialic acid to the Type 1 chain, catalyzed by a sialyltransferase, occurs and that this product has a distinctive specificity. However, Le$^c$, like Le$^d$, is clearly not a product of an allele at the *Lewis* locus, irrespective of whether the specificity arises from the action of the 3-fucosyltransferase on a Type 2 chain glycolipid, from the absence of the action of *Le* and *H*-gene products on a Type 1 precursor glycolipid, or from the action of a sialyltransferase on the same Type 1 chain glycolipid.

## Interrelationships between ABH and Le Gene Products

### Heterogeneity of Carbohydrate Chains

Although most of the work on the acceptor specificities of the *A*, *B*, *H*, and *Le* glycosyltransferases has been carried out with low-molecular-weight substrates of known structure it is possible to extrapolate from these results to the macromolecular-weight glycoproteins and glycolipids and thereby to draw certain inferences concerning the origin of the heterogeneity of the carbohydrate chains. It has been known for many years that the blood-group-specific glycoproteins carry multiple serological specificities on the same molecules (Morgan and Watkins, 1956; Watkins and Morgan, 1957a; Brown et al., 1959). For example, in the secretions of a donor with *A*, *B*, *H*, *Le*, and *Se* genes all five of the blood group specificities A, B, H, Le$^a$, and Le$^b$ may be carried on a single macromolecule. That the nature of the complete carbohydrate chain is preordained by the position in the peptide backbone of the amino acid to which the chain is attached (see Schachter and Tilley, 1978) appears improbable and a more likely explanation of the heterogeneity is competition for the precursor carbohydrate chains by the various enzymes involved in the assembly of the determinant structures (Ginsburg, 1972; Watkins, 1974). The *H*- and *Le*-gene-specified transferases may compete to catalyze the addition of fucose to a Type 1 chain (Fig. 23). An Le$^a$ structure, once formed, is not an acceptor substrate for the A- and B-gene-specified transferases, nor, possibly, to any extent for the *H*-gene-specified enzyme. Therefore the *Le*-gene-catalyzed addition of fucose at this stage, virtually constitutes a chain-terminating step and the Le$^a$ structures remain available for reactivity with Le$^a$ antibodies. An H structure formed on a Type

1 chain, on the other hand, may escape further substitution, or may undergo conversion into either an Le$^b$-active structure or an A- or a B-active structure (Fig. 23). The Le$^b$-active structures are not acceptors for the A- or B-gene-specified transferases and therefore these structures remain available for reactivity with anti-Le$^b$ sera.

Structures with Le$^b$ groupings underlying A and B groupings have not yet been isolated from the degradation products of A- and B-specific glycoproteins although glycolipids with the ALe$^b$ structures (Table X) have been obtained from human small intestine and from human erythrocytes (Karlsson, 1978). Evidence that these structures also exist in A- and B-active glycoproteins was obtained from enzymic degradation experiments (Stealey, 1973). Treatment of B substance with an H-destroying enzyme from *Trichomonas foetus* destroys the preexisting Le$^b$ activity without loss of B activity. If this preparation is then treated with a coffee-bean α-galactosidase to remove the terminal α-galactosyl residue from the B structure, then not only does H develop (Watkins *et al.*, 1962) but there is also a considerable increase in Le$^b$ activity. The most probable explanation of this finding is that removal of the galactose exposes an underlying Le$^b$-active structure. A similar development of Le$^b$ activity can be demonstrated when A-active glycoproteins from either A$_1$ or A$_2$ individuals are treated with an α-$N$-acetylgalactosaminidase (Fig. 24). The sequence of sugar transfer reactions that lead to the formation of the Le$^b$ structures underlying A and B groupings in glycoproteins and glycolipids must be first the transfer of $N$-acetylgalactosamine or galactose, respectively, to H-active structures and secondly the transfer of fucose to $N$-acetylglucosamine catalyzed by the $Le$-gene-specified α-4-fucosyltransferase (Fig. 23). It is assumed that essentially the same pathways are followed for the conversion of Type 2 chain endings in the glycoproteins; the relative timing of the additions controlled by the $H$-gene-specified transferase and the α-3-L-fucosyltransferase would determine the subsequent changes that could occur at the terminal nonreducing ends of the chains. In a group A person with $A$, $H$, $Le$, and $Se$ genes, the secreted glycoproteins, by a combination of incomplete chain synthesis and the formation of structures which are not substrates for any of the biosynthetic glycosyltransferases in the cell, could have some carbohydrate chains ending with the structures shown in Fig. 23 together with some ending with structures (1), (2), and (3) in Fig. 25 and also the Type 2 monofucosyl A and H structures (Fig. 2). In a person carrying both $A$ and $B$ genes even greater diversity of chain endings would be generated.

At the site of synthesis of the Type 1 chain glycolipids that are taken up by the red cells, competition between the *H*- and *Le*-gene-specified transferases would similarly determine whether an Le$^a$- or an H-active structure is formed. Unless the Le$^a$ glycolipid is an acceptor for the *H*-gene-catalyzed transfer of fucose (Prohaska *et al.*, 1978) it would appear that the *H* enzyme competes effectively for the precursor glycolipid, since in individuals with an *H*, *Se*, and *Le* gene the red cells have Le$^b$ activity and seldom any detectable Le$^a$ activity. The formation of the ALe$^b$-active glycolipid in A$_1$, rather than A$_2$, individuals (Crookston, 1978), must be assumed to result from the *A*$^1$ transferase competing more effectively for the *H* glycolipid than the *Le* transferase, resulting in an A structure which is subsequently converted to the ALe$^b$ determinant (Fig. 23). In A$_2$ individuals the *A*$^2$ transferase presumably competes less effectively than the *Le* transferase so that an Le$^b$ structure is synthesized which is not then a substrate for the *A*$^2$ transferase.

The blood-group-active glycolipids which are integral parts of the membrane synthesized by the red cell precursors have less heterogeneity of chain ending because they are built only on Type 2 chains and the 3-fucosyltransferase does not appear to be functional at this site. However, the more complex glycolipids, with branched chains, appear to carry A, H, and I activities on the same macromolecules (Koscielak, 1977; Hakomori *et al.*, 1977).

## Changes in A, B, H, and Lewis Antigens in Neoplasias

Loss of A and B serological activity in human gastric carcinoma tissue was first reported by Masamune *et al.* (1958), and subsequently losses of A, B, and H antigenic activity were demonstrated by the specific red cell adherence test (Davidsohn and Li, 1969; Davidsohn *et al.*, 1969, 1971) and by immunofluorescence and immunoperoxidase techniques (Bonfiglio and Feinberg, 1976) to occur in the majority of squamous and transitional cell carcinomas. Antigens were lost in foci of invasive cancer, were considerably reduced or lost in areas of classic carcinoma *in situ*, and were reduced in most cases of dysplasia. In theory, failure to detect A, B, or H activity could result from the addition of further sugars which mask the original specificity, from breakdown of the carbohydrate chains by glycosidases or from failure to synthesize the specific determinant structures. That loss of activity results from incomplete synthesis of carbohydrate chains of the blood group active glycolipids was suggested by the work of Hakomori *et al.* (1967). These authors described the accumulation of fucose-containing glycolipids in human adenocarcinoma with H and Le$^a$ activities and the associated deletion of blood group A or B activities. The enzymic basis for the loss of A and B antigenic activity was shown to reside in greatly reduced levels of *A* and *B* transferases as compared to normal mucosal tissue (Stellner *et al.*, 1973). The disappearance of glycoprotein-associated blood group A activity in human colonic adenocarcinoma was investigated by Kim *et al.* (1974), and again the *A* transferase activity was found to be greatly diminished in tumor tissue whereas glycosidase activities were similar in the normal and tumor tissues. Increased reactivity of glycoprotein extracts from colonic tumors with anti-I and anti-i sera was also observed (Feizi *et al.*, 1975), indicating the presence of unfinished carbohydrate chains. These findings, together with the immunohistological findings of Szulman (1960) which demonstrated that blood group determinants appeared and disappeared in a certain order during genetic development, and the observation of Pann and Kuhns (1972) that the H determinant is a marker of cellular differentiation, led Watanabe and Hakomori (1976) to suggest that a genetic or epigenetic program for synthesizing blood group determinants and their carrier carbohydrate chains develops step by step during ontogenesis and that the program of synthesis is blocked or modified in the process of oncogenesis. If this is the case the loss of one specificity and the appearance of a new specificity in malignancy might be expected to follow the same pattern of changes as those that occur in the blood group specific glycoproteins upon sequential degradation of the carbohydrate chains with exoglycosidases (Watkins, 1962). In secretors with an *Le* gene loss of A and B, activities should first be accompanied by an increase in H and Le$^b$ activities and then, as H is lost, by an increase of Le$^a$ activity and in reactivity with reagents that recognize unsubstituted Type 2 chain endings, such as Type XIV anti-pneumococcal serum and certain anti-I sera (Figs. 4 and 24). Recently Picard *et al.* (1978) studied the expression of A, B, H, Le$^a$, and I (Ma) antigens in glycoprotein-rich extracts of gastric carcinomas and compared the activities with those found in adjacent uninvolved gastric mucosa of 16 patients with gastric cancer. They found that the levels of the A, B, H, and Le$^b$ antigens in tumor extracts from secretor patients were frequently, but not invariably, decreased, and that occasionally the H and Le$^b$ antigens were increased. Le$^a$ activity was increased in six of the tumor extracts, and in ten out of the fourteen secretor patients the

I (Ma) activity was dramatically increased in the tumor extracts. In two nonsecretor patients Le[a] and I activity were found in the normal tissue and these activities persisted in the tumor extracts. In general these results support the idea of a sequential loss of the capacity to synthesize A, B, and H structures with the consequent availability of precursor structures which react with the appropriate antibodies. The Le-gene-specified α-4-fucosyltransferase appears less susceptible to change than the A, B, and H genes in the oncogenic process and the accumulation of Le[a]-active glycolipids has been reported in gastric (Hakomori, 1971) and colonic (Siddiqui et al., 1978) adenocarcinomas.

By means of the immunofluorescence technique, Häkkinen (1970) claimed to have demonstrated the aberrant expression of A antigen in gastric adenocarcinoma tissues from four group O and two group B patients. These results may indicate derepression of a ubiquitously present A transferase (Boettcher, 1978a; Levine, 1978) or a malignancy-related change in the protein product of a silent O allele, or in the B-gene-specified transferase, which enables these proteins to catalyze the transfer of N-acetylgalactosamine. However, Hakomori et al. (1977b) observed that the Forssman antigen is expressed in neoplasms when it is absent from normal mucosa. The structure of the Forssman glycolipid α-GalNAc(1→3)β-GalNAc(1→3)α-Gal(1→4)β-Gal(1→4)Glc-CER(Siddiqui and Hakomori, 1971) bears resemblances to the A determinant and it has long been known that Forssman and A specificities cross-react under certain conditions (see Wiener, 1943). It is therefore possible that the immunofluorescence tests used by Häkkinen were detecting Forssman and not A antigen. The possibility of cross-reactivity with other A-like precursor structures in the carbohydrate chains of N-acetylgalactosamine containing glycoproteins (see Uhlenbruck, 1979) would also have to be ruled out before the abberant expression of A in group B and O persons could be unreservedly accepted.

Changes in blood group antigenic expression also occur on the red cells of patients with malignant hemopathies (see Salmon, 1978). Deficiencies or complete disappearance of A, B, and H antigens are sometimes observed, but the appearance of neoantigens has not been reported. Examination of the sera of 25 untreated patients with acute myeloid leukemia revealed that all had low H-gene-specified α-2-fucosyltransferase activity when compared to normal control sera of the same ABO group (Kuhns et al., 1976, 1979). Serial investigations on patients during clinical remission following therapy and in relapse showed a consistent pattern: the values reverted to the normal range during at least a portion of the time in remission and fell to a low value again in relapse. In group A and B leukemic patients the A and B transferase levels also increased on remission and fell to a lower value on relapse, but the changes were less marked than those for the H transferase values (Kuhns et al., 1976; Watkins, 1978; and unpublished observations). This is perhaps to be expected in view of the difference in origins of the H from the A and B transferases in serum. Since the H transferase appears to originate mainly from the hemopoietic tissue, whereas only 20–30% of the A transferase is derived from this source, a disease involving hemopoietic tissue might be expected to be reflected in greater changes in the H transferase values than in those of the A and B transferases. Cartron and Ropars (1978) were unable to detect A transferase in the red cell membranes of three group A leukemic patients whose A antigen had completely disappeared from the cell surface.

The H transferase assays on the sera of leukemic patients described by Kuhns et al. (1976, 1979) were carried out with the low-molecular-weight compound phenyl-β-D-galactoside as the fucosyl acceptor (see Section on the H-gene-specified α-2-L-fucosyltransferase). In contrast, using fetuin, from which sialic acid had been removed, as the acceptor substrate Khilanani et al. (1977) and Bauer et al. (1977) reported elevated activities of the α-2-fucosyltransferase in presentation serum samples from leukemic patients with a fall to normal levels on remission. The positional linkages of the added fucose were not established, however, and it now seems most probable that the elevated fucosyltransferase that was measured with this macromolecular substrate was not the H gene product (Kessel, 1979).

## The Lewis System and Renal Transplantation

The possible importance of the Lewis system in renal transplantation was recently suggested by a retrospective study of Oriol et al. (1978b). Actuarial survival of grafts at two years was significantly lower in the le le recipients than in the Le recipients indicating that mismatching of these antigens contributes to rejection of kidney transplants. These authors thought that the effect of mismatching for the Lewis and HLA systems was additive but Williams et al. (1978) suggest that Lewis-mismatching alone may be responsible for graft rejection. Biosynthesis of ABH and

Lewis antigens in kidneys of both normal and transplanted patients was reported by Oriol *et al.* (1978a) to occur locally in the kidney and the relevant glycosyltransferases were identified at different levels of the nephron.

# THE P SYSTEM

## *Serology and Genetics*

The P blood group system was first discovered by Landsteiner and Levine (1927) by testing immune sera prepared by injecting human red cells into rabbits. Suitably absorbed sera detected a new, inherited, blood group character present on the red cells of about 75% of all individuals. For many years the system was considered to be monofactorial and bloods were differentiated simply into $P^+$ or $P^-$. Subsequently, the system was much enlarged (see Race and Sanger, 1975) and five phenotypes, $P_1$, $P_2$, $P_1^k$, $P_2^k$, and p are now recognized (Table XI). The five phenotypes depend upon the presence or absence of three distinct serological specificities $P_1$, P, and $P^k$. The enlargement of the system was a logical development from the observation that the serum formerly called anti-$Tj^a$ was a mixture of anti-$P_1$, anti-P and anti-$P^k$ (Sanger, 1955; Matson *et al.*, 1959) but the implication that the antigens of the system are all alleles at a single locus, or at closely linked loci, is now known to be incorrect. The recent biochemical information on the antigens makes it apparent that genes at two, and possibly three, independent loci are at present included in the P system.

TABLE XI. The P Blood Group System (after Race and Sanger, 1975)

| Phenotype | Antigens on red cells | Antibodies in serum | Approximate frequency |
|-----------|----------------------|---------------------|----------------------|
| $P_1$ | $P_1P$ | None | 75% |
| $P_2$ | P | Anti-$P_1$ | 25% |
| $P_1^k$ | $P_1P^k$ | Anti-P | |
| $P_2^k$ | $P^k$ | Anti-P | Very rare |
| p | None | Anti-P $P_1P^k$ | |

Red cells of the $P^k$ phenotype lack the P antigen and p red cells lack $P_1$, P, and $P^k$ antigens. $P_1$ and P antigens have been detected on skin fibroblasts and lymphocytes and $P^k$ antigen occurs on fibroblasts of individuals with the $P_1$ and $P_2$ phenotype despite its absence from their red cells (Fellous *et al.*, 1974). Neither the $P_1$, $P^k$, nor P antigens occur in human tissue fluids or secretions in amounts measurable by the available techniques.

## Chemistry of $P_1$, P, and $P^k$ Determinants

The earliest evidence indicating the chemical nature of the $P_1$ determinant on the red cell was obtained from inhibition tests with simple sugars. Examination of the effect of many mono-, di-, and trisaccharides on the agglutination of $P_1$ red cells by human and rabbit anti-$P_1$ sera indicated that an α-D-galactose was the immunodominant sugar in the $P_1$ determinant (Watkins and Morgan, 1964). The fact that α-D-galactose was also involved in $P^k$ specificity was indicated by the results of Voak *et al.* (1973) and Furukawa *et al.* (1974).

Human patients with hydatid disease sometimes have strong $P_1$ antibodies and this led Cameron and Staveley (1957) to test hydatid cyst fluid for $P_1$ activity. They found that the contents of hydatid cysts from the livers of sheep infected with *Echinococcus granulosus* strongly inhibited anti-$P_1$ serum. Subsequently Matson *et al.* (1959) showed that the cyst fluids also had $P^k$ activity but not P activity. These cysts therefore provided a water-soluble source of $P_1$- and $P^k$-active material for chemical studies. Previous experience with the antigens associated with the ABH and Lewis systems suggested that, irrespective of whether or not the macromolecules in the cyst fluid were identical with those on the red cell, the structures responsible for $P_1$ and $P^k$ specificities were most probably identical with those in the red cell antigens.

The material with $P_1$ and $P^k$ activity purified from sheep hydatid cyst fluid was found to be a glycoprotein (Morgan and Watkins, 1964). Evidence that D-galactose was the immunodominant sugar in both the $P_1$ and $P^k$ structures in the glycoprotein was obtained by means of an enzyme from *Trichomonas foetus*. The crude preparation destroyed the $P_1$ activity of the glycoprotein and this destruction could be inhibited by D-galactose (Watkins and Morgan, 1964). Despite the similarity with the B determinant, which also has an α-galactosyl residue as the terminal sugar, an α-galactosidase from coffee beans that destroys B serological activity had no detectable action on the $P_1$ preparation. Subsequently *T. foetus* was shown to have three linkage-specific galactosidases, one of them a 1,3-α-galactosidase that inactivates B specificity and another a 1,4-α-galactosidase that inactivates both $P_1$ and $P^k$ specificities (Yates *et al.,* 1975). When subjected to partial acid hydrolysis the $P_1P^k$ glycoprotein yielded a series of diffusible oligosaccharide fragments from which a disaccharide, α-Gal(1→4)Gal (1) and a trisaccharide, α-Gal(1→4)β-Gal(1→4)GlcNAc (2) were isolated and chemically characterized. Trisaccharide (2) was strongly inhibitory with human and rabbit anti-$P_1$ sera and was identified as the $P_1$ determinant (Cory *et al.,* 1974). Both disaccharide (1) and trisaccharide (2) were strongly inhibitory in the $P^k$ system although the disaccharide was very poorly active in the $P_1$ system (Watkins and Morgan, 1976).

Marcus and his colleagues approached the nature of the $P^k$ and P determinants by inhibition tests with purified glycosphingolipids of known structure (Naiki and Marcus, 1974), and made the surprising observation that the well-characterized and relatively abundant glycolipid, globoside (Table XII), constituted the P antigen on the red cell surface. Another well-characterized glycolipid, ceramide trihexoside (Table XII), was found to be responsible for the $P^k$ antigenic activity. In accordance with the results of the inhibition studies with the fragments isolated from the hydatid cyst $P_1P^k$-active glycoprotein the terminal disaccharide in CTH has the structure α-Gal(1→4)Gal.

The $P_1$ activity of red cells was known to be associated with a glycosphingolipid fraction (Marcus, 1971). Extensive purification of the $P_1$ glycolipid (Naiki *et al.,* 1975) established that it was a ceramide pentasaccharide (Table XII). The structure of the trisaccharide at the terminal nonreducing end of the $P_1$-active glycosphingolipid is identical with that of the trisaccharide (2) isolated from the $P_1$ active glycoprotein. Although $P_1$ and $P^k$ have identical terminal disaccharide structures, ceramide trihexoside does not inhibit anti-$P_1$ (Naiki and Marcus, 1975; Watkins and Morgan, 1976). The $P_1$ agglutinins appear to be strongly orientated to the conformation of trisaccharide (2) and have little or no affinity for disaccharide (1). The *N*-acetylglucosamine residue must therefore constitute an important part of the determinant structure. The specificity of anti-$P^k$ sera appears to be less closely delineated than that of anti-$P_1$ sera and a number of compounds containing terminal α-galactosyl residues were inhibitory in the $P^k$–anti-$P^k$ system (Watkins and Morgan, 1976). Since

**TABLE XII. Structures of $P^k$, P, and $P_1$ Glycosphingolipids and Their Precursors**

| Glycolipid | Structure | Specificity |
|---|---|---|
| Lactosyl ceramide | β-Gal(1→4)Glc-CER | — |
| Ceramide trihexoside (CTH) | α-Gal(1→3)α-Gal(1→4)β-Gal(1→4)Glc-CER | $P^k$ |
| Globoside | β-GalNAc(1→3)α-Gal(1→4)β-Gal(1→4)Glc-CER | P |
| Paragloboside (Lacto-$N$-neotetraosyl ceramide) | β-Gal(1→4)β-GlcNAc(1→3)β-Gal(1→4)Glc-CER | Type XIV pneumococcal |
| $P_1$ Glycolipid | α-Gal(1→4)β-Gal(1→4)β-GlcNAc(1→3)β-Gal(1→4)Glc-CER | $P_1$ |

anti-$P^k$ occurs together with anti-P and anti-$P_1$ in the sera of p people, and has to be freed from these two antisera by absorption with $P_1$ cells, it is possible that anti-$P^k$ represents the end of a spectrum of antibodies related to the $\alpha$-Gal(1→4)Gal structure; those remaining after absorption are the ones with a low affinity for the $P_1$ determinant.

Many antibodies that cause paroxysmal cold hemoglobinuria (Donath–Landsteiner antibodies) appear to be directed against the blood group P determinant (Levine *et al.*, 1965). Recently Schwarting *et al.* (1979) demonstrated that these antibodies are also inhibited by globoside although some are inhibited more effectively by the Forssman glycolipid $\alpha$-GalNAc(1→3)$\beta$-GalNAc(1→3)$\alpha$-Gal(1→4)$\beta$-Gal(1→4)Glc-Cer which contains the globoside structure plus an additional terminal nonreducing $N$-acetylgalactosamine residue (Siddiqui and Hakomori, 1971). Schwarting *et al.* (1979) suggested that the antibodies are probably elicited by immunization against Forssman antigens that are widespread in animal tissues and in microorganisms.

Independent evidence for the role of ceramide trihexoside and globoside in $P^k$ and P specificities, respectively, was obtained from analyses of the glycosphingolipids in p red cells (Koscielak *et al.*, 1976c; Marcus *et al.*, 1976). Ceramide trihexoside was missing from the glycolipids and globoside was present only in trace amounts. The amount of lactosyl ceramide was increased and there was an accumulation of glycolipids containing sialic acid, fucose, and $N$-acetylglucosamine. Marcus *et al.* (1976) also found globoside to be absent from $P^k$ red cells, and the amount of ceramide trihexoside was increased. An antibody which reacted preferentially with red cells of individuals with the p phenotype was inhibited specifically by sialoparagloboside, $\alpha$-NeuNAc(2→3)$\beta$-Gal(1→4)$\beta$-GlcNAc(1→3)$\beta$-Gal(1→4)Glc-Cer (Schwarting *et al.*, 1977). The authors postulate that the level of sialoparagloboside is increased in the p phenotype because the block in synthesis of globoside and ceramide trihexoside increases the quantities of precursor glycolipids available for utilization in other biosynthetic pathways.

## Biosynthetic Pathways

The elucidation of the structures of the three antigens $P_1$, P, and $P^k$ in the P system has engendered much speculation on the pathways of biosynthesis and interrelationships of the antigens in this system. Consideration of the structures of ceramide trihexoside and globoside (Table XII) indicates a straightforward precursor–product relationship between them. Globoside differs from ceramide trihexoside only in the presence of one further sugar, $N$-acetylgalactosamine joined in β(1→3) linkage to the nonreducing end of the carbohydrate chain. The P$^k$ antigen is thus a direct precursor of P and hence the two specificites cannot be the products of allelic genes. The gene controlling the completion of a P determinant must code for a β-3-$N$-acetylgalactosaminyltransferase (Fig. 26). Individuals homozygous for a silent allele of this gene would lack the transferase and ceramide trihexoside would occur unchanged on their red cells and be available for reactivity with anti-P$^k$ sera (Naiki and Marcus, 1975; Watkins and Morgan, 1976): Since ceramide trihexoside remains unchanged only in persons who fail to receive from either parent the gene coding for the β-$N$-acetylgalactosaminyltransferase, the recessive pattern of inheritance of P$^k$ is readily understood (see Race and Sanger, 1975). Evidence that fibroblasts from individuals of the P$^k$ phenotype lack β-$N$-acetylgalactosaminyltransferase was presented by Kijimoto-Ochiai *et al.*

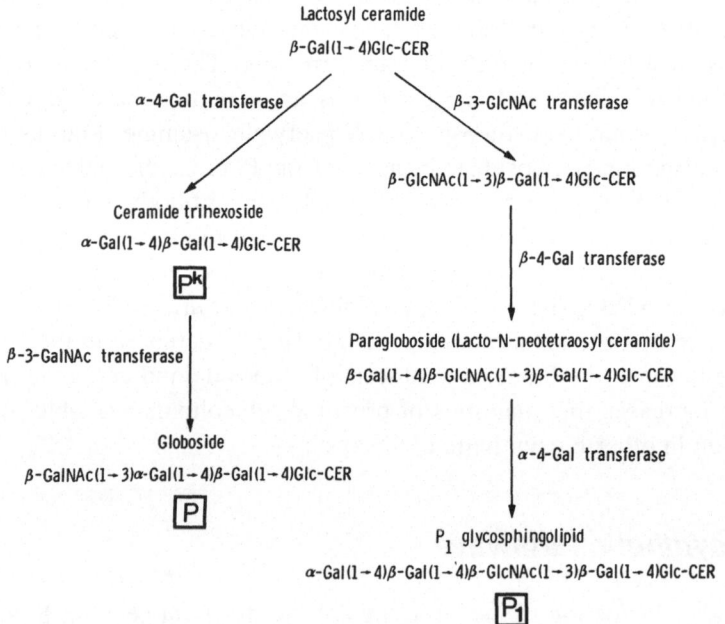

Fig. 26. Possible biosynthetic pathways for the formation of P$^k$, P, and P$_1$ glycolipids from lactosyl ceramide. Abbreviations as in Figs. 1 and 2.

(1977), although the levels found in individuals of the $P_2$ phenotype were low and none was detected in cells of the p phenotype. However, this latter result is difficult to reconcile with the demonstration that P is re-expressed on polykaryon cells obtained by fusion of $P^k$ and p fibroblasts (Fellous *et al.,* 1977) since the most obvious explanation for the complementation is that the p cells supply the gene for the $\beta$-*N*-acetylgalacto-saminyltransferase which converts the ceramide trihexoside, provided by the $P^k$ cells, into globoside. P antigen was not expressed on polykaryon cells from fusion of $P^k \times P^k$ or p $\times$ p fibroblasts. The complementation experiments support the view that the P antigen belongs to a genetic system independent of $P_1$ and $P^k$.

Whether $P_1$, $P^k$ and $p$ are alleles at one genetic locus, or whether an independent locus is responsible for $P_1$ specificity is still not clear. To be satisfactory a genetic scheme must explain 1) the absence of both $P_1$ and $P^k$ activities in the p phenotype (the absence of P follows upon the absence of $P^k$), 2) the existence of two $P^k$ phenotypes, $P_1^k$, in which the red cells have both $P_1$ and $P^k$ activities, and $P_2^k$, in which the red cells have only $P^k$ activity, and 3) the fact that individuals of the $P_2$ phenotype have the capacity to synthesize ceramide trihexoside, the immediate precursor of the P antigen, although they do not make $P_1$ antigen. The simplest explanation, that a single $\alpha$-galactosyltransferase has the capacity to add the terminal galactose unit to both lactosyl ceramide to make the $P^k$ antigen and to paragloboside to make the $P_1$ antigen (Naiki and Marcus, 1974), is rendered improbable by the existence of the two $P^k$ phenotypes and the fact that $P_2$ individuals cannot synthesize $P_1$ antigen. To overcome this anomaly Naiki and Marcus (1975) proposed that the $P_1$ gene perhaps produces a regulatory molecule that alters the acceptor specificity of the $\alpha$-galactosyltransferase to enable it to utilize paragloboside as a substrate in addition to ceramide trihexoside. Another proposal, along somewhat similar lines, is that the $P^k$ gene product is an $\alpha$-galactosyltransferase composed of a single polypeptide chain ($\alpha$) and that the $P_1$ gene produces a $\beta$-polypeptide that must combine with $\alpha$ (to form an $\alpha\beta$ dimer) to function as the $\alpha$-galactosyltransferase for paragloboside (Giblett, 1977). If either of these mechanisms is correct, the reexpression of $P_1$ in the children of a proportion of p $\times$ $P_2$ matings would be expected. In the admittedly limited number of p $\times$ $P_2$ matings studied (3 families with 11 children) none of the offspring was $P_1$ (see Race and Sanger, 1975). A simpler, and hence at the moment the most plausible, hypothesis is one that occurred independently to a number of workers in the blood group field (Greenwell, 1977; Koscielak, 1978; Graham and Williams, 1978). The proposal is that $P^k$, $P_1$, and $p$ are allelic genes. $P^k$ and $P_1$ each code for an α-galactosyltransferase but the enzyme produced by the $P^k$ gene has a strict specificity and can transfer galactose only to lactosyl ceramide whereas the product of the $P_1$ gene is less specific and can utilize both lactosyl ceramide and paragloboside as acceptor substrates. The third allele $p$ is a mutant which does not produce an enzymically active product so that lactosyl ceramide and other larger glycolipids, including sialoparagloboside, accumulate (Fig. 27). The antibodies that react preferentially with p cells would thus be ones that have specificities related to the accumulated precursor glycolipids and they would not be reacting with a specific product of the $p$ gene. The relationship between the $P^k$ and $P_1$ α-galactosyltransferases would be roughly analogous to the situation in *Pseudomonas aeruginosa*, in which the wild-type amidase hydrolyzes acetamide but not *N*-phenylacetamide, whereas an artificially induced mutant enzyme, differing by only one amino acid substitution, hydrolyses both acetamide and *N*-phenylacetamide (Betz *et al.*, 1974).

Until the relevant α-galactosyltransferases have been purified and their acceptor specificities rigorously characterized, or cell hybrid studies have shown that $P_1$ and $P^k$ are nonallelic, no decision can be reached as to whether one or two distinct genetic loci are involved in the final stages of the biosynthesis of the $P^k$ and $P_1$ determinants. The P system badly needs a new and systematic nomenclature that separates the $P$-gene-associated globoside synthetase from $P_1$, $P^k$, and $p$. However, to prevent further confusion it would seem prudent to defer the introduction of new symbols until the biochemical and genetic relationships between the $P_1$, $P^k$, and p phenotypes are unequivocally established.

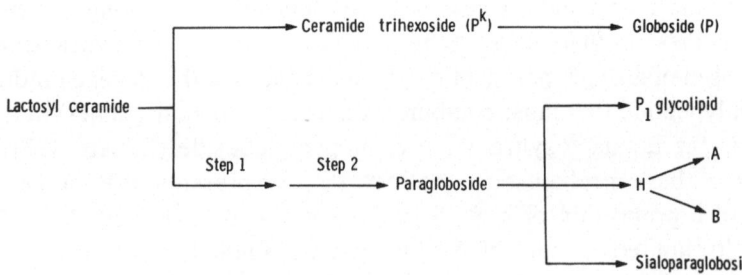

Fig. 27. Summary of pathways for the formation of $p^k$, P, $P_1$, H, A, B, and sialoparagloboside from lactosyl ceramide. Step 1 and step 2 represent the two sugar additions necessary for the synthesis of paragloboside.

## Relationship between ABH and P Systems

The A, B, H, P, $P^k$, and $P_1$ active glycolipids synthesized by the red cell precursors are all based on the dihexosyl glycosphingolipid, lactosyl ceramide (Fig. 27). It is not known, however, whether there is competition for this substrate by the enzymes synthesizing the various blood group determinants. There is evidence that glycosylation of glycosphingolipids, as well as of glycoproteins, occurs in the Golgi apparatus which is part of the endomembrane system of the cell (see Schachter, 1974b). However, it is not yet established whether the carbohydrate chains of different glycolipids each have their own distinct multiglycosyltransferase system, and hence are made on physically separate assembly lines, or whether there is competition for the same glycosyltransferases and pools of precursor substances. Marcus *et al.* (1976) observed that the lactosyl ceramide which accumulates in p cells contained predominantly C22 and C24 fatty acids in contrast to the lactosyl ceramide from normal cells which contains mostly C16 and C18 fatty acids. The authors suggested that this accumulation might arise because the transferase which normally synthesizes ceramide trihexoside is specific for a molecular species of lactosyl ceramide containing long-chain fatty acids. Koscielak *et al.* (1978b), however, considered it more likely that all the glycosphingolipids synthesized by the red cell precursors contained long-chain fatty acids and that the glycosphingolipids in plasma have shorter-chain fatty acids. The high content of shorter-chain fatty acids in lactosyl ceramide from normal red cells was taken as evidence of exchange of the glycolipid between plasma and erythrocytes.

If there is free competition between glycosyltransferases in the cells synthesizing the glycolipids, then the lactosyl ceramide pool can be converted either to ceramide trihexoside ($P^k$) and hence to globoside (P) or, through the sequential addition of N-acetylglucosamine and galactose to paragloboside (lacto-N-neotetraosyl ceramide) (Table 4). Paragloboside once formed can be converted either to a Type 2 H structure, and hence to A and B structures, to a $P_1$ determinant by the addition of an α-galactosyl residue, or to sialoparagloboside by the addition of sialic acid (Fig. 27). It is of interest in this connection that while the levels of H, A, and B activities on the red cells of individuals with normal ABO phenotypes are relatively constant from one person to another there is a considerable variation in the strength of the $P_1$ antigen on the red cells of different individuals. This variation might reflect the ability of the $P_1$ transferase to compete with the *H* transferase, or with a sialyltransferase, for the available paraglobiside. Homozygous $P_1P_1$ individuals are among those whose cells give the strongest reaction with anti-$P_1$ sera, and this observation would be compatible with more transferase being available, but analysis of family data has shown that homo- or heterozygosity is not the only factor involved in determining the strength of the $P_1$ antigen (see Race and Sanger, 1975). Whether the $P_1$ determinant is restricted to the short-chain paraglobiside molecule or whether the specificity is also carried on the longer, more highly branched, glycosphingolipids which carry A, B, H, and I determinants is not yet clear.

Another interesting facet of the $P_1$ determinant structure is the apparently close similarity to the structure of the Type 2 B-active trisaccharide $\alpha$-Gal(1→3)$\beta$-Gal(1→4)GlcNAc. This trisaccharide lacks the fucose substituent on the subterminal galactose residue which is part of the complete determinant (Fig. 2) but nevertheless the trisaccharide is serologically B-active (Painter *et al.*, 1963). Although the B and $P_1$ trisaccharides both have similar sugars with identical anomeric configurations there is no cross-reactivity between them with human or rabbit anti-B or anti-$P_1$ sera. A consideration of conformation of these trisaccharides (Morgan, 1977) indicated that the distinctive profiles could arise from the different positional attachments of the terminal galactoses to their neighboring subterminal galactose units (Fig. 28). In the $P_1$ trisaccharide the terminal galactose is joined by an axial–axial $\alpha$(1→4) linkage to the pen-

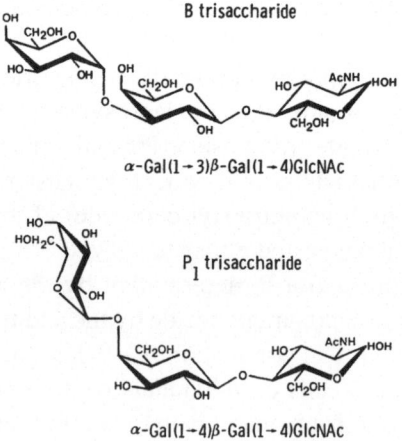

Fig. 28. Suggested conformations for the B and $P_1$ active trisaccharides (after Morgan, 1977).

ultimate galactose whereas in the B trisaccharide the two galactose units are joined $\alpha(1\rightarrow3)$ in the much more common axial–equatorial linkage. The immunodominant galactose residues are therefore positioned very differently with respect to the remainder of the molecule. Hakomori *et al.* (1971) had earlier commented on the absence of serological relationship between the carbohydrate $\alpha$-Gal($1\rightarrow3$)Gal-R structure of rabbit erythrocyte B-active glycolipid and the carbohydrate structure in ceramide trihexoside.

# CONCLUDING REMARKS

The antigenic structures associated with the functional alleles in the ABO, H, Lewis, and P blood group systems are carbohydrate and thus they provide examples of the complex interactions which can occur when the genes code not for the antigens themselves but for enzymes catalyzing the assembly of carbohydrate chains. The elucidation of the chemistry and biosynthesis of the antigens has revealed that a variety of macromolecules may carry determinants belonging to the same system and that the same precursor substrates may be used for the formation of antigens belonging to different systems. The patterns of interaction are determined by the genetic endowment of an individual with respect to the genes controlling the synthesis of the determinants, the location at different sites of the enzymic products of the genes, the presence in the same cells of the requisite glycosphingolipid, glycoprotein, or oligosaccharide acceptor molecules, and the relative timing of the sugar transfers catalyzed by the various enzymes.

Lactosyl ceramide (Table XI) is the key precursor for both the glycosphingolipids that are intrinsic components of the red cell membrane and for those acquired by the cells from the plasma. In the red cell, one biosynthetic pathway leads to ceramide trihexoside (the $P^k$ antigen) and globoside (the P antigen) and the other pathway leads to lacto-$N$-neotetraosyl ceramide (Table IV) which is the precursor glycolipid for the formation of the H, A, B, I, and $P_1$ specific determinants on the erythrocyte surface. Even the highly complex poly(glycosyl) ceramides (Koscielak *et al.*, 1978) are ultimately based on this tetrahexosyl ceramide which has a Type 2 chain ending (Fig. 1). On the other hand, the precursor of the

Le$^a$, Le$^b$, H, ALe$^b$, and BLe$^b$ glycosphingolipids that circulate in the plasma, and are taken up onto red and white blood cells, is lacto-$N$-tetraosyl ceramide (Table X) which has a Type 1 chain ending (Fig. 1).

The glycoproteins synthesized by the mucus-secreting cells have both Type 1 and Type 2 structures as branches (Fig. 3) on the many carbohydrate chains attached to the peptide core. A, B, H, and I determinants may be carried on the Type 2 chains and A, B, H, Le$^a$, Le$^b$, ALe$^b$, and BLe$^b$ determinants on the Type 1 chains. The pathways of biosynthesis of these determinants depends upon the interaction of the four genetic systems *ABO, Hh, Sese,* and *Lele* as originally proposed (Watkins and Morgan, 1959). However, the existence of the two types of chain carrying different determinants was not known at that time. The competition for the Type 1 chains by the *H*- and *Le*-gene-specified glycosyltransferases, and the different stages at which the *Le* gene catalyzes the addition of the fucose to these chains (Fig. 23), renders more complicated attempts to summarize the genetic pathways in a simple comprehensive scheme which shows the sequential formation of the antigens. Boettcher (1978*b*) presented a figure which, in the light of present knowledge, more accurately represents the sequence of events than the original version in that the step controlled by the *H* gene is placed before that controlled by the *Le* gene. However, this scheme is still only a partial truth, and now that the biochemistry has been unraveled it is probably better to express these pathways in terms of the precursor substrates and the biosynthetic steps catalyzed by the glycosyltransferase products of the genes.

The biosynthetic pathways for the formation of the P$^k$, P, and P$_1$ antigens in the P system appear to be straightforward but the genetic relationships are not yet completely clarified. Lactosyl ceramide, P$^k$ (CTH), and P (globoside) are synthesized one from the other by the sequential addition of single sugar residues (Fig. 26) and hence conform to the ABH model. In order to place P$_1$ in the P system, however, a new mechanism has to be proposed (Marcus, 1977). The P$_1$ antigen is assumed to be synthesized by the addition of galactose in $\alpha(1{\rightarrow}4)$ linkage to lacto-$N$-neotetraose and the P$^k$ antigen by the addition of galactose, also in $\alpha(1{\rightarrow}4)$ linkage to lactosyl ceramide (Fig. 26). If, as appears the simplest explanation, the $P_1$ gene is an allele of $P^k$ and $p$ and codes for an $\alpha$-4-galactosyltransferase with a broader acceptor specificity than the product of the $P^k$ gene, there is no parallel for this situation in the glycosyltransferases specified by allelic genes associated with the ABO, H, or Lewis systems. An understanding of the biochemical basis of the formation of blood-group-specific antigens is thus contributing to knowledge on the fine distinctions and range of acceptor specificities of glycosyltransferases in general.

The chemical structures at the terminal nonreducing ends of the carbohydrate chains that confer A, B, H, $Le^a$, $Le^b$, P, $P^k$, and $P_1$ specificities on macromolecules are now firmly established and a number of these determinants have been chemically synthesized. The recent advances in chemical techniques which have permitted the synthesis of blood-group-active oligosaccharides and closely related structures have already given impetus to more detailed studies on the combining sites of naturally occurring blood group antibodies (Kabat et al., 1978; Feizi et al., 1978). The preparation of artificial antigens with single well-defined determinants (see Lemieux, 1978) should also permit the production of monospecific antibodies and enable detailed kinetic investigations to be carried out on the interaction between blood group antigens and antibodies. Although there is probably little further work to be done on the structures of the determinants the influence of neighboring groups on the reactivity of these determinants with antibodies has still to be fully explored.

The biochemical basis of the $A_1$ and $A_2$ subgroups of A remains controversial, but the findings of many workers that only Type 2 chains occur in the glycoproteins or glycolipids extracted from red cell membranes militates against the suggestion that $A_2$ specificity is determined by the Type 1 chain A trisaccharide (Fig. 2) whereas the $A_1$ speçifcity is determined by the Type 1 chain A trisaccharide (Moreno, et al., 1971; Kisailus and Kabat, 1978). Biosynthesis experiments with low-molecular-weight acceptors, H-active glycoproteins, and group O red cells (Table VIII) indicate that it is not possible to extrapolate in a strictly quantitative manner from the low-molecular-weight acceptors to the macromolecules, but there is no evidence to suggest that the $\alpha$-$N$-acetylgalactosaminyl-transferases produced by the $A^1$ and $A^2$ genes have different acceptor specificities. The weight of evidence points to a quantitative difference in the number of H structures which are converted into A structures in glycoproteins or glycolipids. Two isoenzymes differing in their quantitative action on a substrate would conform with the general pattern observed for isoenzymes which are the products of multiple alleles at one gene locus (see Harris, 1975). The difference in behavior of anti-$A_1$ and anti-A reagents could, as suggested by Mäkelä et al. (1969), be ascribed to the requirement of anti-$A_1$ reagents for a high density of A receptors. The profile presented to antibodies by a single A determinant surrounded by neighboring chains terminating with H or I structures, as found in the complex glycosphingolipids from $A_2$ red cells, may be very different from the more closely packed A determinants found in glycosphingolipids from $A_1$ red cells (Koscielak, 1977; Hakomori et al., 1977a). The nonspecific interaction of antibodies with neighboring structures might result in an apparent qualitative difference between the $A_1$ and $A_2$ determinants in antibody binding studies.

Anti-I agglutinins are macroglobulins requiring both low temperature and multivalent binding for agglutination. Since the branched and very complex poly(glycosyl) ceramides have highest I activity, Koscielak (1977) suggested that the I gene can probably be equated with the transferase responsible for the addition of N-acetylglucosamine to the 6-position of an internal β-galactosyl residue to form the branched core structure (Fig. 3a and Table V). This proposal is compatible with the evidence from enzymic degradation experiments and with much of the recent data obtained by inhibition studies and also with the findings of Hakomori et al. (1977a) that the complex glycolipids are present in lower concentrations in cord bloods, which fail to react with anti-I sera, than in adult red cells. On the other hand Ginsburg et al. (1979) suggest that almost any sugar sequence on the erythrocyte surface might be classified as an I or i antigen depending upon characteristic changes in its density during development. Characterization of the relevant β-6-N-acetylglucosaminyltransferase, and demonstration of the levels of this enzyme in normal adults, newborn infants, and adults with the i phenotype might help to resolve these divergent views.

The invariable presence of the appropriate A and B transferases in the serum of individuals with normal ABO groups has enabled the classification of the system to be extended to include the transferases (Table 1). Investigations of the A-, B-, and H-gene-specified transferases in serum and red cells in rare blood groups where there is abnormal expression of A, B, or H antigens on the red cells are helping to clarify the basis of the variant expression in single individuals, and within families. Moreover, examination of the transferase activities in these atypical phenotypes is contributing to a general understanding of the normal distribution, functioning, and regulation of the primary enzymic products of the ABO genes. Regulation by the Se gene of the expression of the H-gene-specified α-2-L-fucosyltransferase in cells producing the secreted glycoproteins has been substantiated by failure to find this enzyme in salivary gland tissue of nonsecretors. The Se gene must also be functional in the cells synthesizing the $Le^b$, $ALe^b$, and $BLe^b$ glycosphingolipids that circulate in the plasma; hence the *Se* gene does not control the formation of H structures only in secreted glycoproteins. Serological and transferase studies make it evident that the expression of the *H*, *A*, and *B* genes at the site of synthesis of the red cell antigens are also subject to control by different regulator genes. The mode of action of the *Se* gene, or of any of the regulator genes, is at present obscure, and they constitute a challenge for future biochemical investigations on the ABO blood group system.

The findings that the *H*, *A*, and *B* transferase levels are depressed in adenocarcinoma tissue and in certain myeloproliferative disorders of the blood suggest their possible potential value as diagnostic or prognostic tools. As additional genetic markers they may also find use in forensic medicine. For these purposes new and more rapid methods are required for the detection and assay of the transferases but it is most important that ascertainment of the anomeric and positional linkage of the transferred sugar is not sacrificed in the interests of speed. For reasons of expediency, that were perfectly valid at the time, much of the earlier work on glycosyltransferases connected with the biosynthesis of glycoproteins was carried out with macromolecules that were not the natural acceptors for the enzyme under investigation (see Roseman, 1970). Frequently these macromolecules were treated with exoglycosidases to sequentially remove terminal residues from the ends of the carbohydrate chains with a view to exposing sugars that were the putative acceptors for the transferred sugar residues. That the transfer does not always take place to the exposed sugar residue has recently been demonstrated (Wilson, *et al.*, 1976) but in any event these macromolecules frequently have several sites for the addition of the same sugar. The homologous blood-group-specific glycoproteins and their precursor, which might appear to be good substrates to use for assay of the *H* or *Le* transferases, can accept L-fucose in at least four different linkages (see Watkins, 1974) and hence measurement of transferred [$^{14}$C]fucose gives only the sum of the action of the different transferases. Unless sufficient enzyme and substrates are available for the activity of the blood group-gene-specified transferases to be assessed by the development of blood group serological activity, low-molecular-weight compounds that accept the transferred sugar in only one positional and anomeric linkage should be the substrates of choice.

With so much knowledge now available on the chemistry, genetics, and biosynthesis of the antigens associated with the ABO, Lewis, and P blood group systems the question might reasonably be asked whether we are any nearer to an understanding of the function of blood group substances or the nature of the selective pressures that maintain the ABO polymorphism. The ABH and Lewis blood group specific glycoproteins undoubtedly have a function as constituents of the mucous layer that protects and lubricates normal epithelial surfaces but the blood group property itself does not appear to be associated with any essential physiological function since the absence of any one blood group character does not lead *per se* to a pathological condition. Similarly, although membrane-bound glycolipids and glycoproteins are believed to mediate a number of functions including cell recognition, differentiation, and growth, and a great variety of cell surface structures would be valuable in the recognition of "self," the variation in carbohydrate chain endings in different individuals would appear to play little part in these functions. The blood group polymorphisms may be a survival of past selections that have outlived their usefulness or the individuality of cell surface may confer advantages or disadvantages under certain environmental conditions, such as attack by bacteria or viruses (see Giblett, 1969; Hakomori and Kobata, 1974). Many microorganisms have cell surface antigens related to the human blood group substances and an individual with an antigen shared by an invading microorganism might be less able to produce antibodies than one who lacks the antigen. However, until recently, explanations for the maintenance of ABO polymorphism have invoked the specific determinants, or the corresponding antibodies as the causative agents. Now that it is recognized that the immunological determinants are the final products in a chain of reactions it is possible to reexamine the problem in terms of the glycosyltransferases which are the intermediate agents between the genes and the determinant structures. These enzymes, or the protein molecules that carry the enzymically specific sites, may have as yet unrecognized functions that hold the key to selection.

## REFERENCES

Anderson, B., Hoffman, P., and Meyer, K., 1963, A serine-linked peptide from chondroitin sulfate, *Biochim. Biophys. Acta* **74**:309–311.

Ando, S., and Yamakawa, T., 1973, Separation of polar glycolipids from human red cells with special reference to blood group A activity, *J. Biochem. Tokyo* **73**:387–396.

Ando, S., Kon, K., Isobe, M., and Yamakawa, T., 1973, Structural study on tetraglycosyl ceramide and gangliosides isolated from human red blood cells, *J. Biochem. Tokyo,* **73**:893–895.

Badet, J., 1976, Activités glycosyltransférasiques sériques associeés à la biosynthèse des antigènes de group sanguins A et B. Application a l'étude de sujets B normaux et Cis AB, *Rev. Franc. Transf. Immuno-Hémat.* **19**:105–116.

Badet, J., Ropars, C., Cartron, J. P., and Salmon, C., 1974, Groups of α-D-galactosyltransferase activity in sera of individuals with normal B phenotype, *Biomedicine* **21**:230–232.

Badet, J., Ropars, C., Cartron, J. P., Doinel, C., and Salmon, C., 1976, Groups of α-D-galactosyltransferase activity in sera of individuals with normal B phenotype. II. Relationship between transferase activity and red cell agglutinability, *Vox Sang.* **30**:105–113.

Badet, J., Ropars, C., and Salmon, C., 1978, α-N-Acetyl-D-galactosaminyl- and α-D-galactosyltransferase activities in sera of *cis* AB blood group individuals, *J. Immunogenet.* **5**:221–231.

Baker, A. P., Griggs, L. J., Munro, J. T., and Finkelstein, J. A., 1973, Blood group A active glycoproteins of respiratory mucus and their synthesis by an *N*-acetylgalactosaminyltransferase, *J. Biol. Chem.* **248**:880–883.

Battey, D. A., Bird, G. W. G., McDermott, A., Mortimer, C. W., Mutchinick, O. M., and Wingham, J., 1974, Case report: Another human chimaera, *J. Med. Genet.* **11**:283–287.

Bauer, C., Köttgen, E., and Reutter, W., 1977, Elevated activities of α-2- and α-3-fucosyltransferases in human serum as a new indication of malignancy, *Biochem. Biophys. Res. Commun.* **76**:488–494.

Bernstein, F., 1924, Ergebnisse einer biostatischen zusammenfassenden Betrachtung über die ehrlichen Blutstrukturen des Menschen, *Klin. Wochenschr.* **3**:1495–1497.

Betz, J. L., Brown, P. R., Smyth, M. J., and Clarke, P. H., 1974, Evolution in action, *Nature* **247**:261–264.

Bhatia, H. M., 1977, Serologic reactions of ABO and O$_h$ (Bombay) phenotypes due to variations in H antigen, in: *Human Blood Groups* (J. F. Mohn, R. W. Plunkett, R. K. Cunningham, and R. E. Lambert, eds.), pp. 293–305, Karger, Basel.

Bhatia, H. M., and Sathe, M. S., 1974, Incidence of 'Bombay' (O$_h$) phenotype and weaker variants of A and B antigen in Bombay (India), *Vox Sang.* **27**:524–532.

Bhende, Y. M., Deshpande, C. K., Bhatia, H. M., Sanger, R., Race, R. R., Morgan, W. T. J., and Watkins, W. M., 1952, A "new" blood-group character related to the ABO system, *Lancet* **i**:903–904.

Bird, G. W. G., Battey, D. A., Greenwell, P., Mortimer, C. W., Watkins, W. M., and Wingham, J., 1976, Case report: Further observations on the Birmingham chimaera, *J. Med. Genet.* **13**:70–71.

Boettcher, B., 1966, Modification of Bernstein's multiple allele theory for the inheritance of the ABO blood groups in the light of modern genetical concepts, *Vox Sang.* **11**:129–136.

Boettcher, B., 1978a, Blood group antigens, in: *The Biochemical Genetics of Man* (D. J. H. Brock and O. Mayo, eds.), pp. 325–363, Academic Press, New York.

Boettcher, B., 1978b, Sequence of action of genes at the secretor, H, ABO and Lewis loci, *Hum. Hered.* **28**:426–430.

Bonfiglio, T. A., and Feinberg, M. R., 1976, Isoantigen loss in cervical neoplasia, *Arch. Pathol. Lab. Med.* **100**:307–310.

Brederode, J. van, and Nigtevecht, G. van, 1974, Dominance relationships between two allelic genes controlling glycosyltransferases with different substrate specificity in *Melandrium, Genetics* **77**:507–520.

Brederode, J. van, and Nigtevecht, G. van, 1975, Dominance relationships between allelic glycosyltransferase genes in *Melandrium*: An enzyme-kinetic approach, *Theor. Appl. Genet.* **46**:353–358.

Brenner, S., 1959, The mechanism of gene action, in: *Ciba Foundation Symposium on*

*Biochemistry of Human Genetics* (G. E. W. Wolstenholme and C. M. O'Connor, eds.), pp. 304–317, Churchill, London.

Brennessel, B. A., and Goldstein, J., 1974, Separation of H-activity from isolated glycoproteins of human O erythrocyte membranes, *Vox Sang.* **26**:405–414.

Brown, P. R., and Clarke, P. H., 1972, Amino acid substitution in an amidase produced by an acetanilide-utilising mutant of *Pseudomonas aeruginosa, J. Gen. Microbiol.* **70**:287–298.

Brown, P. C., Glynn, L. E., and Holborow, E. J., 1959, Lewis[a] substance in saliva; a qualitative difference between secretors and non-secretors, *Vox Sang.* **4**:1–12.

Bush, M., and Sabo, B., 1973, Three generations of AB antigens in *cis* position, *Transfusion* **13**:362 (Abstr.).

Cameron, G. L., and Staveley, J. M., 1957, Blood group P substance in hydatid cyst fluid, *Nature (London)* **179**:147–148.

Carlson, D. M., 1977, Chemistry and biosynthesis of mucus glycoproteins, *Adv. Exp. Med. Biol.* **89**:251–273.

Carlson, D. M., McGuire, E. J. Jourdian, G. W., and Roseman, S., 1973, The sialic acids. XVI. Isolation of a mucin sialyltransferase from sheep submaxillary gland, *J. Biol. Chem.* **248**:5763–5773.

Carne, L. R., and Watkins, W. M., 1977, Human blood group *B* gene specified α-3-galactosyltransferase: Purification of the enzyme in serum by biospecific adsorption onto blood group O erythrocyte membranes, *Biochem. Biophys. Res. Commun.* **77**:700–707.

Carne, L. R., and Watkins, W. M., 1979, Purification of the human blood group *B* gene specified α-3-galactosyltransferase by biospecific adsorption onto group O erythrocyte membranes, in: *Glycoconjugate Research*, Vol. II (J. D. Gregory and R. W. Jeanloz, eds.), pp. 1019–1021, Academic Press, New York.

Cartron, J. P., 1976, Etude des propriétés α-N-acetylgalactosaminyltransferasiques des sérums de sujets A et "A faible," *Rev. Franç. Transf. Immuno-hemat.* **19**:67–88.

Cartron, J. P., 1978, Biosynthesis of human blood group antigens, in: *XVth Congress of the International Society of Blood Transfusion, Paris, 1978*, Plenary Sessions—Main Lectures, pp. 69–86, Librairie Arnette, Paris.

Cartron, J. P., and Ropars, C., 1978, Cited in Cartron, J. P. (1978).

Cartron, J. P., Gerbal, A., Hughes-Jones, N. C., and Salmon, C., 1974, Weak A phenotypes. Relationship between agglutinability and antigen site density, *Immunology* **27**:723–727.

Cartron, J. P., Gerbal, A., Badet, J., Ropars, C., and Salmon, C., 1975, Assay of α-N-acetylgalactosaminyltransferases in human sera. Further evidence for several types of A_m individuals, *Vox Sang.* **28**:347–365.

Cartron, J. P., Mulet, C., Badet, J., Jacquinet, J. C., and Sinäy, P., 1976a, Use of two chemically synthesised H acceptors as substrates for A and B blood group gene-specified glycosyltransferases, *FEBS Lett.* **67**:143–148.

Cartron, J. P., Ropars, C., Calkovska, Z., and Salmon, C., 1976b, Detection of $A_1A_2$ and $A_2A_m^{A1}$ heterozygotes among human A blood group heterozygotes, *J. Immunogenet.* **3**:155–161.

Cartron, J. P., Badet, J., Mulet, C., and Salmon, C., 1978, Study of the α-N-acetylgalactosaminyltransferase in sera and red cell membranes of human A subgroups, *J. Immunogenet.* **5**:107–116.

Ceppellini, R., 1955, On the genetics of secretor and Lewis characters: A family study, in: *Proceedings of the Vth Congress of the International Society of Blood Transfusion, Paris, 1954*, p. 207.

Ceppellini, R., 1959, Physiological genetics of human blood factors, in: *Ciba Foundation Symposium on Biochemistry of Human Genetics* (G. E. W. Wolstenholme and C. M. O'Connor, eds.), pp. 242–261, Churchill, London.

Ceppellini, R., Nasso, S., and Tecilazich, F., 1952, *La Malattia Emolitica del Neonato*, Istituto Sieroterapico Milanese Serafino Belfanti Milano, p. 204.

Chester, M. A., 1971, The role of fucosyltransferases in the biosynthesis of blood group substances, Ph.D. Thesis, University of London.

Chester, M. A., and Watkins, W. M., 1969, α-L-Fucosyltransferases in human submaxillary glands and stomach tissues associated with the H, Le$^a$ and Le$^b$ blood group characters and ABH secretor status, *Biochem. Biophys. Res. Commun.* **34**:835–842.

Chester, M. A., Yates, A. D., and Watkins, W. M., 1976, Phenyl-β-D-galactopyranoside as an acceptor substrate for the blood-group *H* gene associated guanosine diphosphate L-fucose: β-D-galactosyl α-2-L-fucosyltransferase, *Eur. J. Biochem.* **69**:583–592.

Chester, M. A., Yates, A. D., Greenwell, P., Kuhns, W. J., and Watkins, W. M., 1977, Unpublished observations cited in Watkins (1977).

Clamp, J. R., Allen, A., Gibbons, R. A., and Roberts, G. P., 1978, Chemical aspects of mucus, *Br. Med. Bull.* **34**:25–41.

Clarke, P. H., 1974, Evolution in the microbial world, in: *Society of General Microbiologists Symposium 24* (P. M. Meadow and S. J. Pirt, eds.), pp. 183–217, University Press, Cambridge.

Cooper, A. G., and Brown, M. C., 1973, Serum i antigen: A new human blood group glycoprotein, *Biochem. Biophys. Res. Commun.* **55**:297–304.

Cory, H. T., Yates, A. D., Donald, A. S. R., Watkins, W. M., and Morgan, W. T. J., 1974, The nature of the human blood group P₁ determinant, *Biochem. Biophys. Res. Commun.* **61**:1289–1296.

Creeth, J. M., 1978, Constituents of mucus and their separation, *Br. Med. Bull.* **34**:17–24.

Crookston, M. C., 1978, Antigens common to red blood cells and plasma, in: *XVth Congress of the International Society of Blood Transfusion, Paris, 1978*, Plenary Sessions—Main Lectures, pp. 51–61, Librairie Arnette, Paris.

Crookston, M. C., and Tilley, C. A., 1977, A and B and Lewis antigens in plasma, in: *Human Blood Groups* (J. F. Mohn, R. W. Plunkett, R. K. Cunningham, and R. M. Lambert, eds.), pp. 246–256, Karger, Basel.

Crookston, M. C., Tilley, C. A., and Crookston, J. H., 1970, Human blood chimaera with seeming breakdown of immune tolerance, *Lancet* **ii**:1110–1112.

Dahr, W., Uhlenbruck, G., Jansen, E., and Schmalisch, R., 1977, Different N-terminal amino acids in the MN-glycoprotein from *MM* and *NN* erythrocytes, *Hum. Genet.* **35**:335–343.

David, S., and Veyrieres, A., 1975, The synthesis of 3,6-di-*O*-(2-acetamido-2-deoxy-β-D-glucopyranosyl)-D-galactose. A branched trisaccharide reported as a hydrolysis product of blood group substances, *Carbohydrate Res.* **40**:23–29.

Davidsohn, I., and Ni, L. Y., 1969, Loss of isoantigens A, B and H in carcinoma of the lung, *Am. J. Pathol.* **57**:307–334.

Davidsohn, I., Kovarik, S., and Ni, L. Y., 1969, Isoantigens A, B and H in benign and malignant lesions of the cervix, *Arch. Pathol.* **87**:306–314.

Davidsohn, I., Ni, L. Y., and Stejskal, R., 1971, Tissue isoantigens A, B and H in carcinoma of the stomach, *Arch. Pathol.* **92**:456–464.

Dawson, G. and Sweeley, C. C., 1970, *In vivo* studies on glycosphingolipid metabolism in porcine blood, *J. Biol. Chem.* **245**:410–416.

Dejter-Juszynski, M., Harpaz, N., Flowers, H. M., 1978, Blood-group ABH-specific macroglycolipids of human erythrocytes: Isolation in high yield from a crude membrane glycoprotein fraction, *Eur. J. Biochem.* **83**:363–373.

Donald, A. S. R., 1973, The products of pronase digestion of purified blood-group specific glycoproteins, *Biochim. Biophys. Acta* **317**:420–436.

Donald, A. S. R., Creeth, J. M., Morgan, W. T. J., and Watkins, W. M., 1969, The peptide moiety of human blood-group active glycoproteins associated with the ABO and Lewis groups, *Biochem. J.* **115**:125–127.

Dungern, E. von, and Hirszfeld, L., 1910, Über Vererbung gruppenspezifischer des blutes. Strukturen des blutes, *Z. Immun. Forsch.* **6**:284–292.

Dunstone, J. R. and Morgan, W. T. J., 1965, Further observations on the glycoproteins in human ovarian cyst fluids, *Biochim. Biophys. Acta* **101**:300–314.

Dzierzkowa-Borodej, W., Seyfried, H., and Lisowska, E., 1975, Serological classification of anti-I sera, *Vox Sang.* **28**:110–121.

Economidou, J., Hughes-Jones, N. C., and Gardner, B., 1967, Quantitative measurements concerning A and B antigen sites, *Vox Sang.* **12**:321–328.

Edwards J. H. and McKusick V. A. 1978. Report of the committee on unassigned linkage groups. *Cytogenetics and cell genetics*, **22**:129–131.

Feizi, T., 1977, Immunochemistry of the Ii blood group antigens, in: *Human Blood Groups* (J. F. Mohn, R. W. Plunkett, R. K. Cunningham, and R. M. Lambert, eds.), pp. 164–171, Karger, Basel.

Feizi, T., and Kabat. E. A., 1972, Immunochemical studies on blood groups LIV. Classification of anti-I and anti-i sera into groups based on reactivity patterns with various antigens related to the Blood group A, B, H, Le^a, Le^b and precursor substances, *J. Exp. Med.* **135**:1247–1258.

Feizi, T., Kabat, E. A., Vicari, G., Anderson B., and Marsh, W. L., 1971a, Immunochemical studies on blood groups. XLVII. The I antigen complex precursors in the A, B, H, Le^a and Le^b blood group system-hemagglutination-inhibition studies, *J. Exp. Med.* **133**:39–52.

Feizi, T., Kabat, E. A., Vicari, G., Anderson, B., and Marsh, W. L., 1971b, Immunochemical studies on blood groups. XLIX. The I antigen complex: Specificity differences among anti-I sera revealed by quantitative precipitin studies; partial structure of the I determinant specific for one anti-I serum, *J. Immunol.* **106**:1578–1592.

Feizi, T., Turberville, C., and Westwood, H. H., 1975, Blood group precursors and cancer related antigens, *Lancet* **ii**:391.

Feizi, T., Wood, E., Augé, C., David, S., and Veyrieres, A., 1978, Blood group I activities of synthetic oligosaccharides assessed by radioimmunoassay, *Immunochemistry* **15**:733–736.

Fellous, M., Gerbal, A., Thessier, C., Frezal, J., Dausset, J., and Salmon, C., 1974, Studies on the biosynthetic pathway of human P erythrocyte antigens using somatic cells in culture, *Vox Sang.* **26**:518–536.

Fellous, M., Gerbal, A., Nobillot, G., and Weils, J., 1977, Studies on the biosynthetic pathway of human P erythrocyte antigen using genetic complementation tests between fibroblasts from rare p and P^k phenotype donors, *Vox Sang.* **32**:262–268.

Ferguson-Smith, M. A., Aitken, D. A., Turleau, C., and de Grouchy, J., 1976, Localisation of the human ABO: Np-1 : AK-1 linkage group by regional assignment of AK-1 to 9q34, *Hum. Genet.* **34**:35–43.

Finne, J., Krusius, T., and Rauvala, H., 1978, Alkali-stable blood group A- and B-active poly(glycosyl)peptides from human erythrocyte membrane, *FEBS Lett.* **89**:111–115.

Friedenreich, V., 1936, Eine bisher unbekannte Blutgruppeneigenschaft (A₃), *Z. Immun. Forsch.* **89**:409–422.

Fujita, S., and Cleve, H., 1975, Isolation and partial characterisation of two minor glycoproteins from human erythrocyte membranes, *Biochim. Biophys. Acta* **382**:172–180.

Fukuda, M., and Osawa, T., 1973, Isolation and characterisation of a glycoprotein from human group O erythrocyte membrane, *J. Biol. Chem.* **248**:5100–5105.

Furukawa, K., Takizawa, H., Takizawa, H., and Iseki, S., 1974, Examples of blood groups p and P$^k$ in Japanese families, *Jap. J. Hum. Genet.* **19**:127–145.

Ganschow, R. and Paigen, K., 1967, Separate genes determining the structure and intracellular location of hepatic glucuronidase, *Proc. Natl. Acad. Sci. USA.* **58**:938–945.

Gardas, A., 1976a, A structural study on a macro glycolipid containing 22 sugars isolated from human erythrocytes, *Eur. J. Biochem.* **68**:177–183.

Gardas, A., 1976b, Studies on I-blood-group-active sites on macroglycolipids from human erythrocytes, *Eur. J. Biochem.* **68**:185–191.

Gardas, A., 1978, Structure of an (A-blood-group)-active glycolipid isolated from human erythrocytes, *Eur. J. Biochem.* **89**:471–473.

Gardas, A., and Koscielak, J., 1971, A, B and H blood group specificities in glycoprotein and glycolipid fractions of human erythrocyte membrane. Absence of blood group active glycoproteins in the membranes of non-secretors, *Vox Sang.* **20**:137–149.

Gardas, A. and Koscielak, J., 1973, New form of A-, B- and H-blood group active substances extracted from erythrocyte membranes, *Eur. J. Biochem.* **32**:178–187.

Gardas, A. and Koscielak, J., 1974a, Megaloglycolipids—unusually complex glycosphingolipids of human erythrocyte membrane, *FEBS Lett.* **42**:101–104.

Gardas, A. and Koscielak, J., 1974b, I-active antigen of human erythrocyte membrane, *Vox Sang.* **26**:227–237.

Giblett, E. R., 1969, *Genetic Markers in Human Blood*, Blackwell Scientific Publications, Oxford.

Giblett, E. R., 1977, Some perspectives on blood group genetics and immunology, in: *Human Blood Groups* (J. F. Mohn, R. W. Plunkett, R. K. Cunningham, and R. M. Lambert, eds.), pp. 437–448, Karger, Basel.

Ginsburg, V., 1972, Enzymatic basis for blood groups in man, *Adv. Enzymol.* **36**:131–149.

Ginsburg, V., Kobata, A., Hickey, C., and Sawicka, T., 1971, Biochemical basis for blood types in man, in: *Glycoproteins of Blood Cells and Plasma* (G. A. Jamieson and T. J. Greenwalt, eds.), pp. 114–126, Lippincott, Philadelphia.

Ginsburg, V., McGinniss, M. M., and Zopf, D. A., 1979, Biochemical basis for some blood groups, in: *Immunobiology of the Erythrocyte* (S. G. Sandler, J. Nusbacher, and M. S. Schanfield, eds.), *Progress in Clinical and Biological Research Series*, Alan R. Liss, New York (in press).

Goodwin, S. D., and Watkins, W. M., 1974, The peptide moiety of blood-group-specific glycoproteins. Some amino acid sequences in the regions carrying the carbohydrate chains, *Eur. J. Biochem.* **47**:371–382.

Graham, H. A., and Williams, A. N., 1978, A simple genetic model for the P blood group system, in: *XVth Congress of the International Society of Blood Transfusion, Paris, 1978*, Abstract, p. 349.

Graham, H. A., Hirsch, H. F., and Davis, D. M., 1977, Genetic and immunochemical relationships between soluble and cell-bound antigens of the Lewis system, in: *Human Blood Groups* (J. F. Mohn, R. W. Plunkett, R. K. Cunningham, and R. M. Lambert, eds.), pp. 257–267, Karger, Basel.

Graham, H. A., Sinäy, P., Hirsch, H. F., and Jacquinet, J. C., 1978, Inhibition of anti-Le$^{dH}$ and *Ulex* anti-H lectin with oligosaccharides, in: *XVth Congress of the International Society of Blood Transfusion, Paris, 1978*, Abstract, p. 552.

Green, F. A., 1968a, Rh antigenicity: An essential component soluble in butanol, *Nature (London)* **219**:86–87.

Green, F. A., 1968b, Phospholipid requirement for Rh antigenic activity, *J. Biol. Chem.* **243**:5519–5524.

Green, F. A., 1972, Erythrocyte membrane lipids and Rh antigenic activity, *J. Biol. Chem.* **247**:881–887.

Greenbury, C. L., Moore, D. H., and Nunn, L. A. C., 1963, Reaction of 7S and 19S components of immune rabbit antisera with human group A and AB red cells, *Immunology* **6**:421–433.

Greenwell, P., 1977, Personal communication.

Greenwell, P., and Watkins, W. M., 1978, Cited in Watkins (1978).

Grollman, E. F., Kobata, A., and Ginsburg, V., 1969, An enzymatic basis for Lewis blood types in man, *J. Clin. Invest.* **48**:1489–1494.

Grubb, R., 1948, Correlation between Lewis blood group and secretor status in man, *Nature (London)* **162**:933.

Gunson, H. H., and Latham, V., 1972, An agglutinin in human serum reacting with cells from Le(a-b-) non-secretor individuals, *Vox Sang.* **22**:344–353.

Hakkinen, I., 1970, A-like blood group antigen in gastric cancer cells of patients in blood groups O and B, *J. Nat. Cancer Inst.* **44**:1183–1193.

Hakomori, S., 1970, Glycosphingolipids having blood group ABH and Lewis specificities, *Chem. Phys. Lipids* **5**:96–115.

Hakomori, S., 1971, Glycolipid changes associated with malignant transformation, in: *Dynamic Structure of Cell Membranes* (D. F. H. Wallach and H. Fischer, eds.), pp. 65–96, Springer-Verlag, Berlin.

Hakomori, S., 1978, Isolation of blood group ABH-active glycolipids from human erythrocyte membranes, *Methods Enzymol.* **50**:207–211.

Hakomori, S., and Andrews, H. D., 1970, Sphingoglycolipids with Le[b] activity, and the copresence of Le[a]-, Le[b]-glycolipids in human tumor tissue, *Biochim. Biophys. Acta* **202**:225–228.

Hakomori, S., and Kobata, A., 1974, Blood group antigens, in: *The Antigens,* Vol. 2 (M. Sela, ed.), pp. 79–140, Academic Press, New York.

Hakomori, S., and Strycharz, G. D., 1968, Investigations on cellular blood group substances. I. Isolation and chemical composition of blood group ABH and Le[b] isoantigens of sphingoglycolipid nature, *Biochemistry* **7**:1279–1286.

Hakomori, S., and Yang, H., 1971, A sphingolipid having a novel type of ceramide and lacto-*N*-fucopentaose III, *J. Biol. Chem.* **246**:1192–1200.

Hakomori, S., Koscielak, J., Bloch, H., and Jeanloz, R. W., 1967, Studies on the immunological relation between the tumor glycolipids and blood group substances, *J. Immunol.* **98**:31–38.

Hakomori, S., Siddiqui, B., Li, Y-T., Li, S-C., and Hellerqvist, C. G., 1971, Anomeric structures of globoside and ceramide trihexoside of human erythrocytes and hamster fibroblasts, *J. Biol. Chem.* **248**:2271–2277.

Hakomori, S., Stellner, K., and Watanabe, K., 1972, Four antigenic variants of blood group A glycolipid. Examples of highly complex, branched chain glycolipid of animal cell membrane, *Biochem. Biophys. Res. Commun.* **49**:1061–1068.

Hakomori, S., Watanabe, K., and Laine, R. A., 1977a, Glycosphingolipids with blood group A, H and I activity: their status in Group A₁ and A₂ erythrocytes and their changes associated with ontogeny and oncogeny, in: *Human Blood Groups* (J. F. Mohn, R. W. Plunkett, R. K. Cunningham, and R. M. Lambert, eds.), pp. 150–163, Karger, Basel.

Hakomori, S., Wang., M., and Young, W. W., 1977b, Isoantigenic expression of Forssman glycolipid in human gastric and colonic mucosa: Its possible identity with "A-like antigen" in human cancer, *Proc. Natl. Acad. Sci. USA.* **74**:3023–3027.

Hamaguchi, H., and Cleve, H., 1972, Solubilisation of human erythrocyte membrane glycoproteins and separation of the MN glycoprotein from a glycoprotein with I, S, and A activity, *Biochim. Biophys. Acta* **278**:271–280.

Hanfland, P., 1975, Characterisation of B and H blood group active glycosphingolipids from human B erythrocyte membranes, *Chem. Phys. Lipids* **15**:105–124.

Hanfland, P., 1978, Isolation and purification of Lewis blood-group active glycosphingolipids from the plasma of human OLe^b individuals, *Eur. J. Biochem.* **87**:161–170.

Hanfland, P., and Egli, H., 1975, Quantitative isolation and purification of blood group active glycosphingolipids from human B erythrocytes, *Vox Sang.* **28**:438–452.

Harris, H., 1975, *The Principles of Human Biochemical Genetics*, 2nd Ed., North-Holland, Amsterdam.

Hartmann, G., 1941, *Group Antigens in Human Organs*, Munksgaard, Copenhagen.

Haselhorst, G., and Lauer, A., 1931, Zur Blutgruppenkombination Mutter AB-Kind O, *Z. Konstit. Lehre* **16**:227–230.

Hearn, V. M., Smith, Z. G., and Watkins, W. M., 1968, An α-*N*-acetyl-D-galactosaminyltransferase associated with the human blood group A character, *Biochem. J.* **109**:315–317.

Hearn, V. M., Race, C., and Watkins, W. M., 1972, α-*N*-Acetylgalactosaminyl- and α-galactosyltransferases in human ovarian cyst epithelial linings and fluids, *Biochem. Biophys. Res. Commun.* **46**:948–956.

Hirschfeld, J., 1977, Conceptual framework shifts in immunogenetics. I. A new look at *cis* AB antigens in the ABO system, *Vox Sang.* **33**:286–289.

Hirsh. H. F.. and Graham. H. A.. 1977. Adsorption of plasma antigens onto red cells (Abstract S-62). American Association of Blood Banks.

Holborow, E. J., Brown, P. C., Glynn, L. E., Hawes, M. D., Gresham, G. A., O'Brien, T. F., and Coombs, R. R. A., 1960, The distribution of the blood group A antigen in human tissues, *Br. J. Exp. Pathol.* **41**:430–437.

Hosoi, T., Yahara, S., Kunitoms, K., Saji, H., and Ohtsuki, Y., 1977, Blood chimeric twins. An example of blood cell chimerism, *Vox Sang.* **32**:339–341.

How, M. J., Brimacombe, J. S., and Stacey, M., 1964, The pneumococcal polysaccharides, *Adv. Carbohydr. Chem.* **19**:303–358.

Hrubisko, M., 1976, Deficient H types, *Rev. Franç. Transf. Immuno-Hématol.* **19**:157–174.

Hrubisko, M., and Mergancovà, O., 1966, Beobachtungen über Varianten des Blutgruppensystems ABO III. Die neuen Variationen O_Hm und A_Hm. Ein Beitrag zur Frage der Biosynthese der Blutgruppen-Antigene, *Blut* **13**:278–285.

Hrubisko, M., Laluha, J., Mergancovà, O., and Zakovicovà, S., 1970, New variants in the ABO/H blood group system due to interaction of recessive genes controlling the formation of H antigen in erythrocytes: The "Bombay-like" phenotypes O_Hm, O^B_Hm and O^{AB}_Hm, *Vox Sang.* **19**:113–122.

Hummel, K., Badet, J., Bauermeister, W., Bender, K., Duffner, G., Lopez, M., Mauff, G., Pulverer, G., Salmon, C., and Schmidts, W., 1977, Inheritance of Cis-AB in three generations (Family Lam.), *Vox Sang.* **33**:290–298.

Jacquinet, J. C., and Sinäy, P., 1975, Synthèse du 2-acetamido-2-deoxy-4-*O*-α-L-fucopyranosyl α-D-glucopyranose, *Carbohydrate Res.* **42**:251–258.

Jacquinet, J. C., and Sinäy, P., 1976, Synthèse des substances de groups sanguin IV. Synthèse du 2-acetamido-2-deoxy-4-O-[2-O-(α-L-fucopyranosyl)-β-D-galacto-pyranosyl]-D-glucopyranose, porteur de la spécificité H, *Tetrahedron* **32**:1693–1697.

Jarkovsky, Z., Marcus, D. M., and Grollman, A. P., 1970, Fucosyltransferase found in human milk. Product of the Lewis blood group gene, *Biochemistry* **9**:1123–1128.

Jeannet, M., Bodmer, J. G., Bodmer, W. F., and Schapira, M., 1973, Lymphocytotoxic sera associated with the ABO and Lewis red cell blood groups, in: *Histocompatibility Testing, 1972* (J. Dausset and J. Colombani, eds.), pp. 493–499, Munksgaard, Copenhagen.

Jeannet, M., Schapira, M., and Magnin, C., 1974, Mise en évidence d'anticorps lymphocytotoxiques dirigés contre les antigènes A et B et contre des antigènes d'histocompatibilité non HL-A, *Schweitz Med. Wschr.* **104**:152.

Kabat, E. A., 1956, *Blood Group Substances: Their Chemistry and Immunochemistry*, Academic Press, New York.

Kabat. E. A.. 1970, The carbohydrate moiety of the water-soluble human A. B. H, Le$^a$ and Le$^b$ substances, in: *Blood and Tissue Antigens* (D. Aminoff, ed.), pp. 187–198, Academic Press, New York.

Kabat. E. A.. 1973. Immunochemical studies on the carbohydrate moiety of water soluble blood group. A. B. H. Le$^a$ and Le$^b$ substances and their precursor I antigens. in: *Carbohydrates in Solution* (H. Isbell, ed.), Advances in Chemistry Series No. 117, pp. 334–361, American Chemical Society, Washington, D.C.

Kabat. E. A.. 1977. Some perspectives for future immunochemical research with blood group substances. in: *Human Blood Groups* (J. F. Mohn, R. W. Plunkett, R. K. Cunningham, and R. M. Lambert. eds.), pp. 236–245, Karger, Basel.

Kabat. E. A.. and Leskowitz, S.. 1955. Immunochemical studies on blood groups. XVII. Structural units involved in blood group A specificity, *J. Am. Chem. Soc.* **77**:5159–5164.

Kabat. E. A.. Bassett. E. W.. Pryzwansky. K.. Lloyd. K. O.. Kaplan, M. E.. and Layug. E. J.. 1965. Immunochemical studies on blood groups. XXXIII. The effects of alkaline borohydride and of alkali on blood group A, B and H substances, *Biochemistry* **4**:1632–1638.

Kabat. E. A.. Liao. J.. and Lemieux. R. U.. 1978. Immunochemical studies on blood groups. LXVIII. The combining site of anti-I Ma (Group I). *Immunochemistry* **15**:727–731.

Karlsson. K. A.. 1978. Glycolipid patterns of blood and other tissues. in: *XVth Congress of the International Society of Blood Transfusion, Paris, 1978*, Abstract, p. 641.

Kent. S. P.. 1964. The demonstration and distribution of water-soluble blood group O (H) antigen in tissue sections using a fluorescein labelled extract of *Ulex europeaus* seeds. *J. Histochem.* **12**:591–599.

Kessel. D.. 1979. Personal communication.

Khilanani. P.. Chou. T.. Lomen. P. L.. and Kessel. D.. 1977. Variation of levels of plasma guanosine diphosphate L-fucose: β-D-galactosyl α-2-L-fucosyltransferase in acute adult leukaemia. *Cancer Res.* **37**:2557–2559.

Kijimoto-Ochiai. S.. Naiki. M.. and Makita. A.. 1977. Defects of glycosyltransferase activities in human fibroblasts of P$^k$ and p blood group phenotypes. *Proc. Nat. Acad. Sci. USA* **74**:5407–5410.

Kim. Y. S.. Perdomo. J.. Bella. A.. and Nordberg. J., 1971*a*, N-Acetyl-D-galactosaminyltransferase in human serum and erythrocyte membranes. *Proc. Nat. Acad. Sci. USA* **68**:1753–1756.

Kim. Y. S.. Perdomo. J.. and Nordberg. J.. 1971*b*, Glycoprotein biosynthesis in small intestinal mucosa. I. A study of glycosyltransferases in microsomal subfractions. *J. Biol. Chem.* **246**:5466–5476.

Kim. Y. S.. Isaacs. R.. and Perdomo. J. M.. 1974. Alterations of membrane glycopeptides in human colonic adenocarcinomas. *Proc. Nat. Acad. Sci. USA* **71**:4869–4873.

Kisailus. E. C.. and Kabat. E. A.. 1978. Immunochemical studies on blood groups. LXVI. Competitive binding assays of A$_1$ and A$_2$ blood group substances with insolubilised anti-A serum and insolubilised anti-A agglutinin from *Dolichos biflorus*, *J. Exp. Med.* **147**:830–843.

Kishi. K.. Takizawa. H.. and Iseki. S.. 1977. Isoelectric analysis of B-gene associated α-galactosyltransferases in human serum and saliva. *Proc. Jpn. Acad. Ser. B* **53**:172–177.

Kobata, A., 1972, Isolation of oligosaccharides from human milk, *Methods Enzymol.* **28**:262–271.

Kobata, A., and Ginsburg, V., 1970, Uridine diphosphate *N*-acetyl-D-galactosamine: D-galactose α-3-*N*-acetyl-D-galactosaminyltransferase, a product of the gene that determines blood group A in man, *J. Biol. Chem.* **245**:1484–1490.

Kobata, A., Grollman, E. F., and Ginsburg, V., 1968a, An enzymatic basis for blood type B in humans, *Biochem. Biophys. Res. Commun.* **32**:272–277.

Kobata, A., Grollman, E. F., and Ginsburg, V., 1968b, An enzymatic basis for blood type A in humans, *Arch. Biochem. Biophys.* **124**:609–612.

Kogure, T., 1975, The action of group $B_m$ or cis AB sera on group O red cells in the presence of UDP-D-galactose, *Vox Sang.* **29**:51–58.

Kogure, T., and Furukawa, K., 1976, Enzymatic conversion of human group O red cells into group B active cells by α-D-galactosyltransferases of sera and salivas from group B and its variant types, *J. Immunogenet.* **3**:147–154.

Komai, T., 1950, Semi-allelic genes, *Am. Nat.* **84**:381.

Koscielak, J., 1963, Blood group A specific glycolipids from human erythrocytes, *Biochim. Biophys. Acta* **78**:313–328.

Koscielak, J., 1977, Chemistry and biosynthesis of erythrocytic membrane glycolipids with A, B, H and I blood group activities, in: *Human Blood Groups* (J. F. Mohn, R. W. Plunkett, R. K. Cunningham, and R. M. Lambert, eds.), pp. 143–169, Karger, Basel.

Koscielak, J., 1978, Personal communication.

Koscielak, J., Piasek, A., Gorniak, H., Gardas, A., and Gregor, A., 1973, Structure of fucose containing glycolipids with H and B blood group activity and of sialic acid and glucosamine containing glycolipid of human erythrocyte membrane, *Eur. J. Biochem.* **37**:214–225.

Koscielak, J., Miller-Podraza, H., Krause, R., and Piasek, A., 1976a, Isolation and characterisation of poly(glycosyl)ceramides (megaloglycolipids) with A, H and I blood group activities, *Eur. J. Biochem.* **71**:9–18.

Koscielak, J., Pacuszka, T., and Dzierzkowa-Borodej, W., 1976b, Activity of B gene specified galactosyltransferase in individuals with $B_m$ phenotypes, *Vox Sang.* **30**:58–67.

Koscielak, J., Miller-Podraza, H., Krauze, R., and Cedergren, B., 1976c, Glycolipid composition of blood group p erythrocytes, *FEBS Lett.* **66**:250–253.

Koscielak, J., Miller-Podraza, H., and Zdebska, E., 1978a, Isolation of poly(glycosyl)ceramides with A, B, H and I blood group activities, *Methods Enzymol.* **50**:211–216.

Koscielak, J., Maslinski, W., Zielenski, J., Zdebska, E., Brudzynski, T., Miller-Podraza, H., and Cedergren, B., 1978b, Structures and fatty acid compositions of neutral glycosphingolipids, *Biochim. Biophys. Acta* **530**:385–393.

Kossovitch, D., 1929, Les groupes sanguins des français et les règles de l'hérédité, *Révue Anthropol.* **39**:374–379.

Kristiansen, T. and Porath, J., 1968, Studies on blood group substances. I. Purification of active material from hog gastric mucin by specific precipitation with *Vicia cracca* phytohemagglutinin, *Biochim. Biophys. Acta* **158**:351–357.

Krusius, T., Finne, J., and Rauvala, H., 1978, The poly(glycosyl) chains of glycoproteins: Characterisation of a novel type of glycoprotein saccharide from human erythrocyte membrane, *Eur. J. Biochem.* **92**:289–300.

Kuhn, R. and Gauhe, A., 1962, Die konstitution der lacto-*N*-neotetraose, *Chem. Ber.* **95**:518–522.

Kuhn, R., Baer, H. H., and Gauhe, A., 1955, Fucosidolactose, das Trisaccharid der Frauenmilch, *Chem. Ber.* **88**:1135–1146.

Kuhn, R., Baer, H. H., and Gauhe, A., 1958, 2-α-L-Fucopyranosyl-D-galactose und 2-α-L-Fucopyranosyl-D-talose, *Ann. Chem.* **611**:242–249.

Kuhns, W. J., Oliver, R. T. D., and Watkins, W. M., 1976, Alterations of serum and tissue glycosyltransferase enzymes in acute leukaemia, *Am. Soc. Haematol.*, **117**(Abstr.):91.

Kuhns, W. J., Oliver, R. T. D., Greenwell, P., and Watkins, W. M., 1979, Serum glycosyltransferase levels in normal and leukaemic subjects: Experiences with low molecular weight acceptors, in: *Glycoconjugate Research*, Vol. II (J. D. Gregory and R. W. Jeanloz, eds.), pp. 719–721, Academic Press, New York.

Landsteiner, K., 1900, Zur Kenntnis der antifermentativen, lytischen und agglutinierenden Wirkungen des Blutserums und der Lymphe, *Zbl. Bakt.* **27**:357–362.

Landsteiner, K., 1901, Uber agglutinationserscheinungen normalen menschlichen Blutes, *Wien, Klin. Wochenschr.*, **14**:1132–1134.

Landsteiner, K., and Levine, P., 1927, Further observations on individual differences of human blood, *Proc. Soc. Exp. Biol. N.Y.* **24**:941–942.

Lehrs, H., 1930, Über gruppenspezifische Eigenschaften des menschlichen Speichels, *Z. Immunol. Forsch.* **66**:175–192.

Leloir, L. F., 1964, Nucleoside diphosphate sugars and saccharide synthesis, *Biochem. J.* **91**:1–8.

Lemieux, R. U., 1978, Human blood groups and carbohydrate chemistry, *Chem. Soc. Rev.* **7**:423–452.

Lemieux, R. U., and Driguez, H., 1975a, The chemical synthesis of 2-*O*-(α-L-fucopyranosyl)-3-*O*(α-D-galactopyranosyl)D-galactose. The terminal structure of the blood-group B antigenic determinant, *J. Am. Chem. Soc.* **97**:4069–4075.

Lemieux, R. U., and Driguez, H. J., 1975b, The chemical synthesis of 2-acetamido-2-deoxy-4-*O*-(α-L-fucopyranosyl)-3-*O*-(β-D-galactopyranosyl)-D-glucose. The Lewis a blood group antigenic determinant, *J. Am. Chem. Soc.* **97**:4063–4068.

Lemieux, R. U., Hendriks, K. B., Stick, R. V., and James, K., 1975a, Halide ion catalysed glycosidation reactions. Synthesis of α-linked disaccharides, *J. Am. Chem. Soc.* **97**:4056–4062.

Lemieux, R. U., Bundle, D. R., and Baker, D. A., 1975b, The properties of a "synthetic" antigen related to the human blood group Lewis a, *J. Am. Chem. Soc.* **97**:4076–4083.

Levine, P., 1978, Self–nonself concept for cancer and diseases previously known as "autoimmune" diseases, *Proc. Natl. Acad. Sci. USA.* **75**:5697–5701.

Levine, P., Robinson, E., Celano, M., Briggs, O., and Falkenburg, L., 1955, Gene interaction resulting in suppression of blood group substance B, *Blood* **10**:1100–1108.

Levine, P., Celano, M. J., and Falkowski, F., 1965, The specificity of the antibody in paroxysmal cold haemoglobinuria (P.C.H.), *Ann. N. Y. Acad. Sci.* **124**:456–461.

Lindberg, B., Lönngren, J., and Powell, D. A., 1977, Structural studies on the specific Type 14 pneumococcal polysaccharide, *Carbohydrate Res.* **58**:177–186.

Liotta, I., Quintiliani, M., Quintiliani, L., Buzzonetti, A., and Guiliani, E., 1972, Extraction and partial purification of blood group substances, A, B and H from erythrocyte stroma, *Vox Sang.* **22**:171–182.

Lloyd, K. O., Kabat, E. A., Layug, E. J., and Gruezo, F., 1966, Immunochemical studies on blood groups. XXXIV. Structures of some oligosaccharides produced by alkaline degradation of blood group A, B and H substances, *Biochemistry* **5**:1489–1501.

Lloyd, K. O., Kabat, E. A., and Licerio, E., 1968, Immunochemical studies on blood groups. XXXVIII. Structures and activities of oligosaccharides produced by alkaline degradation of blood group Lewis[a] substance. Proposed structure of the carbohydrate chains of human blood group A, B, H, Le[a] and Le[b] substances, *Biochemistry* **7**:2976–2990.

Lopez, M., Liberge, G., Gerbal, A., Brocteur, J., and Salmon, C., 1976, *Cis* AB blood groups. Immunologic, thermodynamic and quantitative studies of ABH antigens, *Biomedicine* **24**:265–271.

Lorusso, D. J., Binette, J. P., and Green, F. A., 1977, Solubilised human erythrocyte membranes and the Rh antigen system, in: *Human Blood Groups* (J. F. Mohn, R. W. Plunkett, R. K. Cunningham, and R. M. Lambert, eds.), pp. 226–235, Karger, Basel.

Lundblad, A., 1970, Blood group specific oligosaccharides in urine, in: *Blood and Tissue Antigens* (D. Aminoff, ed.), pp. 427–436, Academic Press, New York.

Lundblad, A., 1978, Oligosaccharides from human urine, *Methods Enzymol.* **50**:226–235.

Maisonrouge-McAuliffe, F., and Kabat, E. A., 1976, Immunochemical studies on blood groups. Structures and immunological properties of oligosaccharides from two fractions of blood group substance from human ovarian cyst fluid differing in B, I and i activities and reactivity toward Concanavalin A, *Arch. Biochem. Biophys.* **175**:90–113.

Mäkelä, O., and Cantell, K., 1958, Destruction of $M$ and $N$ group receptors of human red cells by some influenza viruses, *Ann. Med. Exp. Biol. Fenn.* **36**:366–374.

Mäkelä, O., and Mäkelä, P., 1956, Le$^b$ antigen. Studies on its occurrence in red cells and plasma and saliva, *Ann. Med. Exp. Biol. Fenn.* **36**:157–162.

Mäkelä, O., Ruoslahti, E., and Ehnholm, C., 1969, Subtypes of human ABO blood groups and subtype-specific antibodies, *J. Immunol.* **102**:763–771.

Marchesi, V. T., Tillach, T. W., Jackson, R. L., Segrest, J. P., and Scott, R. E., 1972, Chemical characterisation and surface orientation of the major glycoprotein of the human erythrocyte membrane, *Proc. Natl. Acad. Sci. USA.* **69**:1445–1449.

Marchesi, V. T., Furthmayr, H., Tomita, M., Silverberg, M., and Cotmore, S., 1977, Molecular features of glycophorin A, the major sialoglycopeptide of the human red cell membrane, in: *Human Blood Groups* (J. F. Mohn, R. W. Plunkett, R. K. Cunningham, and R. M. Lambert, eds.), pp. 374–382, Karger, Basel.

Marcus, D. M., 1971, Isolation of a substance with blood group $P_1$ activity from human erythrocyte stroma, *Transfusion* **11**:16–18.

Marcus, D. M., and Cass, L. E., 1969, Glycosphingolipids with Lewis blood group activity: Uptake by human erythrocytes, *Science* **164**:553–555.

Marcus, D. M., Naiki, M., and Kundu, S. K., 1976, Abnormalities in the glycosphingolipid content of human $P^k$ and p erythrocytes, *Proc. Natl. Acad. Sci. USA.* **73**:3263–3267.

Marr, A. M. S., Donald, A. S. R., Watkins, W. M., and Morgan, W. T. J., 1967, Molecular and genetic aspects of human blood group Le$^b$ specificity, *Nature* **215**:1345–1349.

Marr, A. M. S., Donald, A. S. R., and Morgan, W. T. J., 1968, Two new oligosaccharides obtained from an Le$^a$-active glycoprotein, *Biochem. J.* **110**:789–791.

Marsh, W. L., and Jenkins, W. J., 1960, Anti-i: A new cold antibody, *Nature (London)* **188**:200–209.

Masamune, H., Kawasaki, H., Abe, S., Oyama, K., and Yamaguchi, Y., 1958, Molisch positive mucopolysaccharides of gastric cancers as compared with the corresponding components of gastric mucosa. First report, *Tohoku J. Med.* **68**:81–91.

Matson, G. A., Swanson, J., Noades, J., Sanger, R., and Race, R. R., 1959, A new antigen and antibody belonging to the P blood group system, *Am. J. Hum. Genet.* **11**:26–34.

McClaren, A., 1976, *Mammalian Chimaeras*, Cambridge University Press.

McGuire, E. J., 1970, Biosynthesis of submaxillary mucins, in: *Blood and Tissue Antigens* (D. Aminoff, ed.), pp. 461–478, Academic Press, New York.

McKibbin, J. M., 1978, Fucolipids, *J. Lipid. Res.* **19**:131–147.

Mohn, J. F., Cunningham, R. K., and Bates, J. E., 1977, Qualitative distinctions between subgroups $A_1$ and $A_2$, in: *Human Blood Groups* (J. F. Mohn, R. W. Plunkett, R. K. Cunningham, and R. M. Lambert, eds.), pp. 316–325, Karger, Basel.

Monnet, A., Cartron, J. P., Cabidi, Y., Marty, Y., and Ruffie, J., 1978, Deux familles non apparentées demonstrant l'existence d'un renforcement allélique dans le système ABO, in: *XVth Congress of the International Society of Blood Transfusion, Paris, 1978*, Abstract, p. 688.

Moreno, C., Lundblad, A., and Kabat, E. A., 1971, Immunochemical studies on blood groups LI. A comparative study of the reaction of $A_1$ and $A_2$ blood group glycoproteins with human anti-A, *J. Exp. Med.* **134**:349–457.

Morgan, W. T. J., 1960, A contribution to human biochemical genetics; the chemical basis of blood group specificity, *Proc. Royal Soc. B* **151**:308–347.

Morgan, W. T. J., 1970, Carbohydrate structures responsible for antigenic specificity, in: *British Biochemistry Past and Present* (T. W. Goodwin, ed.), pp. 99–115, Academic Press, London.

Morgan, W. T. J., 1977, Observations on the immunochemical genetics of the human blood group P system, in: *Human Blood Groups* (J. F. Mohn, R. W. Plunkett, R. K. Cunningham, and R. M. Lambert, eds.), pp. 216–225, Karger, Basel.

Morgan, W. T. J., and Heyningen, R. van, 1944, The occurrence of A, B, and O blood group substances in pseudomucinous ovarian cyst fluids, *Br. J. Exp. Path.* **25**:5–15.

Morgan, W. T. J., and Watkins, W. M., 1948, The detection of a product of the blood group *O* gene and the relationship of the so-called O substance to the agglutinogens A and AB, *Br. J. Exp. Path.* **29**:159–173.

Morgan, W. T. J., and Watkins, W. M., 1953, The inhibition of the haemagglutinins in plant seeds by human blood group substances and simple sugars, *Br. J. Exp. Pathol.* **34**:94–103.

Morgan, W. T. J., and Watkins, W. M., 1956, The product of the human blood group *A* and *B* genes in individuals belonging to group AB, *Nature (London)* **177**:521–522.

Morgan, W. T. J., and Watkins, W. M., 1964, Blood group $P_1$ substance. 1. Chemical properties, in: *Proceedings of the 9th Congress of the International Society of Blood Transfusion, Mexico, 1962*, pp. 225–229, Karger, Basel.

Morgan, W. T. J., and Watkins, W. M., 1969, Genetic and biochemical aspects of human blood group A-, B-, H-, $Le^a$ and $Le^b$ specificity, *Br. Med. Bull.* **25**:30–34.

Mulet, C., Cartron, J. P., Badet, J., and Salmon, C., 1977, Activity of 2-$\alpha$-L-fucosyltransferase in human sera and red cell membranes, *FEBS Lett.* **84**:74–78.

Mulet, C., Schenkel-Brunner, H., Cartron, J. P., and Salmon, C., 1978a, *In vitro* conversion of $B_h$ cells into $B^-H^+$ cells and further conversion of the latter into $A^+H^-$ cells by enzymatic treatment in: *XVth Congress of the International Society of Blood Transfusion, Paris, 1978*, Abstract, p. 689.

Mulet, C., Cartron, J. P., Lopez, M., and Salmon, Ch., 1978b, ABH glycosyltransferase levels in sera and red cell membranes from $H_z$ and $H_m$ variant bloods, *FEBS Lett.* **90**:233–238.

Munro, J. R. and Schachter, H., 1973, The presence of two GDP-L-fucose:glycoprotein fucosyltransferases in human serum. *Arch. Biochem. Biophys.* **156**:534–542.

Nagai, M. and Yoshida, A., 1978, Possible existence of hybrid glycosyltransferases in heterozygous blood group AB subjects, *Vox Sang.* **35**:378–381.

Nagai, N., Dave, V., Kaplan, B. E., and Yoshida, A., 1978a, Human blood group glycosyltransferases. I. Purification of N-acetylgalactosaminyltransferases, *J. Biol. Chem.* **253**:377–379.

Nagai, N., Dave, V., Muensch, H., and Yoshida, A., 1978b, Human blood group glycosyltransferases. II. Purification of galactosyltransferase. *J. Biol. Chem.* **253**:380–381.

Naiki, M., and Marcus, D. M., 1974, Human erythrocyte P and $P^k$ blood group antigens, *Biochem. Biophys. Res. Commun.* **60**:1105–1111.

Naiki, M., and Marcus, D. M., 1975, An immunochemical study of the human blood group $P_1$, P and $P^k$ glycosphingolipid antigens, *Immunology* 14:4837–4841.

Naiki, M., Fong, J., Ledeen, R., and Marcus, D. M., 1975, Structure of the human erythrocyte blood group $P_1$ glycosphingolipid, *Biochemistry* 14:4831–4837.

Niemann, H., Watanabe, K., Hakomori, S., Childs, R. A., and Feizi,.T.,.1978, Blood group i and I activities of "lacto-*N*-*nor*hexaosylceramide" and its analogues: The structural requirements for i specificities, *Biochem. Biophys. Res. Commun.* 81:1286–1293.

Oriol, R., Cartron, J. P., Yvart, J., and Cartron, J., 1978a, Biosynthesis of ABH and Lewis antigens in the kidney of normal and transplanted patients, in: *XVth Congress of the International Society of Blood Transfusion, Paris, 1978*, Abstract, p. 645.

Oriol, R., Cartron, J., Yvart, J., Bedrossian, J., Duboust, A., Bariety, J., Gluckman, J. C., and Gagnadoux, M. F., 1978b, The Lewis system: New histocompatability antigens in renal transplantation, *Lancet* i:574–575.

Pacuszka, T. and Koscielak, J., 1972, The biosynthesis of blood-group B character on human O-erythrocytes by a soluble α-galactosyltransferase from milk, *Eur. J. Biochem.* 31:374–377.

Pacuszka, T., and Koscielak, J., 1974, α-1,2-Fucosyltransferase of human bone marrow, *FEBS Lett.* 41:348–351.

Pacuszka, T. and Koscielak, J., 1976, Enzymatic synthesis of two fucose-containing glycolipids with fucosyltransferases of human serum, *Eur. J. Biochem.* 64:499–506.

Pacuszka, T., Koscielak, J., Seyfried, H., and Walewska, I., 1975, Biochemical, serological and family studies in individuals with cis AB phenotype, *Vox Sang.* 29:292–300.

Painter, T. J., Watkins, W. M., and Morgan, W. T. J., 1963, Isolation of two serologically active trisaccharides from human blood group B substance, *Nature (London)* 199:282–283.

Painter, T. J., Watkins, W. M., and Morgan, W. T. J., 1965, Serologically active fucose containing oligosaccharides isolated from human blood group A and B substances, *Nature (London)* 206:594–597.

Pann, C. and Kuhns, W. J., 1972, Differentiation of HeLa cells with respect to blood group H antigen, *Nature (London)* 240:22–24.

Picard, J., Waldron Edward, D., and Feizi, T, 1978, Changes in the expression of the blood group A, B, H, $Le^a$ and $Le^b$ antigens and the blood group precursor associated I (Ma) antigen in glycoprotein rich extracts of gastric carcinomas, *J. Clin. Lab. Immunol.* 1:119–128.

Poretz, R. D. and Watkins, W. M., 1972, Galactosyltransferases in human sub-maxillary glands and stomach mucosa associated with the biosynthesis of blood group B specific glycoproteins, *Eur. J. Biochem.* 25:455–462.

Potapov, M. I., 1970, Detection of the antigen of the Lewis system, characteristic of the erythrocytes of group Le(a-b-) secretor, *Prob. Haematol.* 11:45–49.

Poulik, M. D., and Lauf, P. K., 1965, Heterogeneity of water-soluble structural components of human red cell membrane, *Nature* 208:874–876.

Prieels, J. P., Beyers, T., and Hill, R. L., 1977, Human milk fucosyltransferases, *Biochem. Soc. Transf.* 5:838–839.

Prohaska, R., Schenkel-Brunner, H., and Tuppy, H., 1978, Enzymatic synthesis of blood group Lewis specific glycolipids, *Eur. J. Biochem.* 84:161–166.

Pusztai, A. and Morgan, W. T. J., 1963, Studies in immunochemistry 22. The amino acid composition of the human blood-group A, B, H and $Le^a$ specific substances, *Biochem. J.* 88:546–555.

Putkonen, T., 1930, Über die gruppenspezifischen Eigenschaften verschiedener Körperflüssigkeiten, *Acta. Soc. Med. Fenn. "Duodecim." A* 14:12.

Race, C., and Watkins, W. M., 1969, Properties of an α-D-galactosyltransferase in human tissues obtained from blood group B donors, *Biochem. J.* **114**:86P.

Race, C., and Watkins, W. M., 1970, The biosynthesis of a blood group B active tetrasaccharide, *FEBS Lett.* **10**:279–283.

Race, C., and Watkins, W. M., 1972a, The action of the blood group *B* gene specified α-galactosyltransferase from human serum and stomach mucosal extracts on group O and 'Bombay' $O_h$ erythrocytes, *Vox Sang.* **23**:385–401.

Race, C., and Watkins, W. M., 1972b, The enzymic products of the human *A* and *B* blood group genes in the serum of 'Bombay' $O_h$ donors, *FEBS Lett.* **27**:125–130.

Race, C., and Watkins, W. M., 1974, Inhibition of the blood group $A^1$ and $A^2$ gene-specified *N*-acetyl-α-D-galactosaminyltransferases by uridine diphosphate D-galactose, *Carbohydrate Res.* **37**:239–244.

Race, C., Ziderman, D., and Watkins, W. M., 1968, An α-D-galactosyltransferase associated with the blood group B character, *Biochem. J.* **107**:733–735.

Race, R. R., and Sanger, R., 1975, *Blood Groups in Man*, 6th Ed. Blackwell Scientific Publications, Oxford.

Rege, V. P., Painter, T. J., Watkins, W. M., and Morgan, W. T. J., 1963, Three new trisaccharides obtained from human blood group A, B, H and Le$^a$ substances: Possible sugar sequences in the carbohydrate chains, *Nature (London)* **200**:532–534.

Rege, V. P., Painter, T. J., Watkins, W. M., and Morgan, W. T. J., 1964a, Isolation of serologically active fucose-containing oligosaccharides from human blood-group H substance, *Nature (London)* **203**:360–363.

Rege, V. P., Painter, T. J., Watkins, W. M., and Morgan W. T. J., 1964b, Isolation of a serologically active fucose-containing trisaccharide from human blood group Le$^a$ substance, *Nature (London)* **204**:740–742.

Renton, P. H., and Hancock, J. A., 1962, Uptake of A and B antigens by transfused group O erythrocytes, *Vox Sang.* **7**:33–38.

Renwick, J. H., and Lawler, S. D., 1955, Genetical linkage between the ABO and nail-patella loci, *Ann. Hum. Genet. (London)* **19**:312–320.

Reviron, J., Jacquet, A., and Salmon, Ch., 1968, Un exemple de chromosome "*cis* $A_1B$." Etude immunologique et génétique de phénotype induit, *Nouvelle Revue Française d'Hematologie* **8**:323–328.

Rochant, H., Tonthat, H., Henri, A., Tieux, M., and Dreyfus, B., 1976, Abnormal distribution of erythrocytes $A_1$ antigens in preleukemia as demonstrated by an immunofluorescence technique, *Blood Cells* **2**:237–255.

Roelcke, D., 1974, A review—cold agglutination antibodies and antigens, *Clin. Immunol. Immunopathol.* **2**:266–280.

Romanowska, E., 1959, Studies on blood group antigens M and N. IV. Action of influenza virus enzyme on the blood group substances M and N, *Arch. Immunol. Ter. Dosw.* **7**:749–757.

Roseman, S., 1970, The synthesis of complex carbohydrates by multiglycosyltransferase systems and their potential function in intercellular adhesion, *Chem. Phys. Lipids.* **5**:270–297.

Rovis, L., Anderson, B., Kabat, E. A., Gruezo, F., and Liao. J., 1973a, Structures of oligosaccharides produced by base-borohydride degradation of human ovarian cyst blood group H, Le$^b$ and Le$^a$ active glycoproteins, *Biochemistry* **12**:5340–5354.

Rovis, L., Anderson, B., Kabat, E. A., Gruezo, F., and Liao, J., 1973b, Activity of reduced oligosaccharides isolated from blood group H, Le$^b$ and Le$^a$ substances by alkaline borohydride degradation, *Biochemistry* **12**:5355–5360.

Sabo, B. H., Bush, M., German, J., Carne, L. R., Yates, A. D., and Watkins, W. M., 1978,

The *cis* AB phenotype in three generations of one family: Serological, enzymatic and cytogenetic studies, *J. Immunogenet.* **5**:87–106.

Salmon, C., 1977, The present status of the ABO blood groups, in: *Human Blood Groups* (J. F. Mohn, R. W. Plunkett, R. K. Cunningham, and R. M. Lambert, eds.), pp. 326–334, Karger, Basel.

Salmon, C., 1978, Blood group antigens and malignancy, in: *XVth Congress of the International Society of Blood Transfusion, Paris, 1978,* Plenary Sessions—Main Lectures, pp. 37–50, Librairie Arnette, Paris.

Salmon C. and Cartron, J. P., 1976, Le renforcement allélique, *Rev. Franç. Transf. Immunohématol.* **19**:145–155.

Salmon, C., Lopez, M., Gerbal, A., Bouguerra, A., and Cartron, J. P., 1973, Current genetic problems in the ABO blood group system, *Biomedicine* **18**:375–386.

Sanders, E. M., and Kent, S. P., 1970, The distribution of water-soluble blood group A antigen in the human large intestine: A mosaic pattern, *Lab. Invest.* **23**:74–78.

Sanger, R., 1955, An association between the P and Jay system of blood groups, *Nature (London)* **176**:1163–1164.

Sawicka, T., 1971, Glycosyltransferases of human plasma, *FEBS Lett.* **16**:346–348.

Schachter, H., 1974a, Glycosylation of glycoproteins during intracellular transport of secretory products, *Adv. Cytopharmacol.* **2**:207–218.

Schachter, H., 1974b, The subcellular sites of glycosylation, *Biochem. Soc. Symp.* **40**:57–71.

Schachter, H., and Tilley, C., 1978, The biosynthesis of human blood group substances, in: *International Review of Biochemistry: Biochemistry of Carbohydrates II,* Vol. 16 (D. J. Manners, ed.), pp. 209–246, University Park Press, Baltimore.

Schachter, H., Michaels, M. A., Crookston, M. C., Tilley, C. A., and Crookston, J., 1971, A quantitative difference in the activity of blood group A specific α-N-acetylgalactosaminyltransferase in serum from $A_1$ and $A_2$ human subjects, *Biochem. Biophys. Res. Commun.* **45**:1011–1018.

Schachter, H., Michaels, M. A., Tilley, C. A., Crookston, M. C., and Crookston, J., 1973, Qualitative differences in the N-acetyl-D-galactosaminyltransferases produced by human $A^1$ and $A^2$ genes, *Proc. Natl. Acad. Sci. USA* **70**:220–224.

Schenkel-Brunner, H., and Tuppy, H., 1970, Enzymes from human gastric mucosa conferring blood group A and B specificities upon erythrocytes, *Eur. J. Biochem.* **17**:218–222.

Schenkel-Brunner, H., and Tuppy, H., 1973, Enzymatic conversion of human blood group O erythrocytes into $A_2$ and $A_1$ cells by α-N-acetyl-D-galactosaminyltransferases of blood-group A individuals, *Eur. J. Biochem.* **34**:125–128.

Schenkel-Brunner, H., Chester, M. A., and Watkins, W. M., 1972, α-L-Fucosyltransferases in human serum from donors of different ABO, secretor and Lewis blood group phenotypes, *Eur. J. Biochem.* **30**:269–277.

Schenkel-Brunner, H., Prohaska, R., and Tuppy, H., 1975, Action of glycosyltransferases upon 'Bombay' $O_h$ erythrocytes. Conversion to cells showing blood group H and A specificities, *Eur. J. Biochem.* **56**:591–594.

Schiff, F., and Sasaki, H., 1932, Der Ausscheidungstypus, ein auf serologischem Wege nachweisbares mendelndes Merkmal, *Klin. Woch.* **11**:1426–1429.

Schwarting, G. A., Marcus, D. M., and Metaxas, M., 1977, Identification of sialoparagloboside as the erythrocyte receptor for an 'Anti-p' antibody, *Vox Sang.* **32**:257–261.

Schwarting, G. A., Kundu, S. K., and Marcus, D. M., 1979, Reaction of antibodies that cause paroxysmal cold hemoglobinuria (PCH) with globoside and Forssman glycosphinolipids, *Blood* **53**:186–192.

Schwyzer, M., and Hill, R. L., 1977a, Porcine A blood group-specific N-acetylgalactosaminyltransferase. I. Purification from porcine submaxillary glands, *J. Biol. Chem.* 252:2338–2345.

Schwyzer, M., and Hill, R. L., 1977b, Porcine A blood group specific N-acetylgalactosaminyltransferase. II. Enzymatic properties, *J. Biol. Chem.* 252:2346–2355.

Seaman, M. J., Chalmers, D. G., and Franks, D., 1968, Seidler: An antibody which reacts with A₁Le(a⁻b⁺) red cells, *Vox Sang.* 15:25–30.

Seyfried, H., Walewska, I., and V. erblinska, B., 1964, Unusual inheritance of ABO group in a family with weak B antigens, *Vox Sang.* 9:268–277.

Shen, L., Grollman, E. F., and Ginsburg, V., 1968, An enzymatic basis for secretor status and blood group substance specificity in humans, *Proc. Natl. Acad. Sci. USA.* 59:224–230.

Siddiqui, B., and Hakomori, S., 1971, A revised structure for the Forssman glycolipid hapten, *J. Biol. Chem.* 246:5766–5769.

Siddiqui, B., and Hakomori, S., 1973, A ceramide tetrasaccharide of human erythrocyte membrane reacting with anti-Type XIV pneumococcal polysaccharide antiserum, ·*Biochim. Biophys. Acta* 330:147–155.

Siddiqui, B., Whitehead, J. S., and Kim, Y. S., 1978, Glycosphingolipids in human colonic adenocarcinoma, *J. Biol. Chem.* 253:2168–2175.

Simmons, A., and Twaitt, J., 1975, Another example of a B variant, *Transfusion* 15:359–362.

Smith, E. L., McKibbin, J. M., Karlsson, K. A., Pascher, I., and Samuelsson, B. E., 1975, Characterisation of a human intestinal fucolipid with blood group Leᵃ activity, *J. Biol. Chem.* 250:659–6064.

Sneath, J. S., and Sneath, P. H. A., 1955, Transformation of the Lewis groups of human red cells, *Nature (London)* 176:172.

Solomon, J. M., Waggoner, R., and Leyshon, W. C., 1965, A quantitative immunogenetic study of gene suppression involving A₁ and H antigens of the erythrocyte without affecting secreted blood group substances. The ABH phenotypes Aʰₘ and Oʰₘ, *Blood* 25:470–485.

Springer, G. F., 1958, Blood group active substances of plant origin, in: *Ciba Foundation Symposium on Chemistry and Biology of Mucopolysaccharides* (G. E. W. Wolstenholme and M. O'Connor, eds.), pp. 216–229, Churchill, London.

Springer, G. F., and Ansell, N. J., 1958, Inactivation of human erythrocyte agglutinogens M and N by influenza viruses and receptor-destroying enzyme, *Proc. Natl. Acad. Sci. USA* 44:182–189.

Springer, G. F., Desai, P. R., Yang, H. J., Schachter, H., and Narasimhan, S., 1977, in: *Human Blood Groups* (J. F. Mohn, R. W. Plunkett, R. K. Cunningham, and R. M. Lambert, eds.), pp. 179–187, Karger, Basel.

Sringarm, S., Greenwell, P., and Watkins, W. M., 1979 (in preparation).

Stealey, J. R., 1973, The isolation of an Leᵃ-destroying enzyme from *Trichomonas foetus*, Ph.D. Thesis, University of London.

Stellner, K., Hakomori, S. I., and Wagner, G. A., 1973, Enzymatic conversion of H₁ glycolipid and deficiency of these enzyme activities in adenocarcinoma, *Biochem. Biophys. Res. Commun.* 55:439–445.

Szulman, A. E., 1960, The histological distribution of blood group substances A and B in man, *J. Exp. Med.* 111:785–800.

Szulman, A. E., 1962, The histological distribution of the blood group substances as disclosed by immunofluorescence. II. The H antigen and its relation to A and B substances, *J. Exp. Med.* 115:977–996.

Szulman, A. E., 1966, Chemistry, distribution and function of blood group substances, *Ann. Rev. Med.* 17:307–322.

Szulman, A. E., and Marcus, D. M., 1973, The histologic distribution of the blood group substances in man as disclosed by immunofluorescence, *Lab. Invest.* **28**:565–574.

Takasaki, S., and Kobata, A., 1976, Chemical characterisation and distribution of ABO blood group active glycoprotein in human erythrocyte membrane, *J. Biol. Chem.* **251**:3610–3615.

Takasaki, S., Yamashita, K., and Kobata, A., 1978, The sugar chain structures of ABO blood group active glycoproteins obtained from human erythrocyte membrane, *J. Biol. Chem.* **253**:6086–6091.

Tanner, M. J. A., and Boxer, D. H., 1972, Separation and some properties of the major proteins of the human erythrocyte membrane, *Biochem. J.* **129**:333–347.

Thomsen, O., Friedenreich, V., and Worsaae, E., 1930, Über die Möglichkeit der Existenz zweier neuer Blutgruppen: auch ein Beitrag zur Beleuchtung sogennanter Untergruppen, *Acta Path. Microbiol. Scand.* **7**:157–190.

Tilley, C. A., Crookston, M. C., Brown, B. L., and Wherrett, J. R., 1975, A and B and $A_1Le^b$ substances in glycosphingolipid fractions of human serum, *Vox Sang.* **28**:25–33.

Tilley, C. A., Crookston, M. C., Crookston, J. H., Shindman, J., and Schachter, H., 1978, Human blood group A- and H-specified glycosyltransferase levels in the sera of newborn infants and their mothers, *Vox Sang.* **34**:8–13.

Topping, M. D., 1976, Glycosyltransferases involved in the synthesis of blood group substances, Ph.D. Thesis, University of London.

Topping, M. D., and Watkins, W. M., 1975, Isoelectric points of the human blood group $A^1$, $A^2$ and B gene-associated glycosyltransferases in ovarian cyst fluids and serum, *Biochem. Biophys. Res. Commun.* **64**:89–96.

Tsai, C., Zopf, D. A., Wistar, R., and Ginsburg, V., 1976, A human cold agglutinin which binds lacto-*N*-neotetraose, *J. Immunol.* **117**:717–721.

Tuppy, H., and Schenkel-Brunner, H., 1969a, Occurrence and assay of alpha-*N*-acetylgalactosaminyl transferase in the gastric mucosa of humans belonging to blood group A, *Vox Sang.* **17**:138–142.

Tuppy, H., and Schenkel-Brunner, H., 1969b, Formation of blood group A substance from H-substance by an α-*N*-acetylgalactosaminyltransferase, *Eur. J. Biochem.* **10**:152–157.

Uhlenbruck, G., Reese, I., Vaith, P., and Haugt, H., 1979, Immuno-chemical studies on the alkali-labile carbohydrate chains of human serum glycoproteins, *J. Clin. Chem. Clin. Biochem.* **17**:29–34.

Vicari, G., and Kabat, E. A., 1969, Immunochemical studies on blood groups. XLII. Isolation and characterisation from ovarian cyst fluid of a blood group substance lacking A, B, H $Le^a$ and $Le^b$ specificity, *J. Immunol.* **102**:821–825.

Vicari, G., and Kabat. E. A., 1970. Immunochemical studies on blood groups. XLV. Structures and activities of oligosaccharides produced by alkaline degradation of a blood group substance lacking A, B, H $Le^a$ and $Le^b$ specificities, *Biochemistry* **9**:3414–3421.

Voak, D., and Lodge, T. W., 1968, The role of H in the development of A, *Vox Sang.* **15**:345–352.

Voak, D., Anstee, D., and Pardoe, G., 1973, The α-galactose specificity of anti-P $^k$, *Vox Sang.* **25**:263–270.

Wasniowska, K., Drzeniek, Z., and Lisowska, E., 1977, The amino acids of M and N blood group glycopeptides are different, *Biochem. Biophys. Res. Commun.* **76**:385–389.

Watanabe, K., and Hakomori, S., 1976, Status of blood group carbohydrate chains in ontogenesis and in oncogenesis, *J. Exp. Med.* **144**:644–653.

Watanabe, K., Laine, R. A., and Hakomori, S., 1975, On neutral fucoglycolipids having long branched carbohydrate chains: H-active and I-active glycosphingolipids of human erythrocyte membranes, *Biochemistry* **14**:2725–2733.

Watkins, W. M., 1959, Some genetical aspects of human blood group substances, in: *Ciba Foundation Symposium on Biochemistry of Human Genetics* (G. E. W. Wolstenholme and C. M. O'Connor, eds.), pp. 217–238, Churchill, London.

Watkins, W. M., 1962, Changes in the specificity of blood group mucopolysaccharides induced by enzymes from *Trichomonas foetus*, *Immunology* 5:245–266.

Watkins, W. M., 1966, Blood group substances, *Science* 152:172–181.

Watkins, W. M., 1967, The possible enzymic basis of the biosynthesis of blood group substances, in: *Proceedings of the 3rd International Congress of Human Genetics, 1966* (J. F. Crow and J. V. Neel, eds.), pp. 171–187, Johns Hopkins Press, Baltimore.

Watkins, W. M., 1968, Biochemical and genetical aspects of blood group specificity. XXI. John G. Gibson II Lecture, Columbia University, New York.

Watkins, W. M., 1972, Blood-group specific substances, in: *Glycoproteins: Their Composition, Structure and Function* (A. Gottschalk ed.), pp. 830–891, Elsevier, Amsterdam.

Watkins, W. M., 1974, Genetic regulation of the structure of blood group specific glycoproteins, *Biochem. Soc. Symp.* 40:125–146.

Watkins, W. M., 1977, The glycosyltransferase products of the *A, B, H* and *Le* genes and their relationship to the structure of the blood group antigens, in: *Human Blood Groups* (J. F. Mohn, R. W. Plunkett, R. K. Cunningham, and R. M. Lambert, eds.), pp. 134–142, Karger, Basel.

Watkins, W. M., 1978, Blood group gene specified glycosyltransferases in rare ABO groups and in leukaemia, *Rev. Franç. Trans. Immuno-hématol.* 21:201–228.

Watkins, W. M., and Morgan, W. T. J., 1955a, Some observations on the O and H characters of human blood and secretions, *Vox Sang.* 5:1–14.

Watkins, W. M., and Morgan, W. T. J., 1955b, Inhibition by simple sugars of enzymes which decompose the blood group substances, *Nature (London)* 175:676–677.

Watkins, W. M., and Morgan, W. T. J., 1956, Role of $O$-β-D-galactopyranosyl($1\rightarrow4$)-$N$-acetyl-D-glucosamine as inhibitor of the precipitation of blood group substances by anti-type XIV pneumococcus serum, *Nature (London)* 178:1289–1290.

Watkins, W. M., and Morgan, W. T. J., 1957a, The A and H character of the blood group substances secreted by persons belonging to group $A_2$, *Acta Genet. Statist. Med.* 6:521–526.

Watkins, W. M., and Morgan, W. T. J., 1957b, Specific inhibition studies relating to the Lewis blood group system, *Nature (London)* 180:1038–1040.

Watkins, W. M., and Morgan, W. T. J., 1959, Possible genetical pathways for the biosynthesis of blood group mucopolysaccharides, *Vox Sang.* 4:97–119.

Watkins, W. M., and Morgan, W. T. J., 1962, Further observations on the inhibition of blood-group specific serological reactions by simple sugars of known structures, *Vox Sang.* 7:129–150.

Watkins, W. M., and Morgan, W. T. J., 1964, Blood group $P_1$ substance. II. Immunological properties, in: *Proceedings of the 9th Congress of the International Society of Blood Transfusion, Mexico, 1962*, pp. 230–234, Karger, Basel.

Watkins, W. M., and Morgan, W. T. J., 1976, Immunochemical observations on the human blood group P system, *J. Immunogenet.* 3:15–27.

Watkins, W. M., Zarnitz, M. L., and Kabat, E. A., 1962, Development of H activity by human blood-group B substance treated with coffee bean α-galactosidase, *Nature (London)* 195:1204–1206.

Watkins, W. M., Yates, A. D., Greenwell, P., Bird, G. W. G., Gibson, M., Roy R. C. F., Wingham, J., and Loeb, W., 1978, A human chimaera first suspected from analyses of the blood group gene specified glycosyltransferases, in: *XVth Congress of the International Society of Blood Transfusion, Paris, 1978*, Abstract, p. 443.

Weiner, W., Lewis, H. B. M., Moores, P., Sanger, R., and Race, R. R., 1957, A gene, *y*, modifying the blood group antigen A, *Vox Sang.* **2**:25–37.

Weitkamp, L. R., Sing, F. C., Shreffler, D. S., and Guttormsen, S. A., 1969, The genetic linkage relation of adenylate kinase: Further data on the ABO-AK linkage group, *Am. J. Hum. Genet.* **21**:600–605.

Westerveld, A., Jongsma, A. P. M., Meera Khna, P., van Someren H., and Bootsma, D., 1976, Assignment of the AK₁:Np:ABO linkage group to human chromosome 9, *Proc. Nat. Acad. Sci. USA* **73**:895–899.

Wherrett, J. R., and Hakomori, S. I., 1973, Characterisation of a blood group B glycolipid accumulating in the pancreas of a patient with Fabry's disease, *J. Biol. Chem.* **248**:3046–3051.

Wherrett, J. R., Brown, B. L., Tilley, C. A., and Crookston, M. C., 1971, A and B blood group substances in a glycosphingolipid fraction of human plasma, *Clin. Res.* **19**:784.

Whitehead, J. S., Bella, A., and Kim, Y. S., 1974*a*, An *N*-acetylgalactosaminyltransferase from human blood group A plasma. I. Purification and agarose binding properties, *J. Biol. Chem.* **249**:3442–3447.

Whitehead, J. S., Bella, A., and Kim, Y. S., 1974*b*, An *N*-acetylgalactosaminyltransferase from human blood group A plasma. II. Kinetic and physicochemical properties, *J. Biol. Chem.* **249**:3448–3452.

Whittemore, N. B., Trabold, N. C., Reed, C. F., and Weed, R. I., 1969, Solubilised glycoprotein from human erythrocyte membranes possessing blood group A, B and H activity, *Vox Sang.* **17**:289–299.

Wiener, A., 1943, *Blood Groups and Transfusion*, Thomas, Springfield, Illinois.

Wiener, A. S., Unger, L. J., Cohen, L., and Feldman, J., 1956, Type-specific cold autoantibodies as a cause of acquired hemolytic anemia and hemolytic transfusion reactions: biologic test with bovine red cells, *Ann. Intern. Med.* **44**:221–240.

Williams, M. A. and Voak, D., 1972, Studies with ferritin-labelled *Dolichos biflorus* lectin on the numbers and distribution of A sites on A₁ and A₂ erythrocytes and on the nature of its specificity and enhancement, *Br. J. Haematol.* **23**:427–441.

Williams, G., Pegrum, G. D., and Evans, C. A., 1978, Lewis antigens in renal transplantation, *Lancet* **i**:878.

Wilson, J. R., Williams, D., and Schachter, H., 1976, The control of glycoprotein synthesis: *N*-acetylglucosamine linkage to a mannose residue as a signal for the attachment of L-fucose to the asparagine-linked *N*-acetylglucosamine residue of glycopeptide from α₁-acid glycoprotein, *Biochem. Biophys. Res. Commun.* **72**:909–916.

Winzler, R. J., 1972, Glycoproteins of plasma membranes, chemistry and function, in: *Glycoproteins: Their Composition, Structure and Function* (A. Gottschalk, ed.), pp. 1268–1293, Elsevier, Amsterdam.

Wood, W. A., 1966, Carbohydrate metabolism, *Ann. Rev. Biochem.* **35**:521–558.

Wrobel, D. M., McDonald, I., Race, C., and Watkins, W. M., 1974, "True" genotype of chimeric twins revealed by blood group gene products in plasma, *Vox Sang.* **27**:283–287.

Wu, T. T., Lin, E. C. C., and Tanaka, S., 1968, Mutants of *Aerobacter aerogenes* capable of utilising xylitol as a novel carbon, *J. Bact.* **96**:447–456.

Yamaguchi, H., 1973, A review of cis AB blood, *Jpn. J. Hum. Genet.* **18**:1–9.

Yamaguchi, H., Okubo, Y., and Hazama, F., 1966, Another Japanese A₂B₃ blood-group family with the propositus having O-group father, *Proc. Jpn. Acad.* **42**:417–520.

Yamakami, K., 1926, The individuality of semen with reference to its property of inhibiting specifically isohaemagglutination, *J. Immunol.* **12**:185–189.

Yamakawa, T., and Susuki, S., 1952, The chemistry of the post-hemolytic residue or stroma of erythrocytes. II. Globoside, the sugar containing lipid of human blood stroma, *J. Biochem. Tokyo* **39**:393–402.

Yang, H., and Hakomori, S., 1971, A sphingolipid having a novel type of ceramide and lacto-*N*-fucopentaose III, *J. Biol. Chem.* **246**:1192–1200.

Yates, A. D., Morgan, W. T. J., and Watkins, W. M., 1975, Linkage-specific α-D-galactosidases from *Trichomonas foetus*. Characterisation of the blood group B-destroying enzyme as a 1,3-α-galactosidase and the blood-group $P_1$-destroying enzyme as a 1,4-α-galactosidase, *FEBS Lett.* **60**:281–285.

Yatziv, S., and Flowers, H. M., 1971, Action of α-galactosidase on glycoprotein from human B erythrocytes, *Biochem. Biophys. Res. Commun.* **45**:514–518.

Yazawa, S., 1976, Studies on fucosyltransferases related to the biosynthesis of human blood group substances. 1. Fucosyltransferases in human saliva (in Japanese), *Kitakanto Igaku* **26**:203–214.

Yosida, K., 1928, Über die gruppenspezifischen Unterschiede der Transsudate, Exsudate, Sekrete, Exkrete, Organ Extrakte, und Organzellen des Menschen und ihre rechtsmedizinischen Anwendungen, *Z. Ges. Exp. Med.* **63**:331–339.

Zahler, P., 1968, Blood group antigens in relation to chemical and structural properties of the red cell membrane, *Vox Sang.* **15**:81–100.

Zdebska, E., and Koscielak, J., 1978, Studies on the structure and I-blood group activity of poly(glycosyl)ceramides, *Eur. J. Biochem.* **91**:517–525.

Ziderman, D., Gompertz, S., Smith, Z-G., and Watkins, W. M., 1967, Glycosyltransferases in gastric mucosal linings, *Biochem. Biophys. Res. Commun.* **29**:56–61.

Zopf, D. A. and Ginsburg, V., 1975, Preparation of precipitating antigens by coupling oligosaccharides to polylysine, *Arch. Biochem. Biophys.* **167**:345–350.

Zopf, D. A., Tsai, C-M., and Ginsburg, V., 1977, Studies on the carbohydrate receptors of cold agglutinins using synthetic antigens, in: *Human Blood Groups* (J. F. Mohn, R. W. Plunkett, R. K. Cunningham, and R. M. Lambert, eds.), pp. 172–178, Karger, Basel.

*Chapter 2*

# HLA—A Central Immunological Agency of Man

D. Bernard Amos and D. D. Kostyu

*Division of Immunology*
*Duke University Medical Center*
*Durham, North Carolina 27710*

## INTRODUCTION

> Life is a series of surprises, and would not be worth taking or keeping if it were not.
> —Emerson

This quotation seems particularly appropriate to the way that knowledge of the complexity of human histocompatibility antigens (HLA) has progressed. At one time leukocyte antigens were a tangle of cell surface markers many of which could be identified in only one laboratory; they then took on the appearance of a well-regulated and orderly series of membrane antigens of little interest outside transplantation. With little warning HLA became one of the most precise of all tools for the anthropologist, and now a new horizon of biologic functions and involvements in disease is opening up. Like Topsy, it has "just growed," and like Pandora's box it continues to offer unlooked for and sometimes unwanted surprises.

The most complete early description of lymphocyte antigens was given by van Rood in 1962. An ambitious earlier attempt at systematic family studies by Payne and Hackel (1961) was frustrated by technical problems and because the then available sera were complex mixtures of antibodies. Indeed, few if any genetic studies were possible before 1965. Ceppellini *et al.* (1965) then published a fascinating theoretical treatment of histocompatibility in man, but their arguments were based largely upon skin grafting and the normal lymphocyte transfer test. Serological data were not included. Indeed, at this point the serology was quite confusing as the number of antigens was unknown, as was the number of loci and their linkage relationships to each other. Van Rood carried out family studies and concluded that his antigens 4, 6, 7, and 8 were closely linked but published no detailed data except for one family which appeared to show recombination between antigens 4 and 6 (van Rood and van Leeuwen, 1965) as well as linkage. The inference reached by Dausset *et al.* (1965) that all the antigens detected by them belonged to a single system was based solely upon population studies. Bach and Amos (1967) carried out collaborative studies on 10 families characterized by serology and mixed lymphocyte culture reactions. By these tests they were able to distinguish genotypes, to prove the unit inheritance of HLA and to deduce the relevance of these tests to skin and kidney graft survival. The relatively clear serologic patterns in the studies of Bach and Amos were possible because antibodies of restricted specificity had become available through planned immunization of volunteer subjects and because of the evolution of the microcytotoxicity test. Knowledge of the individual HLA antigens and of their genetic control proceeded rapidly. The existence of two (later three) closely linked loci was predicted and soon confirmed by demonstrating recombination between them and by 1968 a small group of investigators had characterized seven antigens at two loci; the complexity and biologic importance of what was emerging as a remarkable collection of loci, as outlined in Table I, was just beginning to be felt.

HLA is now acknowledged to include five known histocompatibility loci—HLA-A, -B, -C, -D, and -DR. This number is almost certainly an underestimate. Already nearly a hundred antigens have been identified and there is presumptive evidence for at least three other loci. In addition to the components of what is regarded as the functioning supergene HLA, many other components are known to be within the HLA region or closely linked to it. These include genes for complement proteins (both of the classical and alternate pathways), genes determining disease susceptibility, structural genes for red cell enzymes and antigens, regulatory genes, and genes for various types of receptor or binding proteins.

Interest in the human MHC (major histocompatibility complex) has been intensified and broadened in appeal from the remarkable association of particular HLA antigens with certain immunopathological diseases, through innovative methods for the study of the biochemistry of these

TABLE I. Significant Events in the History of HLA[a]

| | |
|---|---|
| 1953–1958 | Leukocyte-agglutinating antibodies are found in the sera of multitransfused patients and many multiparous women. |
| 1958 | The first human lymphocyte antigen Mac (now HLA-A2 and A28) is described. |
| 1962 | By computer analysis, the first allelic lymphocyte antigenic system, 4a and 4b (now Bw4 and Bw6) is identified; others such as 6a, 6b, and 6c, and LA1, LA2, and LA3 soon follow. |
| 1963–1964 | The mixed lymphocyte culture (MLC) assay is developed as an *in vitro* example of primary immune recognition and proliferation. |
| 1964 | Miniaturization of the lymphocytotoxicity test and the introduction of rabbit complement establishes a rapid, reproducible microtechnique, which replaces leukoagglutination. |
| | First International Histocompatibility Workshop is held at Duke University; sequential workshops held in 1965, 1967, 1970, 1972, 1975, and 1977. |
| 1964–1966 | First evidence of the relevance of leukocyte antigens to skin transplantation and the use of HLA matching within families for kidney transplants. |
| 1967 | The first HLA and disease associations: the "4c" antigen with Hodgkins disease and HLA-A2 with acute lymphocytic leukemia. |
| 1968 | Two HLA loci are established, one called the First or LA locus (now HLA-A) and the Second or Four locus (now HLA-B); in 1975, the original connotation HL-A is changed to HLA. |
| 1969 | First demonstration of a third locus, HLA-C, which is also detectable by lymphocytotoxicity. |
| 1970 | First demonstration that a fourth locus, now HLA-D, controls immune recognition in the MLC. |
| 1972–1973 | Discovery of B-cell-specific antigens (HLA-DR). |
| 1974 | Linkage between HLA and the complement component Bf noted; later C2 and C4 are linked. |
| 1953–present | Parallel developments in other species establishes similar MHCs (major histocompatibility complex) in the mouse, rhesus monkey, chimpanzee, pig, rabbit, rat, dog, cattle, etc. |

[a] From references (Amos and Ward, 1975; Albert and Götze, 1977).

antigens as integral membrane components, and from the genetic organization of the supergene. Antigens determined by the MHC are implicated in T-cell-specific and B-cell-specific differentiation; other MHC-linked genes govern the ability to mount a humoral or cellular immune response against bacteria, viruses, or transplanted allogeneic cells or organs. The products of this supergene, both cell-membrane molecules and plasma proteins, are involved in immunologic communication and cell–cell interactions which maintain the integrity and well-being of the immunologic system of an individual, and may possibly represent the mechanism for self-recognition. Similar MHCs have been described in the rat (des-

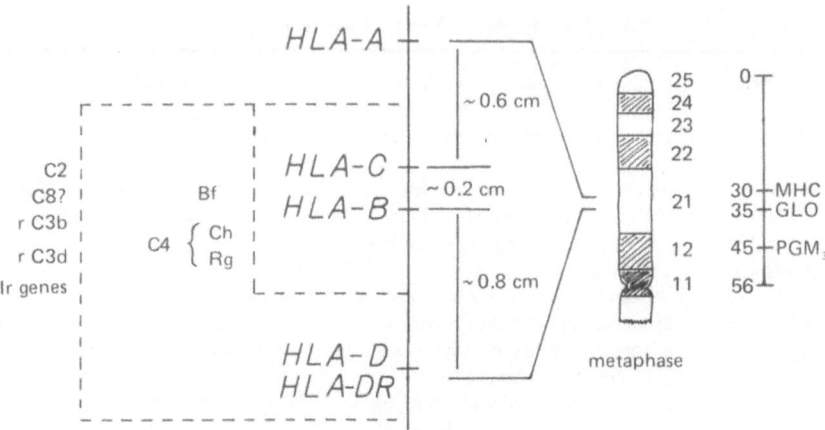

Fig. 1. The HLA complex of genes (or MHC) has been localized to a short segment of
chromosome 6 (6p21-6p22).


ignated AgB), chicken (B), mouse (H-2), Dog (DLA), pig (SL-A), chimpanzee (CHLA), rhesus monkey (RHLA), guinea pig (GPLA) and rabbit
(RL-A) (Götze, 1977).

## HLA: A SUPERGENE

HLA has been localized to the short arm of chromosome 6 by cell
hybridization (Jongsma *et al.*, 1973) and family studies (Lamm *et al.*, 1974;
Breuning *et al.*, 1977). The HLA complex, illustrated in Figure 1, is composed of five major loci, each coding for cell surface membrane antigens.
These loci, designated HLA-A, -B, -C, -D, and -DR (Albert *et al.*, 1978),
are the best understood components of HLA and, as such, will be the
major emphasis of this review.

Many other components now known to be within the HLA region
or closely linked to it will not be discussed in great detail but are listed
here with appropriate references.* C2 and C4, components of the classical
complement pathway, have been linked both by deficiency studies in fam-

---

* For lack of space it is impossible to list all the references that could be given. Where there
  was a choice to be made, we have chosen the most recent or most complete in hopes that
  the interested reader will be able to trace the subject backward with less difficulty.

ilies (Ochs *et al.*, 1977; Cukrova *et al.*, 1977; Hauptman *et al.*, 1977; Ward *et al.*, 1977) and by the familial inheritance of electrophoretic variants (Meo *et al.*, 1977; Teisberg *et al.*, 1977). Rogers (Giles *et al.*, 1976) and Chido (Middleton *et al.*, 1974), once thought to be red cell groups, have recently been described as representing antigenic variants of C4 (O'Neill *et al.*, 1978*a*, 1978*b*) and are regulated by genes near HLA-B. Bf or Factor B of the alternate pathway of complement is also closely linked to C4 and HLA-B (Albert *et al.*, 1977; Arnason *et al.*, 1977; Bender *et al.*, 1977). Receptors for C3b and C3d, the breakdown fragments of C3, may also be HLA-linked (Curry *et al.*, 1976). A C8 deficiency was linked by Merritt *et al.* (1976) to HLA-B, but other studies of C8 deficiency (Giraldo *et al.*, 1977; Jersild *et al.*, 1976) or electrophoretic variants (Alper cited in Hobart, 1977) showed no HLA linkage. Since C8 consists of 3 chains as does C4 (Müller-Eberhard, 1975) it is possible that only one of the chains may be HLA-linked. Other complement components, on the other hand, are not HLA-linked (Lachman and Hobart, 1978). These include Clr deficiency (Mittal *et al.*, 1976; Day *et al.*, 1975), C1 inhibitor deficiency (Rittner, 1976), C3 deficiency (Osofsky *et al.*, 1977) and C3 electrophoretic variants (Gedde-Dahl, Jr. *et al.*, 1974; Lamm *et al.*, 1975), C5 deficiency (Rosenfeld *et al.*, 1977), C6 deficiency (Mittal *et al.*, 1976; Raum *et al.*, 1976), C6 variants (Olving *et al.*, 1977; Hobart *et al.*, 1977) and C7 deficiency (Rittner *et al.*, 1976; Delage *et al.*, 1977).

A locus for congenital adrenal hyperplasia (21-hydroxylase deficiency) is on the B·side of HLA-A (Dupont *et al.*, 1977*a*); another provisional gene is olivopontocerebellar ataxia, OPCA-1 or SCA (Jackson *et al.*, 1977). Glyoxalase (*GLO*), a red cell enzyme, is located approximately 5 cM from HLA-D (Mayr *et al.*, 1976; Olaisen *et al.*, 1976). Phosphoglucomutase-3 ($PGM_3$) is loosely linked to HLA, at a distance of 15 cM in males (Lamm *et al.*, 1970). The reported linkage of urinary pepsinogen 5 to HLA, outside of the HLA-A locus, is doubtful (Weitkamp, 1977). These components, many of which are related to immune function, attest to the complexity of this supergene and may eventually help to give a clearer understanding of the MHC and how it functions.

Other genes assigned to chromosome 6 include superoxide dismutase 2 (SOD-2); malic enzyme 1 (ME1) (van Someren *et al.*, 1974); a receptor for monkey red blood cells (Pellegrino *et al.*, 1975); mitochondrial glutamate oxaloacetate transaminase ($GOT_M$) (Craig *et al.*, 1977); genes for a separate group of cell surface antigens, SA-6, detected with mouse "anti-chromosome 6" sera (Knowles *et al.*, 1977); genes for immunoglobulin heavy chains and alpha-1-antitrypsin (Smith and Hirschhorn, 1978), and for an adenosine-deaminase-complexing protein (Koch and Shows, 1978).

For further information, the reader is directed to earlier reviews on the history and genetics of HLA (Amos, 1969; Ceppellini and van Rood, 1974; Ferrara, 1977; Amos and Ward, 1975; Thorsby, 1974; Ceppellini, 1971; Kissmeyer-Nielsen and Thorsby, 1970; Svejgaard *et al.*, 1975; Snell *et al.*, 1976), HLA and disease (Dausset and Svejgaard, 1977; Murphy, 1977; Ryder and Svejgaard, 1977), HLA and other MHCs (Götze, 1977; Snell *et al.*, 1976), the MHC and fertility (Amos, 1974; Beer and Billingham, 1977), evolution (Bodmer and Thomson, 1977), or aging (Walford *et al.*, 1978), and the early history of transplantation (Saunders, 1972). The greatest concentration of original articles is to be found in the seven International Histocompatibility Testing Workshops (Russell and Winn, 1965; Balner *et al.*, 1966; Curtoni *et al.*, 1967; Terasaki, 1970; Dausset and Colombani, 1973; Bodmer *et al.*, 1978a; Kissmeyer-Nielsen, 1975) or in specialist journals such as *Tissue Antigens* and *Transplantation.*

## HLA TERMINOLOGY

HLA terminology is regulated by a committee under the auspices of the World Health Organization and the International Union of Immunologic Societies. There are, as of 1977, 20 antigens at the HLA-A locus, 33 antigens at HLA-B, 6 antigens at HLA-C, 11 antigens at HLA-D, and 7 antigens at HLA-DR (Albert *et al.*, 1978). About one-fifth of these are well-agreed-upon, easily defined antigens and, as such, are given official HLA numbers, e.g., the first antigen at the A locus is HLA-A1. Other antigens, often not as easily defined due to the absence of monospecific typing reagents, have nevertheless been well recognized by tests carried out during one or more histocompatibility workshops. The "workshops" may be unique to this field. They began modestly as an attempt to standardize techniques and reagents during a three-day practical demonstration. They now take more than a year to complete, and up to 200 laboratories participate by exchanging antisera and homozygous typing cells for *in vitro* tests and by making the data available to a central computer. The final analysis is presented as a Joint Report of the workshop and as a WHO-IUIS report of terminology. The provisional (workshop) antigens, prefixed with a "w," e.g., HLA-Bw35, currently account for the remaining four-fifths of the currently recognized HLA antigens.*

Definition of an HLA antigen proceeds in orderly steps. For example, an antigen called Ao81 at Duke and an antigen called U18 by Dausset in France were found to be identical during the 1972 International Histocompatibility Testing Workshop (Dausset and Colombani, 1973) and were designated Bw16, the next available number. Two antigenic variants of Bw16 were later identified; these in turn have been given new numbers, Bw38 and Bw39.† Thus, the process of "splitting" old antigens and finding new antigens continues. This process is mentioned later in the section on Serology. A complete summary of HLA antigens through 1977 is given in Table II.

## INHERITANCE OF HLA

If the two C6 chromosomes of the father are designated ab and the mother cd, there are four possible combinations in the offspring: ac, ad, bc, and bd, since each child inherits one paternal and one maternal chromosome. The HLA chromosomal complex, including HLA-A, -B, -C, -D, and -DR antigens, is termed a haplotype. For example, in Figure 2, a father who has the HLA phenotype of A1, A3, B7, and B8, etc., may pass on an HLA-A1, B8 haplotype to one child and an A3, B7 haplotype to another. The father's HLA haplotypes and genotype would then be written as A1, B8/A3, B7. HLA-C, -D, and -DR locus antigens and the

---

* The original HLA nomenclature preceded the clear separation of HLA-A from HLA-B. Consequently, antigens at the A and B loci were numbered in order of their recognition, e.g., HL-A1, 2, 3, 5, etc. As other loci were added and the number of antigens increased, this nomenclature was revised (WHO-IUIS Terminology Committee, 1975). The hyphen in HL-A was removed, and each antigen prefixed with its locus, e.g., HL-A 1 is now HLA-A1, and HL-A w22 is now HLA-Bw22. While the A and B series of antigens continue to be numbered jointly, antigens at the newer loci (C, D, and DR) are each numbered consecutively from 1, e.g., HLA-Cw1, HLA-Dw1, etc. Note that the "provisional" designation is usually temporary and does not imply any difference in significance.

† The renumbering of splits is confusing to the nonspecialist, but it has been adopted as the obvious alternative, that of giving symbols indicative of a subdivision. If this had been done in the early days of HLA, for example, Bw4 would be subdivided into some 10 components and some of these, e.g., B5, have been further divided into 3 or more subdivisions. As other races are studied, new subdivisions appear. Thus the present sequential system, although it may require frequent reference to the tables of specificities, has the merit of simplicity.

TABLE II. HLA-A, -B, -C, -D, and -DR Antigens[a]

| HLA-A locus | HLA-B locus | HLA-C locus | HLA-D locus | HLA-DR locus |
|---|---|---|---|---|
| A1 | B5 | Cw1 (T1,AJ) | Dw1 (LD101) | DRw1 (WIA1) |
| A2 | Bw51 (5.1) | Cw2 (T2,SA532) | Dw2 (LD102,LD-7a) | DRw2 (WIA2) |
| A3 | Bw52 (5.2) | Cw3 (T3,UPS) | Dw3 (LD103,LD-8a) | DRw3 (WIA3) |
| A9 | B7 | Cw4 (T4,Rh315) | Dw4 (LD104) | DRw4 (WIA4) |
| Aw23 | B8 | Cw5 (T5) | Dw5 (LD105) | DRw5 (WIA5) |
| Aw24 | B12 | Cw6 (T7) | Dw6 (LD106) | DRw6 (WIA6) |
| A10 | Bw44 (12 not TT*) | | Dw7 (LD107) | DRw7 (WIA7) |
| A25 | Bw45 (TT*) | | Dw8 (LD108) | |
| A26 | B13 | | Dw9 (TB9,OH) | |
| A11 | B14 (Maki) | | Dw10 (LD16) | |
| A28 | B15 (LND) | | Dw11 (LD17) | |
| Aw19 (Li) | Bw16 | | | |
| A29 (w19.1) | Bw38 (16.1) | | | |
| Aw30 (w19.3) | Bw39 (16.2) | | | |
| Aw31 (w19.4) | B17 (Mapi) | | | |

Aw32 (w19.5)
Aw33 (w19.6)
Aw34 (Malay 2)
Aw36 (Mo*,LT)
Aw43 (BK)

B18 (CM)
Bw21
Bw49 (w21.1,SL-ET)
Bw50 (w21.2, ET*)
Bw22 (AA)
B27 (FJH)
Bw35 (W5,R*)
B37 (TY)
B40 (w10,BB)
Bw41 (Sabell,LK,Da34)
Bw42 (MWA)
Bw46 (HS,SIN 2)
Bw47 (407*,Mo66,Cas,Bw40c)
Bw48 (KSO,JA,Bw40.3)
Bw53 (HR)
Bw54 (Sapi, Bw22J)
Bw4 (4a)
Bw6 (4b)

a Previous designations are listed in parentheses.

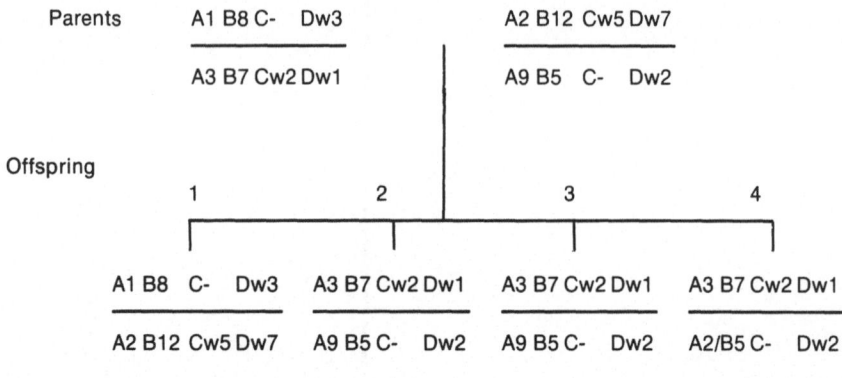

Fig. 2. Family segregation of HLA "haplotypes." Note that child No. 4 possesses the maternal recombinant haplotype, A2/B5,C-,Dw2.

electrophoretic variants of C2, C4, Bf, and glyoxalase, which are also controlled by genes of the haplotype, are sometimes, but not always, distinguishable. They can be of great use in identifying a haplotype or determining the location of an HLA recombination and the full haplotype designation would include this information.

## Recombination

Recombination (crossing-over between homologous chromosomes during meiosis) occurs between all HLA loci. The existence of recombinants has been essential for identifying the component loci of HLA and an estimate of the map distance has been gained by the frequency of recombination between two given loci. Since it is now possible in many instances to thoroughly analyze an HLA haplotype for HLA-A, -B, -C, and -DR antigens by antibody-mediated complement-dependent cytotoxicity assays, HLA-D by MLR, and C2, C4, GLO, and Bf by electrophoretic analysis of variants, mapping in the HLA region is progressing rapidly.

HLA-A/B recombination occurs with a frequency of approximately 0.8% (Bijnen *et al.*, 1976; Belvedere *et al.*, 1975a). Thus, as few as 100 or possibly as many as 2000 genes could exist between the A and B loci. HLA-C is close to -B (Nielsen *et al.*, 1975; Hansen *et al.*, 1975). Estimates of the map distance between HLA-B and -D range from 1 to 2.2 cM (Keuning *et al.*, 1975; Netzel *et al.*, 1975; Lamm *et al.*, 1978). Of 139 individuals studied, no recombination has been seen between B and Chido (Lamm and Kristensen, 1977).

An influence of sex on recombination frequency has been claimed (Weitkamp *et al.*, 1973; Weitkamp, 1976; Belvedere *et al.*, 1975a; Lamm *et al.*, 1977). For linkage between HLA and PGM$_3$, certainly the sex influence is very marked, and linkage is observed only with male parents (Lamm *et al.*, 1975). Specific population differences in recombination frequencies may also exist (Weitkamp, 1976). A recent study has suggested that children who are HLA-B/D recombinants often have parents sharing B locus antigens ($p< 0.00013$) (Dupont *et al.*, 1977b). Interestingly, a number of families include more than one recombinant, not necessarily from the same parent.

# THE HLA-A, -B, AND -C ALLELIC SERIES OF ANTIGENS

The HLA-A and -B antigens are glycoproteins expressed on the plasma membrane of most nucleated cells. Although HLA-C has been less well-studied it is thought to be similar to the A and B molecules.

## Typing Procedures

The A, B, and C antigens are routinely determined by a microlymphocytotoxicity assay, based on an assay by Gorer and O'Gorman (1956), later modified by Terasaki and McClelland (1964). It involves the incubation of 2000–3000 lymphocytes with 0.001 ml of antiserum in wells of a microtiter tray. Following sensitization and an optional wash (Amos *et al.*, 1970), rabbit serum (Walford, 1964) as a source of complement is added. Killing of the target lymphocytes by specific human antibodies in the presence of complement is determined by eosin or trypan blue exclusion or release of markers such as $^{51}$Cr (Rogentine, 1967; Sanderson and Batchelor, 1967) or fluorescein diacetate (Martel *et al.*, 1974; Bodmer *et al.*, 1967; Rotman and Papermaster, 1966). A two-color fluorescent technique allows cytotoxicity of two different cell populations, e.g., B cells and T cells, to be monitored at the same time (van Rood *et al.*, 1976).

The addition of an antiimmunoglobulin may increase sensitivity (dos Reis *et al.*, 1972; Johnson *et al.*, 1972). Lymphocytes are generally isolated from peripheral blood, by passing leukocyte suspensions through nylon wool or by gradient sedimentation on Ficoll–Hypaque (Böyum, 1968).

Peripheral blood lymphocytes can be easily obtained and can be HLA-typed directly by cytotoxicity. Platelets can be typed, albeit not as easily, by $^{51}Cr$ release (Aster *et al.*, 1973; Aster *et al.*, 1977) or by platelet complement fixation (Colombani *et al.*, 1971). In some cases, such as with granulocytes and erythrocytes, the HLA-A and -B antigens are more sparse and have only been demonstrated by absorption (Thorsby, 1969) or through the autoanalyzer. $^{125}I$-labeled protein A from *Staphylococcus aureus* can also be used to directly measure Ab binding (Brown *et al.*, 1977; Dorval *et al.*, 1977; Welsh *et al.*, 1977). Other methods of HLA typing, including leukoagglutination (van Rood and van Leeuwen, 1963; Amos and Peacocke, 1963), mixed hemagglutination (Milgrom *et al.*, 1965), and indirect immunofluorescence (Décary *et al.*, 1975), have been used but are technically difficult, give poorly defined reactions, or may be relatively insensitive. There is no indication, furthermore, that the antigens detected by these methods are the same HLA-A, -B, and -C antigens detected by the usual lymphocytotoxicity assay.*

## Antibodies

HLA antibodies are rarely found without prior sensitization, although exceptions have been noted (Amos and Peacocke, 1963; Collins *et al.*, 1973; Lepage *et al.*, 1976). Sensitization can follow skin grafting (Batchelor and Kennedy, 1973), therapeutic or experimental blood transfusion (Ceppellini *et al.*, 1964; Ferrara *et al.*, 1978a), experimental immunization with lymphocytes (Amos *et al.*, 1973), organ transplantation, and most frequently through pregnancy (Doughty and Gelsthorpe, 1976; Vives *et al.*, 1976; Ahrons, 1971). The route of administration, type of immunizing cell, amount, and interval between exposures will all influence the development of cytotoxic antibodies. A single skin graft, although sufficient

---

* This is not to imply that the definition of HLA as given by the conventional complement-dependent reactions are correct. The present convention for HLA is based upon cytotoxic reactions; a later definition may take into account antibody binding rather than the ability of an antibody to drive the activation of the complement cascade. Cells not lysed by an antibody and complement may be capable of absorbing that antibody (CNAP or CYNAP) (Ceppellini *et al.*, 1965).

to stimulate accelerated rejection of skin (Rapaport *et al.*, 1960), only rarely leads to a detectable humoral response (Batchelor and Kennedy, 1973). Aplastic individuals requiring repeated platelet transfusions often develop HLA antibodies in addition to antiplatelet antibodies. Antibody has been detected as early as the 24th week of a first pregnancy (Ahrons, 1971), and also as a result of miscarriage or spontaneous abortion (Amos and Peacocke, 1963). Depending upon the sensitivity of the test, and the time of testing after delivery, from 20 to 60% of multiparous women will form HLA-A or -B antibodies. Interestingly, some of these antibodies disappear soon after delivery while others persist for 20 years. However, some individuals remain inexplicably refractory to antibody formation despite repeated immunization or repeated pregnancies (Amos *et al.*, 1973; Hattler *et al.*, 1966); American Indian women are one example.

The sera used for HLA typing are from highly selected bleedings from multiparous women, transplant recipients, or experimentally immunized subjects. The antibody is usually of the IgG class. All of the antibodies currently used for typing are lytic in the presence of complement. Other antibodies which are agglutinating without being cytotoxic (van Rood and van Leeuwen, 1965), are noncomplement fixing (Basch, 1974; Colombani *et al.*, 1973*a*), or are active only in ADCC (Tosi *et al.*, 1975), are not used for routine purposes. The great majority of HLA antibodies are active undiluted or only in low dilutions.

## HLA Serology

Serological reactions can have exquisite specificity in identification of antigens (Landsteiner, 1942; Karush, 1962). Landsteiner (1942) has many examples of both specific and cross-reactive interactions. Detailed measurements of the strength of binding between trinitro and dinitro derivatives of benzene and toluene have been given by Little and Eisen (1969) and Eisen and Siskind (1964). Benjamini and co-workers (1969) have shown that while all rabbits immunized to tobacco mosaic virus protein recognized the same decapeptide, individual rabbits reacted against different pentameric sequences within the decapeptide. These studies provide a valuable perspective for studies on the less well-defined histocompatibility antigens. Batchelor and Sanderson (1970) and others (Amos, 1970; Dausset, 1971) have postulated a similar variability in recognition of complex antigens of HLA. Indeed, it is rare for two anti-HLA antibodies to have exactly the same specificity, and a very great deal of selection is necessary before antisera are accepted for use as HLA-typing reagents. With selection, however, great specificity can be attained.

The first "antigens" described by van Rood—4a, 4b, 6a, 6b, 7b, 7c, 7d, 8a—and the 4c antigen of Payne are usually regarded as "supertypic" since each was later found to include a series of subtypic antigens. For example, the antigen first designated 7c "includes" B7, B27, and Bw22, while 4c "includes" B5 (both Bw51 and Bw52), Bw53, B18, and Bw35. Although this process of splitting may seem arbitrary, there are five reasons for supposing that the subtypic definition of specificities in HLA is meaningful. (1) The subtypic specificities segregate clearly and are inherited independently in families. (2) The presence of a subtypic specificity may be associated with susceptibility to disease, e.g., B27 and ankylosing spondylitis, while a highly cross-reactive but clearly different specificity, e.g., B7, shows no such association and may, in fact, have different disease associations (Dausset and Svejgaard, 1977). (3) Very specific antigenic differences, for example, those between the two variants of B5, Bw51, and Bw52, can be clearly distinguished by the fundamentally different process of cell-mediated cytotoxicity (Robinson *et al.*, 1978). (4) Population studies often show that one subtypic antigen, e.g., Bw44, is very common in a Caucasian population, while the other B12 subtype Bw45 is found only in black populations. (See also section on population genetics.) (5) The distinction between *B* locus subtypic specificities is highly correlated with Bw4 or with Bw6.

The reactivities of most "supertypic" sera, such as those defining "4c," indicate similarity between a group of subtypic antigens, often referred to as a cross-reactive group of antigens (Svejgaard and Kissmeyer-Nielsen, 1968; Mittal and Terasaki, 1972; Dausset, 1971; Amos and Yunis, 1969) called a CREG (Colombani *et al.*, 1970). For example, most antisera produced against HLA-B5 will react not only with all cells that are B5 (e.g., Bw51, Bw52, and B5.y), but also with those cells that carry Bw35, B18, Bw53, and sometimes B15, B17, and Bw21. A few of the many CREGs are shown in Figure 3. Cross-reactivity greatly complicates the procurement of "monospecific" sera for HLA typing since the vast majority of unselected sera are cross-reactive.

Supertypic sera, however, can be of great use in identifying new HLA antigens. For example, an individual may not type as a B5, Bw35, or B18, but will react with the longer "4c" sera. This usually indicates that an individual possesses a new antigen belonging to the 4c cross-reactive

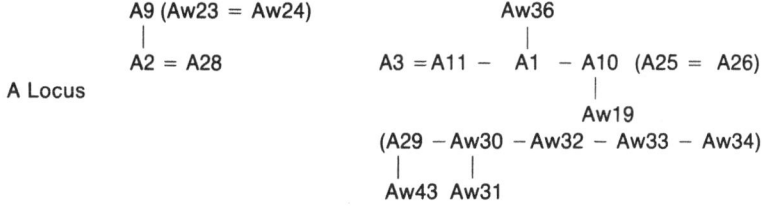

A Locus

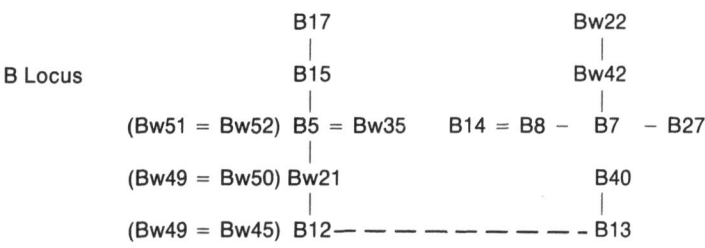

B Locus

Fig. 3. Some cross-reactive groups (CREGs) of HLA antigens. The lines drawn between antigens indicate strength of cross-reactivity: =, extremely strong cross-reactions; –, frequent cross-reactions; ---, occasional cross-reactions.

group. A recent example is the identification of a new antigen of this group, B5.y (Payne *et al.*, 1978).

It is possible to utilize a knowledge of cross-reactivity for the generation of highly specific antibodies by planned immunization since usually, but not necessarily always, the most specific antisera arise from immunization between two individuals carrying antigens of the same CREG. Note, however, that attempts to produce an antibody within certain CREGs have been unsuccessful, suggesting a genetic restriction on antibody production (M. A. Woodbury and D. B. Amos, unpublished).

In many cases, patterns of cross-reactivity extend beyond overt cytotoxicity. For example, of two B5 sera, one may lyse Bw35 cells and the other may not, but both sera can be absorbed by Bw35 cells. This phenomenon, where cytotoxicity is negative but absorption is positive (CYNAP), is an indication of the cross-reactivity of HLA and is a major but frequently ignored pitfall of the HLA cytotoxicity assay. An extreme form of CYNAP in which a maternal serum behaved as a typical anti-B12 when tested on a donor panel but failed to react with the spouse and weakly with two children was reported by Yunis and co-workers (1970). Bias and co-workers (1974) have suggested that CYNAP depends upon the activity of a gene unlinked to HLA, which modifies HLA antigen expression. While this is possible, CYNAP often disappears when a more sensitive technique is used.

Two of van Rood's original antigens, 4a and 4b (now Bw4 and Bw6), are unique and have come back to occupy a very special place in the definition of HLA-B locus antigens. As shown by Ayres and Cresswell (1976) and others (Bernoco *et al.*, 1973; Richiardi *et al.*, 1974; Legrand and Dausset, 1973; Bright, 1974; Ferrone *et al.*, 1978), the HLA-B molecule apparently carries two HLA antigens, a public antigen (which is either Bw4 or Bw6) and a subtypic antigen. As mentioned earlier in discussing the validity of subtypic determinants, the fact that certain B locus antigens are always associated with Bw4 and the remaining with Bw6 is of great practical importance (Bright, 1976; D'Amaro, 1975; Oliver and Festenstein, 1975) (see Table III). Thus, while few laboratories have antisera to Bw45 and so cannot distinguish between the two major variants of HLA-B12, HLA-Bw44 is included in Bw4 while Bw45 is included in Bw6. Even in the absence of subtypic sera, a subject who types as having B12 and who is Bw6 rather than w4 is most probably Bw45, while B12 individuals typing as Bw4 are most probably Bw44. We thus regard w4 and w6 as distinctive diallelic specificities and not as cross-reactivities.

It is thus not surprising that cross-reactivities may cut across the Bw4, Bw6 categories. For example, one of the strongest cross-reactivities is that between B5 and Bw35, another is that between Bw44 and Bw45. Both B5 and Bw44 are associated with Bw4 (4a) while Bw35 and Bw45 are associated with Bw6 (4b). If 4a and 4b are diallelic variants of one cistron, then the reactions of sera to the Bw4 or Bw6 antigen must be regarded as being specific. The subtle differences between different Bw4, Bw6 sera may tell a great deal about the possible configurational complexity of mutational variants of these proteins or about the specificity of immune response genes. Alternatively, one might suggest that if there is a Bw4, Bw6 cistron, recombination must on occasion occur between the gene for Bw4 and the gene for the peptide carrying the subtypic specificity. The tertiary structural change in the protein resulting from this type of recombination will be modified; thus a grouping which would react as Bw44 when intercalated with a Bw4 peptide could react as Bw45 on a w6 background. We are aware that this might not be a complete explanation for the interrelationship between Bw4 and Bw6 and subtypic antigens, but it appears to be consistent with well-categorized variants.

We do not know why a particular serum is cross-reactive while another is subtypic, and we have very limited information about antibodies

TABLE III. HLA-B Antigen Inclusions in Bw4
(4a) or Bw6 (4b)[a]

| Bw4 (4a) | | Bw6 (4b) |
|---|---|---|
| B5 | | Bw35 |
| Bw51 | "4c" | B18 |
| Bw52 | | |
| Bw53 | | |
| Bw49 | Bw21 | Bw50 |
| B "15.2" | B15 | B "15.1" |
| B17 | | Bw46 |
| Bw44 | B12 | Bw45 |
| Bw38 | Bw16 | Bw39 |
| B13 | | B40 |
| Bw47 | | Bw41 |
| | | Bw48 |
| | | B7 |
| B27 | | Bw42 |
| | | Bw22 |
| | | B14 |
| | | B8 |
| B37 | | |

[a] Horizontal lines separate CREGs. Data from
Bodmer et al. (1978a).

formed in different individuals responding to antigen from a common immunizing cell. As one possible explanation, Dausset (Legrand and Dausset, 1973; Dausset, 1971) suggested that the HLA antigens consist of several antigenic determinants or factors, with a complexity similar to that
of the Rh system (Dausset, 1972). The molecular basis for HLA antigenicity has also been discussed by Batchelor and Sanderson (1970), Ceppellini (1971), Duquesnoy (1975), Dausset and Legrand (1974) and by
Waters and Walford (1972); Hirschfeld (1965) has stressed the fact that

both the antigens and antibodies may be complex, thereby affecting the interpretation of serologic specificity. Amino acid sequences as well as conformation can determine "antigenic structure" (Atassi, 1975; Atassi and Lee, 1978). Of particular interest might be the occurrence of cross-reactivity between the A and B loci (Belvedere et al., 1975b; Cresswell and Ayres, 1976; Legrand and Dausset, 1975a) which suggests that "public" antigens exist on both HLA-A and -B molecules. While sequence studies now in progress will undoubtedly help us understand the antigenicity of HLA, it seems probable that as in the lysozyme system (Atassi and Lee, 1978), active sites from a large series of different specificities will be required for a full understanding of cross-reactivity. Thus, definitive answers cannot be expected for some time.

## The Use of Multispecific Sera

The majority of sera from multipara, and even some that are raised by planned immunization or obtained from primipara, are called "multispecific." Multispecificity is due to (1) the presence of more than one antibody population in a serum, e.g., a serum that reacts as an anti-HLA-A3, an anti-Bw35, and an anti-Cw4 and which is likely to be resolved into three component antibodies by absorption; (2) a high level of cross-reactivity, e.g., anti-HLA-B5, Bw35, B18, and Bw53; (3) or both, e.g., an anti-A3, A11, A1, and anti-Bw35, B5, B18. Multispecificity is a serious practical problem since of 100 antisera, 10–20% are too weak to be of value and at least 50% are "multispecific." Some of the latter can be "salvaged" by absorption or dilution.

Absorption consists of adding antigen, usually in the form of platelets or lymphocytes, to serum in suitable proportions (for a description of the quantitative aspects of absorption see Day, 1965 and 1966; and for technical considerations see Eguro et al., 1973; Rodey et al., 1973; Yunis et al., 1972). Elution consists of washing the absorbing cell (to remove unbound antibody) and releasing the specifically bound antibody, usually by changing the pH. Absorption is simplest and most valuable when a multispecific serum contains antibody populations to two antigens of different CREG, e.g., HLA-A3 and B5. Absorption with A3 cells would leave anti-B5 in the supernatant. The A3 antibody could then be recovered by washing the A3 cells, followed by acid elution and neutralization, or by absorbing a fresh sample of serum with B5 cells.

Absorption procedures are most commonly used in removing anti-HLA-A, -B, and -C activity from sera also containing antibodies to HLA-DR (van Rood *et al.*, 1975*a*). Absorption may also be used to narrow the reactivity of a high titered cross-reactive antibody. For example, an anti-HLA-A3 serum which reacts to a titer of 1:8 with HLA-A3 cells may also react with A11 cells, but at a much lower titer. By dilution, a much more specific antiserum can be obtained. Alternatively, absorption of that serum with the cross-reactive antigen, i.e., A11 cells, will reduce A11 reactivity but leave A3 reactivity. Unfortunately, in most instances, anti-A3 activity is also diminished and a trace of residual A11 activity remains and can be demonstrated when more sensitive tests are used. Since many of the cross-reactive antibodies appear to result from the recruitment of a spectrum of antibody producing clones, it is sometimes possible to fractionate them; heteroclitic antibodies, e.g., those reacting preferentially with HLA-A11 even though the immunization was against HLA-A3, can be recovered under appropriate conditions (Dorf *et al.*, 1972). Unfortunately, since this form of fractionation is laborious, it is about as useful in practice as separating gold from sea water. A careful study of cross-reactivity could, however, teach us much about the immune response potential of the antibody producer and of the nature of cross-reactivity and of the antigenic ligands but the analysis is difficult (Nau *et al.*, 1978), and the same end can often be accomplished by obtaining another serum specimen at a later date when the titer (and the cross-reactivity) has fallen. Cross-reactivity can occur even with monoclonal antibodies if a sequence in the ligand is common to two specificities.

Other manipulations of the cytotoxicity test, such as varying the initial time of cell–serum incubation or "sensitization period" (Kostyu *et al.*, 1979), or the addition of diluted antiglobulin (dos Reis *et al.*, 1972; Johnson *et al.*, 1972) to increase the sensitivity can be extremely useful in identification of the components of many sera. The development of monoclonal antibodies by hybridomas (Trucco *et al.*, 1978; Parham and Bodmer, 1978; Barnstable *et al.*, 1978*a*) will undoubtedly increase our knowledge of the MHC antigens, but it will not abolish the problems of cross-reactivity (Lemke *et al.*, 1978).

## *Tissue Distribution*

The HLA-A and -B antigens have been found on all nucleated cells examined, including lymphocytes, platelets, granulocytes, monocytes, neutrophils, basophils, eosinophils, cultured cells, fibroblasts, spleen and heart, liver, lung, intestine, kidney (Amos and Ward, 1975; Albert and Götze, 1977), and endothelial cells (Moraes and Stastny, 1975; Gibofsky et al., 1975). The most thoroughly studied cells are the lymphocytes, which appear to have $10^3-10^4$ HLA molecules per specificity per cell (Sanderson and Welsh, 1974; Giphart et al., 1975; Dumble and Whittingham, 1975). Cultured lymphoblastoid cell lines have 5–13 times as many HLA molecules as do peripheral blood lymphocytes (Papermaster et al., 1972; McCune et al., 1975).

Erythrocytes appear to have some HLA antigens, but the quantity is very low and only detectable on the autoanalyzer (Seaman et al., 1967; Doughty et al., 1973; Nordhagen and Orjasaeter, 1974); conceivably those antigens that are present are restricted to the reticulocyte or are, as in the case of Lewis antigen, adsorbed. Morton and co-workers (1971) have shown that three Bennett–Goodspeed antigens are either HLA antigens or are highly correlated with them, e.g., $Bg^a$ with HLA-B7, $Bg^b$ with HLA-B17, and $Bg^c$ with HLA-A28.

HLA-A and -B have also been detected in saliva, plasma, and serum (Billing et al., 1977; Pellegrino et al., 1974; Albert and Götze, 1977), urine Reisfeld et al., 1977; Bernier et al., 1976), seminal plasma (Singal et al., 1971; Mittal, 1975), and colostrum and milk (Dawson et al., 1974; Kachru and Mittal, 1975). The exact time of appearance of the antigens during development is unknown, but they were present on the youngest (6-week) fetus tested (Seigler and Metzgar, 1970; Mattiuz et al., 1973). The placenta appears to be rich in HLA (Bruning et al., 1964; Faulk and Temple, 1976), but not the trophoblast, the only component of the placenta in direct contact with maternal tissues (Faulk et al., 1977). Tumors originating from some fetal membranes, e.g., chorion, do express HLA (Loke et al., 1971).

Although most tissues have HLA as shown by absorption or direct testing, the amount varies greatly. Little detailed information is available as most of the studies were performed before highly specific antisera became available and when the existence of HLA-C and HLA-DR was unknown. Further, it seems unlikely that all of the cells in a complex tissue carry equivalent amounts of antigen and the contribution of contaminating lymphocytes and vascular endothelial cells to antigenicity was not often assessed.

The HLA antigens are usually codominantly expressed, the amount being a function of the regulation of the structural gene activity in the particular tissue (the location of the regulator genes is unknown). There are, however, some interesting exceptions. There is reported to be enhanced expression of $\beta_2$-microglobulin and HLA on cells treated with interferon (Heron *et al.*, 1978). Duquesnoy and co-workers (1977; Aster *et al.*, 1977) and others (Dausset *et al.*, 1970; Svejgaard *et al.*, 1970) have found that some normal individuals expressing HLA-B12, Bw4, or Bw6 on their lymphocytes lack the antigens on their platelets. While some have reported the haploid expression of HLA-A, -B, and -DR antigens on sperm (Halim *et al.*, 1974), others are sceptical; $\beta_2$-microglobulin is present (Fellous *et al.*, 1976). Other rare but important anomalies have been found. Van Rood and his colleagues (Van Rood *et al.*, 1977*b*; Schurmann *et al.*, 1979) describe in a Turkish family two children with severe hypogammaglobulinemia. Both children lacked HLA antigens on lymphocytes, platelets, and uncultured fibroblasts. A similar finding was described by Betuel and co-workers (1978). Mayr found antigens in three children which were absent from the mother but expressed on the somatic tissues of their maternal grandmother. Gonadal mosaicism was suspected in the mother (Mayr *et al.*, 1979). Mosaicism of another type or chimerism, was reported by Ceppellini (1971). His subject, who had severe juvenile diabetes among a number of other abnormalities, had both HLA haplotypes of both parents and thus resembled the tetraparental mice of Mintz (1971). HLA-A, -B, and -C deficiency secondary to absence of $\beta_2$-microglobulin, is observed on occasional tissue culture lines, e.g., Daudi (Poulik *et al.*, 1974; Arce-Gomez *et al.*, 1978).

## Biochemistry

The HLA-A and -B molecules, figuratively shown in Figure 4, are transmembrane glycoproteins of molecular weight 44,000 (gp44) existing independently in the lipid bilayer (Barnstable *et al.*, 1978*b*; Walsh and Crumpton, 1977). They are noncovalently bound to $\beta_2$-microglobulin, a small polypeptide of molecular weight 11,500 which by sequence and intrachain disulfide bridge structure is homologous with a single domain of immunoglobulin (Cunningham and Berggard, 1974; Peterson *et al.*, 1972). The 44,000-molecular-weight chain carries the serologically detected antigens (HLA-A, -B, or -C) and is coded by a gene(s) within the HLA complex on chromosome 6. $\beta_2$m is determined by a gene on the 15th chromosome (Goodfellow *et al.*, 1975; Zeuthen *et al.*, 1977).

Detailed structural studies and amino acid sequencing of the A and

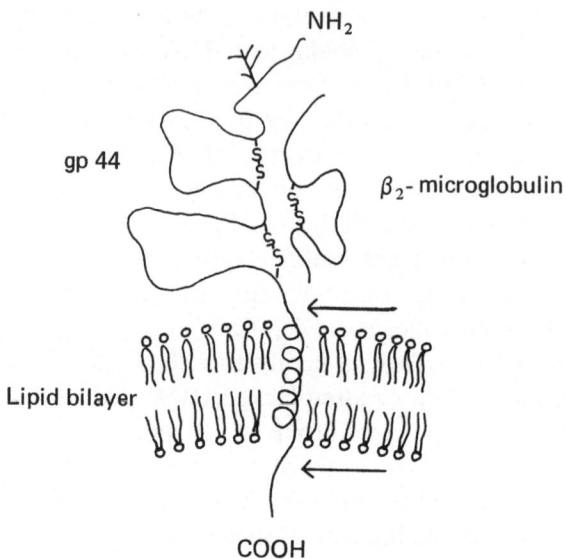

Fig. 4. A schematic drawing of the HLA-A, B, and C molecule. The arrows designate papain cleavage sites.

B molecules suggest that there is a strongly hydrophilic, intracellular C terminal end, a short hydrophobic segment responsible for membrane insertion, and a long extracellular segment (Springer and Strominger, 1976; Terhorst et al., 1976; Pober et al., 1978). The HLA molecule carries a carbohydrate side chain of molecular weight 3000 which does not show any antigenic properties or heterogeneity (Parham et al., 1977; Terhorst et al., 1976). HLA-A and -B antigens have been isolated by a variety of different procedures. Detergent solubilization (Springer et al., 1974; Dawson, 1976; Cresswell and Dawson, 1975; Springer and Strominger, 1976) and papain solubilization, taking advantage of a papain-sensitive site close to the membrane (Cresswell et al., 1973, 1974; Turner et al., 1975) give the most consistent yields.

The amino acid composition of purified HLA molecules of different A or B specificity have shown a high degree of similarity (Terhorst et al., 1976; Tanigaki et al., 1975; Bridgon et al., 1976). Sequencing shows that approximately 13 of the first 20 N-terminal residues are constant (Allison et al., 1978a). Papain-solubilized antigens contain four half-cystine residues, with a fifth present in detergent-solubilized preparations (Terhorst et al., 1976). The cystines suggest that the molecule may be structured into two domains, similar to immunoglobulins, although no cysteines have been found within the first 40 positions. Other data on internal sequencing around the cysteines suggest that the immunoglobulin homology may hold up (Robb *et al.*, 1978). Biochemical and amino acid sequence homology appear to confirm the theory that the A and B loci arose from a common ancestral gene by duplication (Bodmer, 1972).

Reports on the biochemical analysis of the HLA-C antigens suggest that they have the same molecular weight as the A and B antigens (Rask *et al.*, 1974) and are also associated with $\beta_2$-microglobulin (Snary *et al.*, 1977*a*; Rask *et al.*, 1974). However, they are more easily degraded, more difficult to isolate, and the carbohydrate moiety is more heterogeneous (Snary *et al.*, 1977*a*; Barnstable *et al.*, 1978*b*). Because HLA-C products cannot be detected in many individuals nor have antibodies been made against them by planned immunization, Ferrara *et al.* (1978*b*) has suggested the existence of HLA-C null.

# HLA-D

When lymphocytes from two HLA-disparate individuals are cultured together for 5–7 days, a small number of lymphocytes are stimulated to undergo blast transformation and to proliferate (Hirschhorn *et al.*, 1963; Dupont *et al.*, 1976). This proliferation is easily quantitated by incorporation of [$^3$H]thymidine. This mixed lymphocyte response (MLR) was originally thought to be a reflection of histocompatibility at HLA-A and -B, since HLA-A and -B identical sibs usually will not "stimulate" each other in a mixed lymphocyte culture (MLC). However, the findings that a small number of HLA-A and -B identical sibs would stimulate in an MLC (Bach and Amos, 1967; Plate *et al.*, 1970; Eijsvoogel *et al.*, 1970) and some parent–child combinations which would not (Seigler *et al.*, 1971), led Yunis and Amos (1971) to postulate genes called MLR-S and MLR-R, linked to but separate from the HLA-A and HLA-B loci, which would determine reactivity in MLC. The MLR-S locus could be mapped close to HLA-B since stimulation by a recombinant was produced where there was a "B-end" difference but not by a difference at HLA-A. The existence of an MLR-S (stimulator) locus has been repeatedly confirmed by other investigators (Dupont *et al.*, 1976) and is now placed 0.8 cM to the left of HLA-B. Consistent with the A, B, C nomenclature, it is designated HLA-D. The 11 detectable HLA-D antigens, Dw1–Dw11, are definable only by MLR.

## Homozygous HLA-D Stimulator Cells and MLR Typing

In a two-way MLR both allogeneic populations are capable of responding. In the more usual one-way MLR, one population of lymphocytes is inactivated by treatment with mitomycin C or $\gamma$- or X-irradiation (Bach and Bach, 1972), usually denoted by the subscript m or x. A simple MLC between individuals A and B would be set up as shown in Figure 5. After 5–6 days, a radioactive label, usually [³H]thymidine, is added and the cells are "harvested" 12–24 hr later. The amount of [³H]thymidine incorporated is a reflection of the extent of cellular proliferation, and gives some measure of genetic distance. HLA identical siblings fail to stimulate

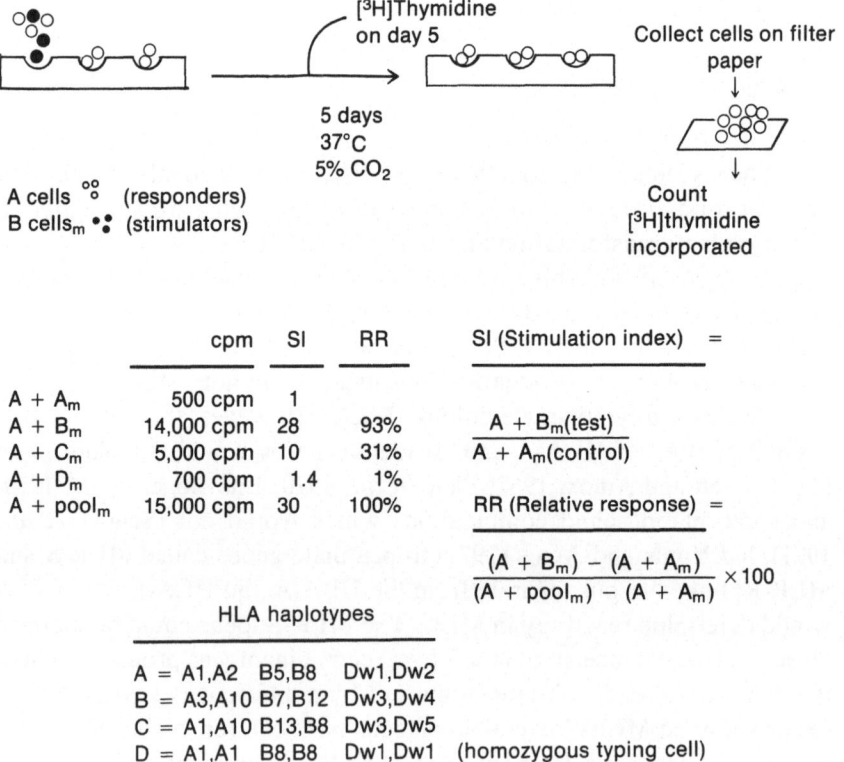

|          | cpm        | SI  | RR   |
|----------|-----------|-----|------|
| A + A_m  | 500 cpm   | 1   |      |
| A + B_m  | 14,000 cpm | 28  | 93%  |
| A + C_m  | 5,000 cpm | 10  | 31%  |
| A + D_m  | 700 cpm   | 1.4 | 1%   |
| A + pool_m | 15,000 cpm | 30  | 100% |

SI (Stimulation index) $=$

$$\dfrac{A + B_m(\text{test})}{A + A_m(\text{control})}$$

RR (Relative response) $=$

$$\dfrac{(A + B_m) - (A + A_m)}{(A + pool_m) - (A + A_m)} \times 100$$

HLA haplotypes

A = A1,A2  B5,B8   Dw1,Dw2
B = A3,A10 B7,B12  Dw3,Dw4
C = A1,A10 B13,B8  Dw3,Dw5
D = A1,A1  B8,B8   Dw1,Dw1  (homozygous typing cell)

Fig. 5. Procedure for a mixed lymphocyte culture (MLC).

while pairs differing at both haplotypes on the average give stronger stimulation than pairs differing by only one haplotype.

Early studies could only describe the relationship of individuals within a nuclear family. Mixtures of cells from unrelated individuals from outbred populations almost invariably gave strong stimulation. Since the number of alleles appeared to be very large and HLA-D alleles are codominantly expressed, no definition of alleles in a heterogeneous population was possible. The finding that some individuals in a more homogeneous population as in many geographic isolates failed to stimulate, especially if they were phenotypically identical for the HLA-A and -B alleles, led to the realization that lymphocytes from HLA-D homozygotes could provide reference standards (van den Tweel et al., 1973; Jorgensen et al., 1973). Children from first-cousin marriages have an appreciable chance of inheriting two copies of the same HLA haplotype from one of the great grandparents. Such homozygotes can provide cells for "typing" other family members, members of other families, and even unrelated panels (Bradley et al., 1973; van den Tweel et al., 1973). Unfortunately, homozygotes inheriting two copies of the same haplotype from a known common ancestor are rare. Most typing cells are selected by screening the MLR capacity of individuals homozygous for HLA-B. This approach has been successful in a number of instances because of the linkage disequilibrium between HLA-B and HLA-D.

HLA-D typing is, however, not a simple procedure. There appear to be at least three main sources of difficulty, one technical, one immunological, and the other due to the genetic complexity of HLA-D. There are many sources of technical error. Cell density, minor variations in temperature, and of pH during culture, contamination of lymphocyte cultures with polys, and the composition of the medium (especially in the serum needed to support proliferation), and sensitivity to the antibiotics added to prevent contamination can all affect the response. Immunological complexities are legion. The reaction itself is believed to be a consequence of the proliferation of helper T cells in response to stimulator B cells (Lohrmann et al., 1974; Kuntz et al., 1976). The proportion of B cells in the stimulator population may thus be critical. The responder population includes helper and suppressor cells; lymphocyte activation leads to the production of a variety of lymphokines which can themselves induce or suppress proliferation (Janis et al., 1970; Jorgensen et al., 1974; Sasazuki et al., 1976). Granulocytes can depress (Mardiney et al., 1972; Ragab and Cowan, 1973) the response. Under certain conditions cytotoxic effector cells are generated and these cells also incorporate thymidine in their proliferation (Kristensen and Jorgensen, 1978). Thus the thymidine uptake only gives a measure of the overall reactivity of a complex mixture of reactions by different cell types. Lymphocytes from a single subject alone or after mixing with autologous cells manipulated by X-irradiation or mitomycin and washing, have a very variable "spontaneous" level of incorporation which may be quite high (Vande-Stouwe et al., 1977). Finally there are major fluctuations in the responsiveness of cells from an individual collected on different occasions.

To compensate for these many sources of variability, a number of technical precautions are required and certain special conventions have been adopted in data processing. The test conditions are standardized as far as possible and all determinations are made at least in triplicate and often at more than one time point. Results can be expressed as raw counts per minute (cpm), or occasionally converted to disintegrations per minute (dpm), per unit number of responding cells, or in the form of a ratio, e.g., a stimulation index (SI), or relative response (RR) (see Fig. 5).

Stimulator cells from some donors are almost always more stimulatory than cells from other individuals, also some responders are always more reactive. To conpensate for this, the data may be double normalized, averaging the sum of all responses of the cell, first as stimulator, then as responder (Ryder et al., 1975; Mendell et al., 1978); a similar method is an interaction index (Mickey et al., 1975). Such procedures are only possible when a large matrix of tests is performed and, optimally, when each cell in the panel serves as stimulator of all others and responder to all others. Other methods which have been used are cluster analysis (Piazza and Galfre, 1975; Mendell et al., 1977), the kurtosis statistic (Mendell et al., 1977), and specific analyses of homozygous typing cells (Jensen et al., 1977).

Even with such elaborate precautions only a proportion of HTC give ideal reactions. An ideal reaction is one in which the HTC fails to stimulate cells carrying the same HLA-D antigen as the HTC, but will strongly stimulate all cells which do not carry the HLA-D allele. There should be no overlap in values between responders and nonresponders. Some stimulator cells do behave in this manner. There are, however, well-documented exceptions which implicate the genetic complexity of HLA-D.

There is evidence for subdivision of the D antigens as has been found with the HLA-A and -B antigens (van den Berg-Loonen, 1977; Suciu-Foca et al., 1978b). Several closely linked loci may be found in the HLA-

D region (Fuller *et al.*, 1978; Kallen *et al.*, 1977; Hsu *et al.*, 1977; Suciu-Foca *et al.*, 1978*b*), and some of these may elicit suppression (Hirschberg and Thorsby, 1977; Hanes *et al.*, 1978). A separate MLR-S locus, possibly adjacent to HLA-A, has been reported to induce weak stimulation (Dupont *et al.*, 1975; Suciu-Foca and Dausset, 1975; Bijnen *et al.*, 1977; Johnson *et al.*, 1975; Eijsvoogel *et al.*, 1972; Thorsby *et al.*, 1973). Histocompatibility antigens not linked to HLA may also be able to trigger a slight MLC response; the MLS system in the mouse is an example of a non-MHC-linked MLR-S locus (Festenstein, 1976).

   HLA-D typing is currently limited because of the large number of stimulator reference cells necessary for the determination of an HLA-D type and because of the scarcity of homozygous individuals (especially those with low-frequency D alleles). HLA-D typing performed with human lymphoblastoid cell lines derived from HTCs may at some future time alleviate this problem (Gatti and Leibold, 1979) but high levels of nonspecific stimulation by cell lines have been frequently encountered (Bauscher and Smith, 1973). A more unusual method of D typing is that of sperm lymphocyte culture (SLC) (Festenstein and Halim, 1977).

## Tissue Distribution

   The D antigens are by definition expressed on cells which will stimulate in MLC. These include B lymphocytes and B-cell lymphoblastoid cell lines (Lohrman *et al.*, 1974; Han *et al.*, 1977; Corley *et al.*, 1976; Bausher and Smith, 1973), epidermal cells (Hirschberg and Thorsby, 1975), probably Langerhans cells (Thorsby *et al.*, 1977), monocytes and macrophages (Kaakinen and Hirschberg, 1977), endothelial cells (Hirschberg *et al.*, 1974), and spermatozoa (Festenstein and Halim, 1977), although for the most part genetic studies have been restricted to lymphocytes. Subcellular fractions of cell lines will stimulate (Corley *et al.*, 1975). Cells which do not stimulate in MLR include erythrocytes and platelets (Bain *et al.*, 1964), fibroblasts, neutrophils (Bain and Pshyk, 1972), and, questionably, T cells (Sondel *et al.*, 1975).

   For more complete listings of source articles on the MLR, reference is made to specialized reviews (Sorensen, 1972; Dupont *et al.*, 1976; Bach and Bach, 1974; Bradley and Festenstein, 1978; Thorsby, 1974; Nabholtz and Miggiano, 1978).

## Primed Lymphocyte Typing (PLT)

A primed MLR response is based on the observation that lymphocytes primed in culture will proliferate more rapidly upon secondary culture with the original stimulating cell, e.g., will reach a peak response at
24–48 hr instead of 120–148 hr. Primed lymphocyte typing, or PLT
(Sheehy and Bach, 1976; Mawas *et al.*, 1975; Fradelizi and Dausset, 1975)
allows a lymphocyte population to be primed to a selected D specificity,
then retested against a panel of test lymphocytes. Those individuals stimulating a secondary response must then carry the same D allele(s) as the
original stimulating cell. For example, a father (Dw1/Dw2) stimulated with
his daughter (Dw1/Dw3), can be primed to give a PLT response only to
cells carrying Dw3. Similarly, priming can be used to generate a PLT
detecting "X," a previously unknown specificity.

|  MLR combination  | | Specificity of |
| --- | --- | --- |
| Responding cell | Stimulating cell | PLT response |
| Father Dw1/Dw2 | Daugher Dw1/Dw3 | Dw3 |
| Father Dw1/Dw2 | Son Dw1/"X" | "X" |

It should be noted that the PLT and the MLR test for HLA-D operate
in opposite directions. A typing response in MLR is a *lack* of response;
a typing response in PLT is an *accelerated* and possibly an augmented
response. While the PLT and MLR both detect specificities on the HLA
haplotype and there is a high correlation between them, it is not entirely
certain that they detect the same elements (Termijtelen *et al.*, 1977; Thomsen *et al.*, 1976; Wank *et al.*, 1977; Bach *et al.*, 1977; Fradelizi *et al.*,
1976; Sasportes *et al.*, 1978; Bradley *et al.*, 1977; Alter *et al.*, 1977; Hartzman *et al.*, 1978).

## CELL-MEDIATED LYMPHOLYSIS (CML)

In addition to the strong proliferative response of T helper cells in
an MLR, a second proliferative response leads to the generation of specific cytotoxic effector lymphocytes (CTLs) (Bach *et al.*, 1976; Kristensen, 1978). The ability of these cells to specifically lyse cells against which
they are primed, as well as other cells which share the same "target"

antigens, is measured in a cell-mediated lympholysis or CML assay. The responding cell population after a 6-day MLR is added directly to $^{51}$Cr-labeled target cells, with the release of $^{51}$Cr after 4 hr a sensitive indicator of cell death (Long *et al.*, 1976). The CTLs generated and studied *in vitro* are probably the same cells responsible for cell-mediated immunity *in vivo* and therefore are directly concerned with allograft rejection and graft-versus-host reactions. The specificity of a CTL is consequently of much interest.

From studies in the mouse, the apparent "target" of CTLs produced against allogeneic lymphocytes was either an H-2D or H-2K molecule, and initial studies in man attempted to demonstrate similar specificity, e.g., for HLA-A or B. Eijsvoogel *et al.* (1973) described an unusual family which included two recombinants. By skillful manipulation, they were able to show that specificity for killing resided with the HLA-B portion of the recombinant haplotype. Ward *et al.* (1969) studied skin graft rejection in three cases of recombinants within the HLA region. In two instances the most rapid rejection was with an HLA-B incompatibility (Ward *et al.*, 1969; Yunis *et al.*, 1973) and in one with the HLA-A end (Ward and Seigler, 1973). *In vitro* experiments by Robinson *et al.* (1978) attest to the specificity of CTL against human targets. They were able to generate CTL that could discriminate between HLA-Bw51 and Bw52; indeed, they were later able to identify an HLA-B5 cell as neither Bw51 nor Bw52 and have the atypical cell independently confirmed as a new specificity recognized by Payne *et al.* (1978) as B5.y. Goulmy and co-workers have described a female patient who had rejected a bone marrow graft from an HLA-identical brother; her CTLs killed cells from A2$^+$ individuals but only those from males, (Goulmy *et al.*, 1977). However, examples such as these are unique, despite attempts to develop other CTLs with such precise specificity (Mawas *et al.*, 1973; Geha *et al.*, 1977; Kristensen and Grunnet, 1975; Mowas *et al.*, 1976; Schendel *et al.*, 1978; Grunnet *et al.*, 1976; Sondel and Bach, 1975; Goulmy *et al.*, 1976). Many of these failures are attributable to multiple antigenic differences between stimulating and responding cells, or to an inability to detect subtle HLA antigenic variants with existing antisera. Even when the A and B locus antigens are carefully matched, HLA-C or other markers may not have been identifiable and could contribute to undetected incompatibility at these antigens.

An alternative hypothesis was raised by Yunis and Amos, who suggested that a new locus, HDR, closely linked to but separate from HLA-

B, could be responsible for stimulating cytotoxic or skin-graft reactivity (Yunis and Amos, 1971; Long *et al.*, 1976). This locus would be analogous to HLA-D and could bear the same relationship to other loci in the HLA complex as HLA-D does to HLA-DR. Even in cases such as that of Schendel, where no relationship to any known HLA could account for variations in sensitivity to lysis, reactivity segregated with the HLA hap-lotype in families (Schendel *et al.*, 1978). Possibly the B locus antigens alone can provide cytotoxic sensitization, or HDR in linkage disequili-brium with B locus antigens or a grid involving several structures will eventually be identified (see also p. 177).

## HLA-DR

While miniaturization of the MLC test and improved methods of isolating and freezing lymphocytes have helped improve HLA-D typing, the procedure is still expensive, time consuming, and subject to consid-erable variability. Consequently, there has been a strong impetus to de-velop nonbiological procedures for HLA-D. Van Rood and his colleagues, struck by observations from their and other laboratories that some sera from multipara would specifically block an MLR, showed by fluores-cence that the blocking sera reacted specifically with only a small pro-portion of cells from the stimulating donor (van Leeuwen *et al.*, 1973). These observations and similar findings from other laboratories (reviewed in Walford, 1977) soon led to reliable serological procedures for detecting the antigens of the stimulating cell. This stimulator cell turned out to be the B lymphocyte, but the antigens detected by the antisera are probably not HLA-D. However, since their distribution is very similar to HLA-D they are classed as D-related or DR.

### HLA-DR Typing

During the 1977 Histocompatibility Testing Workshop, seven HLA-DR specificities were provisionally defined corresponding in their pop-ulation distribution in Caucasians to Dw1–7 (Bodmer *et al.*, 1978*b*). As with antisera to the HLA-A, -B, -C antigens, the sera used to detect DR specificities come from planned immunization and pregnancy. Conse-quently, many of them also contain antibodies to the A, B, or C locus products and must be made specific for B cells by absorption with platelets (van Rood *et al.*, 1975a). Since it may take the platelets from many milliliters of blood to absorb 1 ml of serum for use in DR typing (especially where the HLA-A, -B, -C titer is high), other sources of reagent are being sought. A few individuals known to have had circulating antibodies to A or B locus antigens have lost this reactivity with time while still retaining activity to DR antigens. Immunization of rabbits with B lymphocytes results in antisera with allospecificity (Cresswell and Geier, 1975; Welsh and Turner, 1976; Klareskog *et al.*, 1978), but these reagents as presently prepared require even more extensive absorption to make them specific. More recently, immunization with highly purified, solubilized antigen has given sera with allospecificity requiring very little absorption. With increasing ability to orient and protect the antigen against proteolytic digestion, as by the use of specially prepared beads (Cresswell, 1979), the immunization of primates (Liberi, 1978), rabbits, or the production of HLA antibodies in mouse hybridomas (Parham and Bodmer, 1978) would appear to be the procedure of the future.

Two basic cytotoxicity assays are used for DR typing. One is a two-dye immunofluorescence assay on peripheral blood lymphocytes developed by van Rood (van Rood *et al.*, 1976). In this method, which does not require the separation of B from T cells, B lymphocytes are labeled with an FITC-coupled antiimmunoglobulin. The cells are then exposed to serum and complement, and the dead cells are stained with ethidium bromide. The reactions can be monitored by using a filter allowing red (ethidium bromide) and green (FITC-anti-IgG) fluorescence to be observed simultaneously.

A second approach is a direct cytotoxicity assay using a B-cell-enriched population and B-cell-specific antisera. Since B cells represent only 10–20% of the total of peripheral blood mononuclear cells, the rest being mainly monocytes and T cells, it is desirable for two reasons to remove non-B cells. The most obvious reason for enrichment is to have a uniformly sensitive population for ease of reading, especially necessary for weak sera. There is a second, more subtle reason. Some of the reagents now in use are unreliable if the enriched population contains less than 85% B cells (Zmijewski *et al.*, 1977). The cause of the difficulty is not completely clear, but it seems probable that some human T cells, like some mouse T cells, have low numbers of B cell antigens on their surfaces. The presence of monocytes, which may comprise up to 40% of T-cell-depleted populations (Moraes *et al.*, 1975), can also significantly affect typing. The enrichment procedure should therefore ideally produce over 90% B cells.

Several methods of enrichment are practical. Since T cells specifically rosette with sheep erythrocytes, the addition of sheep erythrocytes to peripheral blood lymphocyte preparations, followed by centrifugation on Ficoll–Hypaque, will sediment the T cells and leave a nearly pure B cell layer (Mendes *et al.*, 1973). The rosetting procedure is most successful when the sheep red blood cells are treated with papain (Wilson *et al.*, 1975) or neuraminidase (Ting *et al.*, 1976).

In another procedure, the crude lymphocyte suspension is absorbed onto Ig-coated sheep erythrocyte monolayers. A different, but also DR-positive, population is absorbable onto a plastic surface previously coated with affinity-purified rabbit or goat anti-human (Fab')$_2$ (Grier *et al.*, 1977). In the first case, Fc positive cells adhere to the antibody–antigen complex on the monolayer; in the second, only SIg ( + ) cells will stick. In both cases the T cells are easily washed off and the Fc-positive or SIg-positive cells are eluted with whole human serum. The detection system for identifying DR antigens in an enriched population is through a modified cytotoxicity test. The major modifications are that the complement used must be very carefully selected to avoid cytolysis by naturally occurring xenoantibodies in the rabbit serum, and the incubation times are (arbitrarily) lengthened. This latter step was occasioned by the weak reactivity of many of the earlier sera; as stronger sera became available incubation times are being decreased and one peculiar problem of B-cell typing, overlysis, is thereby being eliminated.

Other methods which have been used include indirect immunofluorescence (van Leeuwen *et al.*, 1975), blockage of the Fc receptor with B-cell antisera to inhibit the formation of rosettes with antibody-coated sheep erythrocytes (Carpenter *et al.*, 1975; Solheim *et al.*, 1976), and capping of the SD determinants (i.e., HLA-A, -B, and -C) with anti-$\beta_2$-microglobulin (Bernoco *et al.*, 1976; Hunter *et al.*, 1978).

## Tissue Distribution

The DR molecules are expressed on B lymphocytes and B cell lymphoblastoid cell lines (Kissmeyer-Nielsen, 1975; Bodmer, 1978*b*; Halper *et al.*, 1978; Winchester *et al.*, 1977), macrophages (Moraes *et al.*, 1977; Albrechtson, 1977; Snary *et al.*, 1977*b*), epidermal cells, especially cells of Langerhans (Klareskog *et al.*, 1977*b*), monocytes (Cicciarelli *et al.*, 1978), endothelial cells (Moraes *et al.*, 1977) and sperm (Kamoun *et al.*, 1977). They are not present on platelets (van Rood *et al.*, 1975*a*), nor probably K cells (Kovithavongs *et al.*, 1978): they may be present on some "activated" T cells (Suciu-Foca *et al.*, 1978*a*; Albrechtsen *et al.*, 1977; Fu *et al.*, 1978). Variant cell lines such as Daudi which do not bear HLA-A, -B, or -C antigens, nor possess β$_2$-microglobulin, nevertheless express HLA-DR (Pious *et al.*, 1974). The HLA-deficient cells previously referred to gave equivocal results when tested for DR antigens. DR antigens are readily detected on cells from most patients with chronic lymphocytic leukemia (Walford *et al.*, 1975), on many patients with combined immunodeficiency disease and in some forms of myelocytic leukemia (Cline and Billing, 1977), and also on cultured malignant melanoma cell lines (Winchester *et al.*, 1978).

## *Serology*

Typing for HLA-DR is in its infancy and the Joint Report issued after the 1977 Histocompatibility Testing Workshop, in which seven DR antigens were defined, gives only an approximation of the probable complexity of DR specificities. Technical problems and ill-defined sera give results reminiscent of those of the early days of HLA-A, -B and -C. With more standard protocols, more precise serum characterization, suitable absorptions, and population studies, the number of DR antigens and the precision of their definition are sure to increase.

It is not yet clear whether typing for DR will provide a speedy alternative to the MLR. To some extent, this will depend upon the type of information required. The correspondence between DR and D is close, so in the great majority of (Caucasian) individuals, D and DR alleles coincide (Bodmer *et al.*, 1978*a,b*). Clear exceptions, though, have been noted (Hartzman *et al.*, 1978; Suciu-Foca *et al.*, 1978*b*). There is strong evidence for another DR-like locus segregating at the A end of the haplotype in recombinants (Mann *et al.*, 1976*a*; Johnson *et al.*, 1977). The B-cell system "Merritt" of Walford has 22 antigens defined by two loci, one near HLA-D and the other possibly near HLA-A (Walford, 1977; Naeim *et al.*, 1978). Two B-cell loci have also been described by Ting *et al.* (1976) and van Rood *et al.* (1975*b*, 1977*a*). Tosi *et al.* (1978) have shown by specific binding assays and immunochemical analysis the existence on the Daudi cell line of two molecules, DRw6 and DC-1, which are controlled by separate HLA-linked loci. Furthermore, there is evidence of B-cell systems unlinked to HLA (Legrand and Dausset, 1975b; Mann et al., 1976b). A similar situation is known for the mouse Ia genes, which are in both the I-A and IC-E regions of H-2.

## Biochemistry

DR molecules are also integral membrane proteins, consisting of two noncovalently bound glycoprotein chains, one a 33,000-molecular-weight and the other a 28,000-molecular-weight chain, forming a 61,000-molecular-weight complex (gp 28,33) (Cresswell, 1977; Snary et al., 1977b; Springer et al., 1977b; Klareskog et al., 1977a) (Fig. 6). Both polypeptides are thought to span the membrane (Barnstable et al., 1978b). Antigenic specificity is thought to reside in the protein rather than the carbohydrate portion of the molecule (Snary et al., 1976), although a glycolipid substance with Ia-like antigenicity has been isolated from urine and cells in the mouse (Parish et al., 1978). B-cell antigens appear to be shed spon-

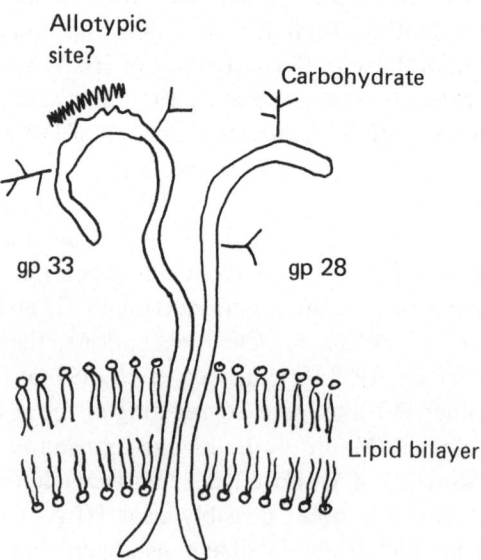

Fig. 6. A schematic drawing of the HLA-DR molecule (modified from Barnstable et al., 1978b).

taneously into the medium, whereas HLA-A and B are not (Wernet *et al.*, 1975), although HLA antigens are detectable in low concentrations in serum, HLA-A9 being present in greatest concentration (Reisfeld *et al.*, 1977).

Sequencing has shown that in comparison with the murine equivalent, the Ia antigens, the first six of nine positions sequenced in the larger chain are identical, while no homology has been found to date between the murine and human 28,000-molecular-weight chains (Allison *et al.*, 1978*b*; Springer *et al.*, 1977*a*). Control of the 28,000-molecular-weight chain by a chromosome other than number 6 has been reported from cell fusion studies; it appears to be nonpolymorphic (Barnstable *et al.*, 1976).

## POPULATION GENETICS

While our knowledge of the HLA antigens is still far from complete, HLA typing is already one of the most powerful tools for the study of population genetics. This is due to the highly polymorphic nature of HLA as well as to the linkage disequilibria characteristic of HLA. It is not possible to describe in detail the many populations studied; reference will be made to general trends giving source materials and to some highlights, sometimes of microcosms.

Some studies have been highly imaginative, such as those leading to the deduction of the haplotypes of a Tuareg leader of the 17th century (Colombani *et al.*, 1973*b*), and some have led to rather desperate and uncomfortable adventures such as those of Albert *et al.* (1973), who lost much of their equipment over a precipice in Nepal, or of MacQueen *et al.* (1978), who stored their reagents in the ice of a semiderelict fishing boat to preserve them on her trip to Mauki in the South Pacific, or of Corley and Spees (1973) in a remote Ixil village in Guatemala where electricity only flowed for an hour at noon to supply the mayor's radio and at night to power the solitary street light. More prosaic was the characterization of Tibetans, not in the wilds of Tibet but in the less arduous setting of Switzerland where the Dalai Lama and his followers had sought refuge, but did not escape the needles of Jeannet (Jeannet *et al.*, 1973).

Generalities can be made about the major ethnic divisions, Caucasian, Black African, American Indian, Oriental, Oceanian (Melanesian and Polynesian) (Dausset and Colombani, 1973; Kissmeyer-Nielsen, 1975;

Bodmer and Bodmer, 1978). Some HLA antigens are found in nearly all populations studied, e.g., HLA-A2 and Bw35, while others are restricted to only some ethnic groups. Some, such as A1, A3, and B8, are frequent in Caucasians and Blacks, but are very rare in Orientals. Some (HLA-Aw43 and Bw42) are found only in Black populations. Orientals have increased frequencies of A9, B5, and B40 and American Indians of A2, A9, Aw31, and Bw35. Many of the newer HLA antigens (Aw43, Bw47, Bw53) have been characterized only through the studies of non-Caucasian ethnic groups in which unusual specificities are common. Current gene frequencies of HLA-A, -B, -C, -D and -DR, compiled from the 1977 Histocompatibility Workshop, are given in Table IV.

Until very recently, almost all studies were conducted with antisera raised in Caucasian donors against Caucasian lymphocytes. The development of HLA typing in Japan and Malaysia, India, the U.S.S.R., Africa, and Latin America, using local as well as shared reagents, will add greatly to our knowledge of the distribution of HLA antigens and will thus refine our information about the prehistoric migrations of peoples. Menozzi *et al.* (1978) have recently combined HLA and non-HLA gene frequencies to plot synthetic maps of Europe and compare these with the growth and spread of populations in the early European farming period. An even more imaginative but unconvincing attempt has been made to characterize the antigens of Peruvian mummies (Stastny, 1974). Future studies will give clearer indications of genetic drift, of the extent of consanguinity, and of tribal and racial intermarriage than has been possible with the lesser polymorphisms of other genetic markers.

Examination of the HLA antigens in many diverse populations has emphasized the extraordinary polymorphisms of the A, B, C, D, and DR loci. More than 300,000,000 genetically different individuals could be expected on the basis of existing HLA alleles; of these, 30,000,000 individuals would be antigenically distinguishable (Bodmer and Bodmer, 1978).

Obviously, the differences must have arisen by mutation. We know nothing about "hot spots" as far as HLA is concerned, but "hot spots" have been demonstrated in the mouse. Of 22 known mutants (observed under laboratory conditions), not less than 11 originated from a single allele, $H-2K^b$. Similarly, recombination within the H-2 complex appears to be nonrandom, crossing over (or gene conversion, we cannot really distinguish between them) appears to be highest where the mother is a $H-2^b \times H-2^dF_1$ hybrid and lowest with $H-2^b \times H-2^k$. The only HLA "mutants" described to date resulted in the loss of expression of the

TABLE IV. HLA-A, B, C, D, and DR Gene Frequencies[a]

| | European Caucasians | N. American Caucasians | American Blacks | African Blacks | Japanese | American Indians |
|---|---|---|---|---|---|---|
| HLA-A | (228)[b] | (290) | (128) | (102) | (195) | (89) |
| A1 | 15.8 | 16.1 | 8.1 | 3.9 | 1.2 | 2.5 |
| A2 | 27.0 | 28.0 | 16.3 | 9.4 | 25.3 | 45.3 |
| A3 | 12.6 | 14.1 | 7.0 | 6.4 | 0.7 | 0.6 |
| Aw23 } A9 | 2.4 | 1.9 | 10.6 | 10.8 | 37.2 | 23.2 |
| Aw24 } A9 | 8.8 | 7.3 | 5.1 | 2.4 | | |
| A25 } A10 | 2.0 | 2.6 | 0.4 | 3.5 | 12.7 | 0.6 |
| A26 } A10 | 3.9 | 3.4 | 2.3 | 4.5 | | |
| A11 | 5.1 | 5.1 | 2.8 | — | 6.7 | — |
| A28 | 4.4 | 4.2 | 5.8 | 8.9 | — | 2.8 |
| A29 | 5.8 | 3.6 | 2.3 | 6.4 | 0.2 | 0.6 |
| Aw30 | 3.9 | 2.9 | 13.0 | 22.1 | 0.5 | 1.1 |
| Aw31 | 2.3 | 4.5 | 2.8 | 4.2 | 8.7 | 19.9 |
| Aw32 | 2.9 | 3.7 | 1.9 | 1.5 | 0.5 | 1.1 |
| Aw33 | 0.7 | 1.2 | 5.1 | 1.0 | 2.0 | 0.6 |
| Aw43 | —[c] | — | — | 4.0 | — | — |
| Blank | 2.2 | 1.3 | 16.5 | 11.0 | 4.2 | 1.8 |
| HLA-B | (228) | (290) | (128) | (102) | (195) | (89) |
| B5 | 5.9 | 5.9 | 4.9 | 3.0 | 20.9 | 14.0 |
| B7 | 10.4 | 10.5 | 12.6 | 7.3 | 7.1 | 0.6 |
| B8 | 9.2 | 10.4 | 5.5 | 7.1 | 0.2 | 1.7 |
| B12 | 16.6 | 13.8 | 14.0 | 12.7 | 6.5 | 1.7 |
| B13 | 3.2 | 2.6 | 0.4 | 1.5 | 0.8 | — |
| B14 | 2.4 | 5.1 | 4.6 | 3.6 | 0.5 | — |
| B18 | 6.2 | 3.1 | 3.6 | 2.0 | — | 0.6 |
| B27 | 4.6 | 5.6 | 0.8 | — | 0.3 | 6.2 |
| B15 | 4.8 | 5.9 | 4.7 | 3.0 | 9.3 | 13.7 |
| Bw38 } Bw16 | 2.0 | 2.5 | 0.4 | 1.5 | 1.8 | 14.5 |
| Bw39 } Bw16 | 3.5 | 1.4 | 0.4 | | 4.7 | |
| B17 | 5.7 | 4.9 | 11.2 | 16.1 | 0.6 | — |
| Bw21 | 2.2 | 3.8 | 4.4 | 1.5 | 1.5 | — |
| Bw22 | 3.6 | 2.3 | 3.9 | — | 6.5 | 0.6 |
| Bw35 | 9.9 | 8.6 | 12.5 | 7.2 | 9.4 | 22.1 |
| B37 | 1.1 | 1.7 | 1.2 | — | 0.8 | — |
| B40 | 8.1 | 9.2 | 3.9 | 2.0 | 21.8 | 16.6 |
| Bw41 | — | — | — | 1.5 | — | — |
| Bw42 | — | — | — | 12.3 | — | — |
| Blank | 3.6 | 2.8 | 11.0 | 17.9 | 7.6 | 7.8 |
| HLA-C | (321) | (271) | (107) | (101) | (203) | (89) |
| Cw1 | 4.8 | 3.7 | 1.9 | — | 11.1 | 10.1 |
| Cw2 | 5.4 | 6.0 | 9.2 | 11.4 | 1.4 | 4.6 |
| Cw3 | 9.4 | 11.4 | 8.8 | 5.5 | 16.3 | 16.6 |

(Continued)

TABLE IV. (*Continued*)

| | European Caucasians | N. American Caucasians | American Blacks | African Blacks | Japanese | American Indians |
|---|---|---|---|---|---|---|
| Cw4 | 12.6 | 10.2 | 12.9 | 14.2 | 4.3 | 23.4 |
| Cw5 | 8.4 | 5.2 | 1.4 | 1.0 | 1.2 | 1.1 |
| Cw6 | 12.6 | 11.3 | — | 17.7 | 2.1 | — |
| Blank | 46.7 | 52.1 | 65.8 | 50.2 | 53.5 | 44.2 |
| | | | | | | |
| HLA-D | (99) | (125) | | | | |
| Dw1 | 7.9 | 6.8 | | | | |
| Dw2 | 9.5 | 11.7 | | | | |
| Dw3 | 9.5 | 9.0 | | | | |
| Dw4 | 5.1 | 5.2 | | | | |
| Dw5 | 9.0 | 6.1 | | | | |
| Dw6 | 11.5 | 8.9 | | | | |
| Dw7 | 5.8 | 9.8 | | | | |
| Dw8 | 2.5 | 1.6 | | | | |
| Blank | 39.1 | 40.9 | | | | |
| | | | | | | |
| HLA-DR | (334) | (273) | (110) | (77) | (164) | (69) |
| DRw1 | 6.2 | 5.2 | 7.3 | — | 4.5 | — |
| DRw2 | 11.2 | 13.9 | 13.8 | 8.7 | 16.5 | 8.4 |
| DRw3 | 8.9 | 11.8 | 12.4 | 11.7 | — | 9.1 |
| DRw4 | 7.8 | 16.5 | 7.2 | 3.5 | 14.4 | 21.5 |
| DRw5 | 15.1 | 11.9 | 15.4 | 7.4 | 5.4 | 6.0 |
| DRw6 | 8.6 | 11.5 | 19.1 | 9.9 | 6.7 | 5.9 |
| DRw7 | 15.6 | 12.4 | 12.0 | 6.6 | — | 3.7 |
| WIA8 | 5.6 | 4.2 | 7.5 | 7.2 | 7.2 | 12.9 |
| Blank | 21.2 | 12.6 | 5.3 | 45.0 | 45.3 | 32.5 |

[a] From Bodmer *et al.* (1978*a*).
[b] Number of individuals typed.
[c] (—) indicates alleles not present.

antigens on lymphocytes, but not on fibroblasts, and so probably involve errors of regulation rather than mutation of a structural gene. It is tempting to speculate that the HLA hot spots will involve antigens of the HLA-B series and especially of the 4c CREG, since so many variants are known, even in American Indian populations where gene drift and inbreeding have reduced the heterozygosity of other loci. Attrition from increased susceptibility to infectious diseases, especially virus diseases where MHC interactions have been repeatedly demonstrated in mice and are now being documented for man, would be greatest in populations where the reservoir of potential response was small.

Alternatively and in a different line of reasoning, heterozygosity and variety may be important in maintaining maternal–fetal tolerance. Since the HLA-A, -B, -C, and -DR antigens are quite capable of eliciting antibodies, it would be possible for these antibodies to play a "blocking" role during fetal development and for the HLA-D alleles to induce local GVH reactions in the placenta and to inhibit massive cell migration by production of lymphokines.

Considering the phenomenal number of alleles at the HLA-A, -B, -C, -D, and -DR loci, one of the most unusual facets is the tendency for certain alleles at different loci to occur together more often on the same chromosome (haplotype) than what would be expected by chance. Such "linkage disequilibrium" is characteristic of particular HLA alleles. In Caucasians, the best known example is the A1, B8 haplotype. With the frequency of HLA-A1 at 0.17 and HLA-B8 at 0.11, the expected frequency of both occurring on a haplotype would be $0.17 \times 0.11$ or 0.019. The observed frequency, however, is 0.088. The difference between the observed and expected is a measure of the linkage disequilibrium between two alleles and is usually referred to as delta.

Examples of linkage disequilibrium are given in Table V. Other than A1-B8, the most frequent Caucasian haplotypes involving HLA-A and

TABLE V. Examples of Linkage Disequilibrium[a]

| HLA | European Caucasian | African Black | Japanese | American Indians |
|-----|-----|-----|-----|-----|
| B8-DRw3 | 440[b][c] | — | — | — |
| A29-B12 | 273* | — | — | — |
| B17-DRw6 | — | 420 | — | — |
| Aw24-B7 | — | — | 349* | — |
| B15-Cw1 | — | — | — | 676* |
| B17-Cw6 | 354* | 698* | — | — |
| B17-DRw7 | 238* | 238 | — | — |
| B40-Cw3 | 245* | — | 567* | 585* |
| Bw35-Cw4 | 842* | 557* | 105 | — |
| B12-Cw5 | 402* | — | — | 89* |
| A1-B8 | 572* | — | 25 | 108* |
| Bw22-Cw1 | 114* | — | 472* | — |

[a] Data from Bodmer et al. (1978a).
[b] $\Delta \times 10^4$.
[c] (*) Denotes $p < 0.001$.

-B are A3-B7, A2-Bw44, and A29-Bw44. Only about half of the known HLA-B alleles are in linkage disequilibrium with HLA-A, while all the HLA-C alleles are closely associated with HLA-B. Some are in linkage disequilibrium with several, e.g., Cw6 with B13, B17, and Bw37. Such examples are not restricted to known CREGs, e.g., Cw4 is usually found with Bw35 and not with Bw51 or Bw52 in Caucasians. Interestingly, linkage disequilibrium may be characteristic of only one population, e.g., Bw35-Cw4 in Caucasians, Bw35-Cw3 in Japanese, B7-Cw4 in African Blacks and B12-Cw4 in Brazilian Indians. HLA-DR and B alleles show much the same pattern. Dausset, in investigating the haplotypes of 53 French families for alleles at A, B, C, DR, Bf, C2, and Glo, found that linkage disequilibrium encompassed the whole distance from HLA-A to Glo, the strongest disequilibrium concerning the HLA-C to Bf, or C to DR, segment (Dausset *et al.*, 1978).

There have been innumerable arguments on the reasons for linkage disequilibrium—natural selection (Bodmer, 1972, 1973) or migration and admixture (lack of equilibration) (Degos and Dausset, 1974) being the most frequently advanced hypotheses. Lack of equilibration could account for HLA-B and C associations but is unlikely to account for all of the observed disequilibria between A–B and B–DR. It may well be that, as pointed out by Thomson (1977), linkage disequilibrium between HLA loci is the result of selection operating not on A, B, C directly, but on other closely linked loci. The linked ''selected'' loci might well be immune response genes. Such genes are being identified in the mouse H-2 region, with presumptive evidence of them in man.

## THE HLA "SUPERGENE" AND TRANSPLANTATION

From many family studies, we know that the HLA complex functions as a powerful transplantation "antigen," but despite nearly 20 years of investigation, we do not yet know which of the components of the MHC are the "true" histocompatibility antigens. While the B series antigens and probably the A can serve as targets in CML, it also appears that an additional and highly potent factor is more complex. The MHC molecules may not be simple antigens in the way that the ABO or Rh blood group antigens are, but consist of molecular groupings on the cell surface which are recognized as foreign or as self by complementary groupings on other cells. The first evidence for the existence of an MHC macromolecular structure came from the work of Boyse who noted that antibodies to Tl$^a$ antigens depressed the apparent antigenicity of H-2D locus antigens but not the H-2K antigens (Boyse *et al.*, 1968). H-2D lies close to Tl$^a$ on chromosome 17, while H-2K is more remote, implying a spatial relationship on the surface of the cell as well as on the chromosome. Other antigenic complexes were provided by Lyt-1 and K, and by Lyt-2 and H-2D. Yunis and Amos (1971) applied similar reasoning to HLA and Ceppellini (1971) gave an excellent summary of the lines of evidence of the functioning of an antigenic grid. Nicolson (1976) has shown how a macromolecular structure might depend upon both microfilaments and microtubular arrangements, and drugs which impair the function of either of these cytoskeletal components tend to abolish MHC related immune functions. Flaherty and Zimmerman (1979) have confirmed the findings of Boyse on the spatial complexing of H-2D, H-2K, and Tl$^a$ and have extended them by showing that this complexing does not occur if the cells are pretreated with dilute paraformaldehyde. Interestingly, a second form of complexing also appears to exist on the cell surface. Antibodies to the gene products of Ly and H-2 (which are determined by genes of separate chromosomes) sterically inhibit antibody binding just as do H-2D and Tl$^a$ (Boyse *et al.*, 1968), but this steric blocking is not inhibited by prior fixation. At least some forms of complexing occur only as a result of an outside influence. In the examples of Boyse and Flaherty, the attracting force is antibody. In cell–cell interactions, the cell membranes presumably fulfill the same function at the points of contact. Any products involved in H-2 restriction (H-Y, some viruses) may therefore be subsequently shown to be grid components while antigens not showing H-2 restriction would not be.

In confirmation of the concept of macromolecular complexes, no single component of the MHC has been shown to be solely responsible for histoincompatibility reactions. Solubilized glycoproteins provoke only feeble immune responses. There is no simple relationship between MLC responses and the response to a transplant. In the mouse, where recombinants at the D end or the K end of H-2 are available, immunity to D or to K can cause rejection, the response to K usually being rather stronger than the response to D. Similarly, in skin grafts in man, there is no consistant rapid rejection either by A-end or B-end differences (Ward *et al.*, 1978). Also, no single H-2 antigen and no single HLA antigen has been shown to be uniquely associated with rapid rejection of skin or kidney grafts. Thus, the target for cellular immunity appears to be an HLA or H-2 molecule but the trigger for the initiation of immunity appears to be a grid and components of the grid can function as targets.

The association of suppressor loci in the H-2J region of H-2 of the mouse and of immune response genes with the outcome of transplantation cannot be ignored in any attempts to understand the vagaries of human transplantation. Many years ago the senior author wrote "there is no way the investigator can reach into a group of Swiss (outbred) mice and select two which will be compatible." This unfortunately is true of outbred man. Matching for A, B, and C loci does make a contribution. It is currently believed that matching for HLA-DR may make an even more significant contribution, but this remains to be proved. Environmental factors are peculiarly strong in transplantation—cross-reactivity with microbial antigens, prior exposure to blood transfusion, and subtle variations in the balance of subsets of antigen reactive cells may all play a role in the outcome of graft survival. If compatibility for DR is contributory to graft success, then histocompatibility will come to have a different meaning. If not, and if the hypothetical HDR locus cannot be substantiated and identified, immunologic rather than genetic approaches will appear to offer greater benefits, except for the intrafamilial graft, the monozygotic twin or the HLA-identical sib being the ideal to be sought after. The deliberate induction of specific suppression, the provocation of specific enhancing antibodies, or the presentation of histocompatibility antigen in the form of a toleragen all offer potential benefits to the recipient.

## EVOLUTION AND MAINTENANCE OF THE MHC— FUNCTION?

The evolution of the MHC remains a mystery. Its existence is evident as far back as the clawed toad (reviewed in Götze, 1977). Primitive chronic allograft reactions first appear in advanced invertebrates, e.g., Annelida and Echinodermata, while "acute," specific, and second-set responses are seen in the more advanced anuran amphibians, e.g., *Rana pipiens*. Although a functional MHC homologue appears to be absent from primitive fishes, primitive amphibians or reptiles, a cluster of genes, perhaps minor H loci, may exist which serve to distinguish self from nonself, either by immunological or nonimmunological means. Of the mammalian species studied, the mouse, rat, rabbit, rhesus, chimp, guinea pig, dog, pig, and cow, the MHCs all appear to contain genes for serologically defined gp 44 antigens, gp 33,28 B-cell-specific antigens, LAD or lymphocyte-activating determinants, and for complement components. The chicken has a similar gene complex suggesting that (a) the evolution of the "supergene" preceded separation of the mammalian and avian classes and that (b) there must be a unique evolutionary advantage in retaining genes of diverse functions on the same chromosomal segment. In our view this can only be explained by postulating essential intergenic interactions.

It has been suggested that the present "MHC" evolved by gene duplication (Shreffler *et al.*, 1971; Bodmer, 1972; Klein, 1975). Biochemical evidence showing sequence and structure homology between structural MHC components in several species (reviewed by Klein, 1978) would confirm this. What may be a further clue to the evolution of the MHC is the similarity of the serologically defined gp 44 HLA-A and B antigens to immunoglobulins (Gally and Edelman, 1972; Tragardh *et al.*, 1978). The HLA-A, -B, and -C molecules are associated with $\beta_2$-microglobulin, which by structure and sequence shows homology with a single Ig domain, notably the $C^H3$ domain of IgG (Cunningham and Berggard, 1974; Peterson *et al.*, 1972). HLA-B7 has been isolated and sequenced: four intrachain disulfide bonds appear to divide the molecule into two fragments or "domains," each the size of a single immunoglobulin domain (Parham *et al.*, 1977; Terhorst *et al.*, 1977). Strong sequence homology with a variety of mouse and human V regions was found in the carbohydrate attachment region and around the intrachain disulfide bridges (Parham *et al.*, 1977; Terhorst *et al.*, 1977). Also reminiscent of immunoglobulins, the two "domains" of the HLA molecule share common amino acid sequences (Strominger *et al.*, 1977).

Thus, there appear to have been two distinct forms of gene duplication. One form would have involved the primordial gene that evolved into the immunoglobulins and the structural membrane proteins of the MHC, the other would have been a simpler form of gene duplication that specified that, in mice and primates at least, there would be at least two copies of the gp 44 product and at least two copies of the gp 33,28 (Ia-like) antigens. In the mouse, the latter are called IA and IC-E antigens; in man the second allelic series comparable to HLA-DR has not yet been named.

In the mouse, genes linked to H-2 determine other cell membrane components which have a structure similar to HLA-ABC. The T (Vitetta *et al.*, 1975a), Tl (Ostberg *et al.*, 1975; Vitetta *et al.*, 1975b), and Qa

(Michaelson *et al.*, 1977) antigens are two-chain structures, one of which is a heavy chain of molecular weight 44,000 and the other $\beta_2$-microglobulin. Recently, the H-Y male antigen, present on human lymphoid cell lines and on differentiated mouse teratocarcinoma cell lines, has been shown to be associated with $\beta_2$-microglobulin as well (Fellous *et al.*, 1978). The possibility remains that other gp 44-$\beta_2$-microglobulin membrane components exist. As with HLA-ABC, they are structures in search of a function.

The association of HLA alleles with particular diseases is one of the most intriguing aspects of the MHC and one which may ultimately help map MHC functions (for specific references see Dausset and Svejgaard, 1977; Murphy, 1977; Batchelor and Morris, 1978). The most remarkable associations have been with autoaggressive and inflammatory diseases, and with diseases in which a receptor abnormality is implicated. In these disease states, the associations can be extraordinarily high. In some cases, an actual "disease gene" in close linkage to HLA can be defined as a result of family studies. The two most outstanding diseases in this category are ankylosing spondylitis (AS) and hemochromatosis.

Ankylosing spondylitis, a deforming inflammatory disease which preferentially attacks males rather than females has an overwhelming association with HLA-B27. Indeed, 90% and in some series 100% of affected individuals have the B27 specificity, in contrast to the antigen frequency in control populations which is about 5%. While there is as yet no formal evidence for a disease gene in AS, the probability is high. Current thinking is that the reason why the disease attacks males preferentially is that most affected males also have chronic prostatitis and AS may be an aberrant response to the prostatitis or the infectious agent that shows up in B27 subjects. This possibly explains the link to another rheumatoid condition, Reiter's disease, which includes urethritis and monoarticular arthritis in its manifestations. Whether a person develops Reiter's syndrome or AS may be a reflection of the pleiotropy of the same disease, phenotypic modification by another gene, or possibly allelism of a disease gene linked to HLA-B and in high linkage disequilibrium with it. The difference between Caucasians and Blacks (90% B27 vs. 60% B27) may be due to differences in linkage disequilibrium in the two populations, to differential racial susceptibility to the infecting organism, or to heterogeneity of the disease.

The other disease in which linkage to a disease gene seems to be certain is hemochromatosis. Affected persons have abnormal iron storage and may accumulate over 20 grams of iron, mainly in the liver, although heart, adrenal glands, and skin may be affected. The onset is insidious and the disease may present in different ways so the diagnosis may only become apparent when the appropriate studies are performed or at autopsy. Since the most effective treatment is phlebotomy, the disease is less severe in menstruating females. The genetic model appears to be intermediate recessive with the gene in very high linkage disequilibrium with HLA-A3. About 20% of heterozygotes carrying the allele have abnormalities of iron metabolism. Family studies in other ethnic groups would be of extreme interest.

If hemochromatosis is the disease having the strongest association with the A locus and ankylosing spondylitis with B, psoriasis has the strongest association with HLA-C, in this case Cw6 (McMichael *et al.,* 1978). Multiple sclerosis, celiac disease, and juvenile diabetes mellitus appear to be more associated with HLA-D, and rheumatoid arthritis and Goodpasture's syndrome with DR antigens. HLA-Dw3 and therefore presumably DRw3 are strongly associated with gluten-sensitive enteropathy.

Where family studies have been performed, these and other diseases appear to be associated with a particular HLA haplotype: multiple sclerosis with HLA-A3-B7-Dw2, Graves disease with A1-B8-Dw3, and hemochromatosis with A3-B14. In all these cases, a high degree of linkage disequilibrium exists between these antigens in the normal as well as in the diseased group. A deficiency of the second component of complement (C2) is also HLA-haplotype associated, but with the more infrequent haplotype Aw25-B18-Dw2. Many of the individuals with a total C2 deficiency are Aw25-B18-Dw2 homozygous and appear to show signs of immune insufficiency often associated with diseases such as systemic lupus erythematosus (SLE) and SLE-like diseases, anaphylactoid purpura, chronic vasculitis, dermatomyositis, rheumatic disease, and glomerulonephritis.

Most of the disease studies are on populations. This is unfortunate, since loose linkage tends to be missed in population studies and few polygenic diseases with one gene linked to HLA would be picked up. An example is provided by leprosy. DeVries *et al.* (1976) in family studies found the form of the disease (lepromatous or tuberculoid) to be a function of the HLA haplotype segregating in the family. They and others, however, have failed to show an association with a specific HLA antigen.

While associations between HLA and malignancy have, with the exception of acute lymphocytic leukemia, not so far been significant, such linkage is seen in the mouse. Linked to H-2 are several genes for susceptibility or resistance to cancer, including several leukemias—Gross, Friend, Tennant—and the mammary cancer virus of Bittner (Klein, 1975). The very high susceptibility of some mouse strains and the resistance of others is apparent solely because any other genes modifying resistance to oncogenesis are fixed in the inbred animals. From appropriate crosses at least three distinct genes have been identified as being involved in the resistance to Gross virus. An association with H-2 in an outbreeding population would probably be missed or at best would be weak. An association could also be identifiable in some populations and not in others, especially if the marker were linked to but at some distance from the MHC. This may be a partial explanation for the early report of association between HLA and Hodgkins disease which could not be confirmed in other studies.

Thus, HLA-disease associations can fall into several categories: (1) malignant diseases, for which there is no definitive evidence as yet, (2) autoaggressive and inflammatory diseases such as ankylosing spondylitis, (3) metabolic diseases such as hemochromatosis and the polyglandular diseases, (4) immune deficiency diseases such as C2 deficiency, (5) abnormal differentiation, e.g., congenital neutropenia (Hansen et al., 1977), and (6) others which are haplotype-linked but not obviously associated with a particular HLA antigen, e.g., leprosy. In some instances, HLA-associated genes may affect the development of a disease, or an individual's resistance to it.

Numerous hypotheses accounting for such disease associations exist and are reviewed extensively elsewhere (Dausset and Svejgaard, 1977). Three predominant theories include (1) the HLA molecules themselves might act as receptors for viruses or other infectious agents, (2) mimicry— the similarity of structure between the HLA molecules and the structure of an infectious agent which could make immune recognition impossible, or (3) other genes closely linked to but separate from the HLA genes themselves. In this last category would be the complement genes as well as genes which determine the specific recognition of foreign antigens, viruses, bacteria, or allogeneic cells, thereby determining the ability of an individual to produce antibody or a cell-mediated immune response. Such immune response (Ir) genes have been identified within the murine MHC H-2.

Numerous attempts have been made to identify human Ir genes using a variety of antigens including the synthetic polypeptides GLT and TGAL (Scher et al., 1975), tetanus toxoid (Sasazuki et al., 1978), vaccinia (de

Vries *et al.*, 1977), influenza A (Spencer *et al.*, 1976), and measles (Haverkorn and Norrby, 1978; Spencer *et al.*, 1977), most of them without any convincing positive findings. Some of the reasons for failure are trivial: inadequate knowledge of the proper discriminating dose, reliance on population studies instead of family studies, inability to control for previous exposure, etc., and the question remains open.

Exceptions in which Ir genes have been thought to be expressed include the report of Greenberg *et al.* (1975) that HLA-B5 subjects tended to be high responders to streptococcal antigen and the division of leprous sibs into tuberculoid and lepromatous on the basis of HLA haplotype (de Vries *et al.*, 1976). Shaw and Biddison (1979) have reported HLA-linked genetic control of *in vitro* cellular responses to influenza virus. The anaphylactic response to allergens may also be HLA-linked. Levine (Levine *et al.*, 1972), confirmed by Blumenthal (Blumenthal *et al.*, 1974) and later by Marsh (Marsh and Bias, 1977), have shown haplotype associations with atopy in families and a gene for sensitivity to ragweed, SRW, has been mapped to chromosome 6 (Marsh and Bias, 1977). There is no proof that this is an *Ir* gene, or that IgE levels per se are MHC-linked. Hsia *et al.* (1977) and Buckley and Roseman (1976) analyzed the same set of data from large Amish families in whom antibody levels to common viruses had been determined. Hsia concluded that there was little evidence for HLA involvement; Buckley concluded there was. In a sense, both could be right, Hsia in the sense that HLA-linked Ir genes are most unlikely to be the sole regulators of immunity and Buckley in the sense that by using multivariate analysis the contribution of other Ir genes can be accounted for and the contribution of the HLA-linked gene(s) detected. From more sophisticated studies in mice, polygenic control appears likely.

## WHAT OF THE FUTURE?

In practical terms, many developments can be expected with confidence. As more family studies are conducted, more diseases will be shown to be HLA-linked. The most favorable families for study are obviously those in which more than one member is involved. Another outcome will be separation of some diseases which are now classified together, as being separate entities but with a similar phenotype. For localization of disease entities to discrete regions of the chromosome, glyoxalase, PGM3, and other external markers will be of use as will the C4 and other internal markers. When the location of the gene is known, transcription with recombinant DNA will permit production of the abnormal gene product *in vitro* and thus lead to an understanding of the etiology of the disease.

At the theoretical level, we will learn more about the mode of action of structural components of the membrane. For example, the $K^b$ allele of the K region of H-2 is the most mutable gene known with a mutation rate of $2 \times 10^{-4}$. The $K^b$ mutant will reject skin or tumor, stimulate strongly in MLR, cause severe graft-vs.-host disease, stimulate the development of cytotoxic lymphocytes (CTL), and serve as a target for CTL (Klein, 1978). Qualitative and quantitative serologic differences between wild type and mutant have also been reported. All these activities are believed to come from a single mutation of a glycoprotein. Furthermore, this molecule has been relegated to the category of "serologically defined" or SD antigen (as opposed to antigens that are "lymphocyte defined" or LD). Since the MHC gp 44 polypeptide may have at least two domains, one can postulate that these domains are functionally separate. Thus, many of the functions ascribed to the Ia region of the mouse may at least in part be attributes of a domain of the H-2K molecule itself.* Similarly, the hypothetical HDR locus that Yunis and Amos postulated to explain certain anomalous reactions of the MHC may indeed be a domain of the gp44 molecule with a relatively low degree of polymorphism, or it may be an interaction product involving one or more domains. We know that varying degrees of polymorphism are found on the same molecule. The HLA-B subtypic antigens are highly polymorphic, Bw4, Bw6 are diallelic, and other "public" antigens, e.g., LHe, may be moderately polymorphic (Kostyu *et al.,* 1980).

We have to admit, at this point, that we do not know how many loci relevant to the supergene are included in it. For HLA, we know that there are the ABC loci and that there may be more gp $44$-$\beta_2$-microglobulin

---

* There is a further point of complexity here. Recombination between K and I is rare—on the order of $2 \times 10^4$. Congenic lines may include over 10 cM of DNA from the second parental line. Several H genes have been mapped between D and Tl$^a$ and at least one H gene lies between D and K. In view of the reported activities of the $K^b$ mutants and the possibility of recombination including unsuspected genes close to but outside H-2, or of double recombination (the recombinant fraction between H-2D and K is on the order of 0.005), the probability of double recombination approaches that of recombination between K and I and assigning functions to the K-I region must, at this point, be somewhat tenuous. Certainly the SD-LD terminology should be abandoned.

molecules. We are certain there are at least two gp 33,28 molecules. We do not know how D and DR are interrelated. At one time we were convinced that the D locus and the DR locus were separate and we suspected that both were duplicated. This would give a minimum of four loci. However, because of the reported multitudinous activities of H-2k$^b$, we wonder if (1) the gp 33,28 molecules have more than one functional domain, or (2) if the gp 33 has one set of functions and the gp 28 another. The essential argument is that a gp 33,28 couplet may give both lymphocyte stimulation and serve as a target for anti-DR sera. Most of the difficulties in the interpretation of MLR data and of DR serotyping disappear once it is accepted that both are duplicated. Thus, we may have two DR loci or two D–DR complexes but the minimum number of each is two. Structural integrity of the membrane is essential for HLA-D and H-2 MLR-S functioning. This could be because HLA-D and MLR-S are not gene products but interactive effects, or because structural conformation is essential for function.

One final topic we cannot resist relates to the functional unity of the haplotype and the interrelationships of the components, including the complement components. Obviously, mammalian genetics are orders of magnitude more complex than viral or bacterial genetics and the regulatory steps are probably very different. At least four forms of regulation are likely, *cis* regulation by adjacent genes, *cis* regulation by distant genes, *trans* regulation by genes on the homologous chromosome, and interactions between unlike genes. Important genetic studies by Popp (1978) have shown linkage between the graying and aging process in mice and the H-2 supergene. Boyse and his colleagues have made equally important discoveries on the relationship between H-2 and mate preference, probably mediated by pheromone-like substances controlled by H-2-linked genes (Yamazaki *et al.*, 1976). H-2-linked restriction of cell–cell interaction (Doherty *et al.*, 1976) is so firmly established there can be no residual doubt but that cell–cell communication in the immunological system (and possibly in other systems) and response to nonself is centrally regulated by these genes. Obviously there must be extensive collaboration between the components of the supergene, and one of the consequences is that certain combinations of alleles on the haplotype must be advantageous and other combinations, disadvantageous. There are very few examples of *cis–cis* interactions in mammals (as yet). The int-temp-rec action in the mouse regulating the appearance of H-2 antigens is the best known (Boubelik *et al.*, 1975). It seems inconceivable that the MHC would be preserved in birds and mammals in essentially identical manner unless either (1) regulation required proximity, or (2) functioning required the simultaneous presence of certain combinations of alleles. The fine genetics and regulation of the HLA supergene still hold many surprises.

ACKNOWLEDGMENTS. Grateful thanks must be given to our colleagues Frances Ward and Peter Cresswell, who read the manuscript and kept us (reasonably) honest; to Ken Paigen and Igor Egorov for generous sharing of ideas; and to Janice Kerber, who slaved over the product on her typewriter. This work was supported by the following grants from the National Institutes of Health: GM-10356, AI-18399 (RCDA), and CA-09058 (training grant).

# REFERENCES

Ahrons, S., 1971, HL-A antibodies: Influence on the human foetus, *Tissue Antigens* 1:129–136.

Albert, E. D., and Götze, D., 1977, The major histocompatibility system in man, in: *The Major Histocompatibility System in Man and Animals* (D. Götze, ed.), pp. 7–77, Springer-Verlag, New York.

Albert, E. D., McClelland, J. D., Hammer, C., Zink, R., and Brendel, W., 1973, Study of the HL-A system in the Nepalese Sherpa population, in: *Histocompatibility Testing, 1972* (J. Dausset and J. Colombani, eds.), pp. 227–232, Munksgaard, Copenhagen.

Albert, E. D., Rittner, C., Scholz, S., Kuntz, B., and Mickey, M. R., 1977, Three point association of HLA-A, B, Bf haplotypes deduced in 200 parents of 100 families, *Scand. J. Immunol.* 6:459–464.

Albert, E., Amos, D. B., Bodmer, W. F., Ceppellini, R., Dausset, J., Kissmeyer-Nielsen, F., Mayr, W., Payne, R., van Rood, J. J., Terasaki, P. I., Trnka, Z., and Walford, R. L., 1978, Nomenclature for factors of the HLA system—1977, *Tissue Antigens* 11:81–86.

Albrechtsen, D., 1977, HLA-D-associated "Ia-like" antigens on human macrophages, *Scand. J. Immunol.* 6:907–912.

Albrechtsen, D., Solheim, B. G., and Thorsby, E., 1977, The presence of Ia-like determinants on a subpopulation of human T lymphocytes, *Immunogenetics* 5:149–159.

Allison, J. P., Ferrone, S., Walker, L. E., Pellegrino, M. A., Silver, J., and Reisfeld, R. A., 1978a, Partial amino acid sequence of HLA-A9 antigen purified with a specific xenoantiserum, *Transplantation* 26:451–454.

Allison, J. P., Walker, L. E., Russell, W. A., Pellegrino, M. A., Ferrone, S., Reisfeld, R. A., Frelinger, J. A., and Silver, J., 1978b, Murine Ia and human DR antigens: Homology of amino-terminal sequences, *Proc. Nat. Acad. Sci. USA* 75:3953–3956.

Alter, B. J., Bach, F. H., Jaramillo, S., and Wernet, P., 1977, Typing an unrelated panel with PLT cells: association with Dw clusters, *Scand. J. Immunol.* **6**:485–488.

D'Amaro, J., 1975, W4(4a) and W6(4b) in diverse human populations. Demonstration of their genetic identity in population and segregation studies, *Tissue Antigens* **5**:386–394.

Amos, D. B., 1969, Genetic and antigenic aspects of human histocompatibility systems, *Adv. Immunol.* **10**:251–297.

Amos, D. B., 1970, Genetic aspects of Human HL-A transplantation antigens, *Fed. Proc.* **29**:2018–2025.

Amos, D. B., 1974, HL-A, fertility and natural selection, in: *Karolinska Symposia on Research Methods in Reproductive Endocrinology* (E. Diczfalusy, ed.), pp. 318–335, Karolinska, Copenhagen.

Amos, D. B., and Peacocke, N., 1963, Leucoagglutination. A modified technique and preliminary results of absorption with tissues, in: *Proceedings of the Ninth Congress of the European Society of Haematology, Lisbon.* p. 1132, Karger, Basel.

Amos, D. B., and Ward, F. E., 1975, Immunogenetics of the HL-A system, *Physiol. Rev.* **55**:206–246.

Amos, D. B., and Yunis, E., 1969, Human leukocyte antigenic specificity HL-A 3: Frequence of occurrence, *Science* **165**:300–302.

Amos, B., Cabrera, G., Bias, W. B., MacQueen, J. M., Lancaster, S. L., Southworth, J. G., and Ward, F. E., 1970, The inheritance of human leukocyte antigens. III. The organization of specificities, in: *Histocompatibility Testing, 1970* (P. I. Terasaki, ed.), pp. 259–275, Munksgaard, Copenhagen.

Amos, D. B., Corley, R. B., and Kostyu, D. D., 1973, The production of antibody against HL-A antigen, *Symp. Ser. Immunobiol. Standardization Intern, Symp. HL-A Reagents, 1972,* **18**:1–10.

Arce-Gomez, B., Jones, E. A., Barnstable, C. J., Solomon, E., and Bodmer, W. F., 1978, The genetic control of HLA-A and B antigens in somatic cell hybrids: Requirement for $\beta_2$-microglobulin, *Tissue Antigens* **11**:96–112.

Arnason, A., Larsen, B., Marshall, W. H., Edwards, J. H., Mackintosh, P., Olaisen, B., and Teisberg, P., 1977, Very close linkage between HLA-B and Bf inferred from allelic association, *Nature* **268**:527–528.

Aster, R. H., Miskovich, B. H., and Rodey, G. E., 1973, Histocompatibility antigens of human plasma, *Transplantation* **16**:205–210.

Aster, R. H., Szatkowski, N., Liebert, M., and Duquesnoy, R. J., 1977, Expression of HLA-B12, HLA-B8, w4 and w6 on platelets, *Transplant. Proc.* **9**:1695–1696.

Atassi, M. Z., 1975, Antigenic structure of myoglobin: The complete immunochemical anatomy of a protein and conclusions relating to antigenic structures of proteins, *Immunochemistry* **12**:423–438.

Atassi, M. Z., and Lee, C-L., 1978, The precise and entire antigenic structure of native lysozyme, *Biochem. J.* **171**:429–434.

Ayres, J., and Cresswell, P., 1976, HLA-B specificities and w4, w6 specificities are on the same polypeptide, *Eur. J. Immunol.* **6**:794–799.

Bach, F. H., and Amos, D. B., 1967, HU-1: Major histocompatibility locus in man, *Science* **156**:1506–1508.

Bach, F. H., and Bach, M. L., 1972, Comparison of mitomycin C and x-irradiation as blocking agents in one-way mixed leukocyte cultures, *Nature (New Biol.)* **235**:243–244.

Bach, M. L., and Bach, F. H., 1974, Immunogenetic disparity and graft-versus-host reactions, *Semin. Hematol.* **11**:291–303.

Bach, F. H., Bach, M. L., and Sondel, P. M., 1976, Differential function of major histocompatibility complex antigens in T-lymphocyte activation, *Nature (London)* **259**:273–281.

Bach, M. L., Jarret-Toth, E., Benike, C., Shih, C. Y., Valentine, E., Alter, B. J., and Bach, F. H., 1977, Primed lymphocyte typing in the assay of HLA-D region disparity, *Transplant. Proc.* **9**:405–409.

Bain, B., and Pshyk, K., 1972, Enhanced reactivity in mixed leukocyte cultures after separation of mononuclear cells on ficoll-hypaque, *Transplant. Proc.* **4**:163–164.

Bain, B., Vas, M. R., and Lowenstein, L., 1964, The development of large immature mononuclear cells in mixed leukocyte cultures, *Blood* **23**:108–116.

Balner, H., Cleton, F. J., and Eernisse, J. G. (eds.), 1966, *Histocompatability Testing, 1965*, 288 pp., Williams and Wilkins Co., Baltimore.

Barnstable, C. J., Jones, E. A., Bodmer, W. F., Bodmer, J. G., Arce-Gomez, B., Snary, D., and Crumpton, M., 1976, Genetics and serology of HLA linked human Ia antigens, *Cold Spring Harbor Symp. Quant. Biol.* **XLI**:443–456.

Barnstable, C. J., Bodmer, W. F., Brown, G., Galfre, G., Milstein, C., Williams. A. F., and Ziegler, A., 1978a, Production of monoclonal antibodies to group A erythrocytes, HLA and other human cell surface antigens—new tools for genetic analysis, *Cell* **14**:9–20.

Barnstable, C. J., Jones, E. A., and Crumpton, M. J., 1978b, Isolation, structure and genetics of HLA-A, -B, -C, and -DRw (Ia) antigens, *Br. Med. Bull.* **34**:241–246.

Basch, R. S., 1974, Effects of antigen density and non-complement fixing antibodies on cytolysis by alloantisera, *J. Immunol.* **113**:554–562.

Batchelor, J. R., and Kennedy, L. A., 1973, HL-A antibody response in volunteers immunized with skin grafts and leucocytes, *Symp. Ser. Immunobiol. Standardization Intern. Symp. HL-A Reagents, 1972*, **18**:33–38.

Batchelor, J. R., and Morris, P. J., 1978, HLA and Disease, in *Histocompatibility Testing, 1977* (W. F. Bodmer, J. R. Batchelor, J. G. Bodmer, H. Festenstein, and P. J. Morris, eds.), pp. 205–258, Munksgaard, Copenhagen.

Batchelor, J. R., and Sanderson, A. R., 1970, Implications of cross-reactivity in the HL-A system, *Transplant. Proc.* **2**:133–143.

Bausher, J. C., and Smith, R. T., 1973, Studies of the Epstein–Barr virus–host relationship: Autochthonous and allogeneic lymphocyte stimulation by lymphoblast cell lines in mixed cell culture, *Clin. Immunol. Immunopathol.* **1**:270–281.

Beer, A. E., and Billingham, R. E., 1977, Concerning the origins and scope of the immunobiology of mammalian reproduction, *Transplant. Proc.* **9**:1357–1361.

Belvedere, M. C., Curtoni, E. S., Dausset, J., Lamm, L. U., Mayr, W., van Rood, J. J., Svejgaard, A., and Piazza, A., 1975a, On the heterogeneity of linkage estimations between LA and FOUR of the HL-A system, *Tissue Antigens* **5**:99–102.

Belvedere, M., Mattiuz, P., and Curtoni, E. S., 1975b, An antibody cross-reacting with LA and FOUR antigens of the HL-A system, *Immunogenetics* **1**:538–548.

Bender, K., Mayerová, A., Frank, R., Hiller, C., and Wienker, T., 1977, Haplotype and analysis of the linkage group HLA-A:HLA-B:Bf and its bearing on the interpretation of linkage disequilibrium, *Hum. Genet.* **36**:191–196.

Benjamini, E., Shimizu, M., Young, J. D., and Leung, C. Y., 1969, Immunochemical studies on tobacco mosaic virus protein. IX. Investigations on binding and antigenic specificity of antibodies to an antigenic area of tobacco mosaic virus protein, *Biochemistry* **8**:2242–2246.

Bernier, I., Dautigny, A., Colombani, J., and Jolles, P., 1976, Investigations on human leukocyte antigens (HLA) from urine, *FEBS Lett.* **63**:320–322.

Bernoco, D., Cullen, S., Scudeller, G., Trinchieri, B., and Ceppellini, R., 1973, HL-A molecules at the cell surface, in: *Histocompatibility Testing, 1972* (J. Dausset and J. Colombani, eds.), pp. 527–537, Munksgaard, Copenhagen.

Bernoco, D., Bernoco, M., Ceppellini, R., Poulik, M. D., van Leeuwen, A., and van Rood, J. J., 1976, B cell antigens of the HLA system: A simple serotyping technique based on non-cytotoxic anti β-microglobulin reagents, *Tissue Antigens* 8:253–260.

Betuel, H., Touraine, J. L., Souillet, G., and Jeune, M., 1978, Absence of cell-membrane HLA antigens in an immunodeficient child, *Tissue Antigens* 11:68–70.

Bias, W. B., Hopkins, K. A., Hutchinson, J. K., and Hsu, S. H., 1974, Evidence for an unlinked gene which modifies HL-A antigen expression, *Tissue Antigens*, 4:36–41.

Bijnen, A. B., Schreuder, I., Meera Khan, P., Allen, F. H., Giles, C. M., Los, W. R. T., Volkers, W. S., and van Rood, J. J. 1976, Linkage relationships of the loci of the major histocompatibility complex in families with a recombination in the HLA region, *J. Immunogenet.* 3:171–183.

Bijnen, A. B., Schreuder, I., Volkers, W. S., Parlevliet, J., and van Rood, J. J., 1977, The lymphocyte activating influence of the HLA-A region, *J. Immunogenet.* 4:1–5.

Billing, R. J., Safani, M., and Peterson, P., 1977, Soluble HLA antigens present in normal human serum, *Tissue Antigens* 10:75–82.

Blumenthal, M. N., Amos, D. B., Noreen, H., Mendell, N. R., and Yunis, E. J., 1974, Genetic mapping of Ir locus in man: Linkage to second locus of *HL-A*, *Science* 184:1301–1303.

Bodmer, W. F., 1972, Evolutionary significance of the HL-A system, *Nature* 237:139–145.

Bodmer, W. F., 1973, Population genetics of the HL-A system: Retrospect and prospect, in: *Histocompatibility Testing, 1972* (J. Dausset and J. Colombani, eds.), pp. 611–617, Munksgaard, Copenhagen.

Bodmer, W. F., and Bodmer, J. G., 1978, Evolution and function of the HLA system, *Br. Med. Bull.* 34:309–316.

Bodmer, W., and Thomson, G., 1977, Population genetics and evolution of the HLA system, in: *HLA and Disease* (J. Dausset and A. Svejgaard, eds.), pp. 280–295, Munksgaard, Copenhagen.

Bodmer, W., Tripp, M., and Bodmer, J., 1967, Application of a fluorochromatic cytotoxicity assay to human leukocyte typing in: *Histocompatibility Testing, 1967* (E. S. Curtoni, P. L. Mattiuz, and R. M. Tosi, eds.), pp. 341–350.

Bodmer, W. F., Batchelor, J. R., Bodmer, J. G., Festenstein, H., and Morris, P. J. (eds.), 1978a, *Histocompatibility Testing, 1977*, 612 pp., Munksgaard, Copenhagen.

Bodmer, J. G., Pickbourne, P., and Richards, S., 1978b, Ia serology, in: *Histocompatibility Testing, 1977* (W. F. Bodmer, J. R. Batchelor, J. G. Bodmer, H. Festenstein, and P. J. Morris, eds.), pp. 35–82, Munksgaard, Copenhagen.

Boubelík, M., Lengerová, A., Bailey, D. W., and Matousek, V., 1975, A model for genetic analysis of programmed gene expression as reflected in the development of membrane antigens, *Dev. Biol.* 47:206–214. –

Boyse, E. A., Old, L. J., and Stockert, E., 1968, An approach to the mapping of antigens on the cell surface, *Proc. Nat. Acad. Sci. USA* 60:886–893.

Böyum, A., 1968, Separation of leukocytes from blood and bone marrow, *Scand, J. Clin. Lab. Invest. Suppl.* 97:21.

Bradley, B. A., and Festenstein, H., 1978, Cellular typing, *Br. Med. Bull.* 34:223–232.

Bradley, B. A., Edwards, J. M., and Franks, D., 1973, Histocompatibility phenotyping by the mixed lymphocyte reaction, *Tissue Antigens* 3:340–347.

Bradley, B. A., Termijtelen, A. M., Franks, D., and van Rood, J. J., 1977, Interpretation of data obtained from primed lymphocyte tests (PLTs), *Transpl. Proc.* 9:421–424.

Breuning, M. H., van den Berg-Loonen, E. M., Bernini, L. F., Bijlsma, J. B., van Loghem, E., Khan, P. M., and Nijenhuis, L. E., 1977, Localization of HLA on the short arm of chromosome 6, *Hum. Genet.* 37:131–139.

Brigdon, J., Snary, D., Crumpton, M. J., Barnstable, C., Goodfellow, P., and Bodmer, W. F., 1976, Isolation and N-terminal amino acid sequence of membrane bound human HLA-A and HLA-B antigens, *Nature (London)* 261:200–205.

Bright, S., 1974, Comparative studies on the rates of re-expression of human histocompatibility antigens after papain treatment, *Tissue Antigens* 4:306–312.

Bright, S., 1976, Second locus HL-A antigens and 4a or 4b, *Tissue Antigens* 7:23–34.

Brown, J. P., Klitzman, J. M., and Hellstrom, K. E., 1977, A microassay for antibody binding to tumor cell surface antigens using $^{125}$I-labelled protein A from *Staph. aureus*, *J. Immunol. Methods* 15:57–66.

Bruning, J. W., van Leeuwen, A., and van Rood, J. J., 1964, Purification of leukocyte group substances from human placental tissue, *Transplantation* 2:649–654.

Buckley, C. E., III, and Roseman, J. M., 1976, Immunity and survival, *J. Am. Ger. Soc.* 24:241–248.

Carpenter, C. B., D'Apice, A. J. P., Soulilou, J. P., Fagan, G., and Garovoy, M. R., 1975, The EA rosette inhibition test for human B-cell antibodies, in: *The First HLA Workshop of the Americas*, NIH Publ. No. 76–1064, pp. 194–196.

Ceppellini, R., 1971, Old and new facts and speculations about transplantation antigens of man, *Progr. Immunol.* 1:973–1025.

Ceppellini, R., and van Rood, J. J., 1974, The HL-A system. I. Genetics and molecular biology, *Semin. Hematol.* 11:233–251.

Ceppellini, R., Celada, F., Mattiuz, P. L., and Zanalda, A., 1964, Study of the possible correlation between blood antigens and histocompatibility in man. I. Production of leukoagglutinins by repeated transfusions from one donor, *Ann. N.Y. Acad. Sci.* 120:335–347.

Ceppellini, R., Curtoni, E. S., Leigheb, G., Mattiuz, P. L., Miggiano, V. C., and Visetti, M., 1965, An experimental approach to genetic analysis of histocompatibility in man, in: *Histocompatibility Testing, 1965* (H. Balner, F. J. Cleton, and J. G. Eernisse, eds.), pp. 13–22, Munksgaard, Copenhagen.

Cicciarelli, J. C., Bernoco, D., Terasaki, P. I., and Shirahama, S., 1978, Studies of HLA-A, B, C, and D antigens on monocytes, *Trans. Proc.* 10:863–865.

Cline, M. J., and Billing, R., 1977, Antigens expressed by human B lymphocytes and myeloid stem cells, *J. Exp. Med.* 146:1143–1145.

Collins, Z. V., Arnold, P. F., Peetoom, F., Smith, G. S., and Walford, R. L., 1973, A naturally occurring monospecific anti-HL-A 8 isoantibody, *Tissue Antigens* 3:358–363.

Colombani, J., Colombani, M., and Dausset, J., 1970, Cross-reactions in the HL-A system with special reference to Da6 cross-reacting group, in: *Histocompatibility Testing, 1970* (P. I. Terasaki, ed.), pp. 79–92, Munksgaard, Copenhagen.

Colombani, J., D'Amaro, J., Gabb, B., Smith, G., and Svejgaard, A., 1971, International agreement on a microtechnique of platelet complement fixation (Pl. c. fix), *Transplant. Proc.* 3:121–126.

Colombani, J., Colombani, M., and Dausset, J., 1973a, Non-complement-fixing IgM antibodies with anti-HL-A 2 specificity and blocking activity, *Transplantation* 16:257–260.

Colombani, J., Degos, L., Pétrignani, C., Chaventré, A., Lefèvre-Wittier, P., and Jacquard, A., 1973b, HL-A gene structure of Kel-Kummer Twareg, in: *Histocompatibility Testing, 1972* (J. Dausset and J. Colombani, eds.), pp. 153–162, Munksgaard, Copenhagen.

Corley, R. B., Spees, E. K., Cabrera, M. G., Swanson, J. L., and Amos, D. B., 1973, HL-A antigens of the Guatemalan Ixils, in: *Histocompatibility Testing, 1972* (J. Dausset and J. Colombani, eds.), pp. 351–357, Munksgaard, Copenhagen.

Corley, R. B., Dawson, J. R., and Amos, D. B., 1975, Lymphocyte stimulation *in vitro*: generation of cytotoxic effector lymphocytes using subcellular fractions of a lymphoid cell line, *Cell. Immunol.* 16:92–105.

Corley, R. B., Dawson, J. R., and Amos, D. B., 1976, Stimulation of lymphocytes by allogeneic lymphocytes and lymphoblasts in the presence of anti-HLA antisera, *Eur. J. Immunol.* **6**:235–240.

Craig, I. W., Tolley, E., and Bobrow, M., 1977, Assignment of a gene necessary for the expression of mitochondrial glutamate oxaloacetate transaminase in human-mouse hybrid cells, IVth International Workshop ⌐n Human *Gene Mapping,* Winnipeg, Canada.

Cresswell, P., 1977, Human B-cell alloantigens: Separation from other membrane molecules by affinity chromatography, *Eur. J. Immunol.* **7**:636–639.

Cresswell, P., 1979, Deoxycholic acid-coupled poly(L-lysyl) agarose. An amphipathic matrix with binding affinity for integral membrane proteins, *J. Biol. Chem.* **254**:414–419.

Cresswell, P., and Ayres, J. L., 1976, HLA antigens: rabbit antisera reacting with all A series or all B series specificities, *Eur. J. Immunol.* **6**:82–88.

Cresswell, P., and Dawson, J. R., 1975, Dimeric and monomeric forms of HL-A antigens solubilized by detergent, *J. Immunol.* **114**:523–525.

Cresswell, P., and Geier, S. S., 1975, Antisera to human B-lymphocyte membrane glycoproteins block stimulation in mixed lymphocyte culture, *Nature (London)* **257**:147–149.

Cresswell, P., Turner, M. J., and Strominger, S. J. L., 1973, Papain solubilized HL-A antigens from cultured human lymphocytes contain two peptide fragments, *Proc. Nat. Acad. Sci. USA.* **70**:1603–1608.

Cresswell, P., Robb, R. J., Turner, M. J., and Strominger, J. L., 1974, Papain solubilized HL-A antigens. Chromatographic and electrophoretic studies of the two subunits from different specificities, *J. Biol. Chem.* **249**:2828–2832.

Cukrová, V., Rychlíková, M., and Démant, P., 1977, Defective MLR capacitation in the human: low xenogeneic MLR capacity associated with HLA antigens Aw25-B18-Dw2, *Immunogenetics* **4**:531–540.

Cunningham, B. A., and Berggård, I., 1974, Structure, evolution and significance of $\beta_2$-microglobulin, *Transplant. Rev.* **21**:3–14.

Curry, R. A., Dierich, M. P., Pellegrino, M. A., and Hoch, J. A., 1976, Evidence for linkage between HLA antigens and receptors for complement components C3b and C3d in human-mouse hybrids, *Immunogenetics* **3**:465–471.

Curtoni, E. S., Mattiuz, P. L., and Tosi, R. M. (eds.), 1967, *Histocompatibility Testing, 1967,* 458 pp., Munksgaard, Copenhagen.

Dausset, J., 1971, The polymorphism of the HL-A system, *Transplant, Proc.* **3**:1139–1146.

Dausset, J., 1972, Similarities between the HL-A system and other immunogenetic systems, *Vox Sang.* **23**:153–164.

Dausset, J., and Colombani, J. (eds.), 1973, *Histocompatibility Testing, 1972,* 778 pp., Munksgaard, Copenhagen.

Dausset, J., and Legrand, J., 1974, The complexity of the HL-A gene product. I. Study of a serum produced against HL-A 5 in an HL-A semi-identical situation, *Tissue Antigens* **4**:329–345.

Dausset, J., and Svejgaard, A., (eds.), 1977, *HLA and Disease,* 316 pp., Munksgaard, Copenhagen.

Dausset, J., Ivanyi, P., and Ivanyi, D., 1965, Tissue alloantigens in humans: Identification of a complex system (Hu-1), in: *Histocompatibility Testing, 1965* (H. Balner, F. J. Cleton, and J. G. Eernisse, eds.), pp. 51–62, Munksgaard, Copenhagen.

Dausset, J., Colombani, J., Legrand, L., and Fellous, M., 1970, Genetics of the HL-A system. Deduction of 480 haplotypes, in: *Histocompatibility Testing, 1970* (P. I. Terasaki, ed.), pp. 53–75, Munksgaard, Copenhagen.

Dausset, J., Legrand, L., Lepage, V., Contu, L., Marcelli-Barge, A., Wildloecher, I., Benajam, A., Meo, T., and Degos, L., 1978, An haplotype study of HLA complex with special reference to the HLA-DR series and to Bf. C2 and glyoxalase I polymorphisms, *Tissue Antigens* **12**:297–307.

Dawson, J. R., 1976, The solubilization of HLA antigens with detergents and partial characterization of the antigen-detergent complexes, *Immunochemistry* **13**:671–679.

Dawson, J. R., Shasby, S. S. and Amos, D. B., 1974, The serological detection of HL-A antigens in human milk. *Tissue Antigens* **4**:76–82.

Day, E. D., 1965, *The Immunochemistry of Cancer, American Lecture Series*, p. 148, Charles C. Thomas, Springfield.

Day, E. D., 1966, *Foundations of Immunochemistry*, pp. 162–171, Williams and Wilkins Co., Baltimore.

Day, N. K., Rubenstein, P., deBracco, M., Moneada, B., Hansen, J. A., Dupont, B., Thomsen, M., Svejgaard, A., and Jersild, C., 1975, Hereditary Clr deficiency: Lack of linkage to HLA in two families, in: *Histocompatibility Testing, 1975* (F. Kissmeyer-Nielsen, ed.), pp. 960–962, Munksgaard, Copenhagen.

Decary, F., Vermeulen, A., and Engelfriet, C. P., 1975, A look at HL-A antisera in the indirect immunofluorescence technique (IIFT), in: *Histocompatibility Testing, 1975* (F. Kissmeyer-Nielsen, ed.), pp. 380–390, Munksgaard, Copenhagen.

Degos, L., and Dausset, J., 1974, Human migrations and HL-A linkage disequilibrium, *Immunogenetics* **1**:195–210.

Delage, J.-M., Bergeron, P., Simard, J., Lehner-Netsch, G., and Prochazka, E., 1977, Hereditary C7 deficiency. Diagnosis and HL-A studies in a French-Canadian family, *J. Clin. Invest.* **60**:1061–1069.

Doherty, P. C., Blanden, R. V., and Zinkernagel, R. M., 1976, Specificity of virus-immune effector T cells for H-2D or H-2K compatible interactions: Implications for H-antigen diversity, *Transplant. Rev.* **29**:89–124.

Dorf, M. E., Eguro, S. Y., Dawson, J. R., Rauckman, E. J., and Amos, D. B., 1972, Cross-reactions of HL-A antibodies. II. Continuous pH gradient elution, *J. Immunol.* **109**:681–685.

Dorval, G., Welsh, K. I., Nilsson, K., and Wigzell, H., 1977, Quantitation of $\beta_2$-microglobulin and HLA on the surface of human cells. I. T and B lymphocytes and lymphoblasts, *Scand. J. Immunol.* **6**:255–263.

Doughty, D. W., and Gelsthorpe, K., 1976, Some parameters of lymphocyte antibody activity through pregnancy and further eluates of placental material, *Tissue Antigens* **8**:43–48.

Doughty, R. W., Goodier, S. R., and Gelsthorpe, K., 1973, Further evidence for HL-A antigens present on adult peripheral red blood cells, *Tissue Antigens* **3**:189–194.

Dumble, L., and Whittingham, S., 1975, Quantitative differences in histocompatibility antigens (HL-A) in populations of lymphocytes, in: *Histocompatibility Testing, 1975* (F. Kissmeyer-Nielsen, ed.), pp. 761–766, Munksgaard, Copenhagen.

Dupont, B., Yunis, E. J., Hansen, J. A., Reinsmoen, N., Suciu-Foca, N., Mickelson, E., and Amos, D. B., 1975, Evidence for three genes involved in the expression of the mixed lymphocyte culture reaction, in: *Histocompatibility Testing, 1975* (F. Kissmeyer-Nielsen, ed.), pp. 547–551, Munksgaard, Copenhagen.

Dupont, B., Hansen, J. A., and Yunis, E. J., 1976, Human mixed lymphocyte culture reaction: genetics, specificity and biological implications, *Adv. Immunol.* **23**:108–187.

Dupont, B., Oberfield, S. E., Smithwick, E. M., Lee, T. D., and Levine, L., S., 1977a, Close genetic linkage between HLA and congenital adrenal hyperplasia (21-hydroxylase deficiency), *Lancet* **ii**:1309–1312.

Dupont, B., Hansen, J. A., Braun, D. W., Jr., Reinsmoen, N., and Yunis, E. J., 1977b, Nonrandom selection of HLA-B/D recombinant gametes, *Transplant. Proc.* **9**:1853–1854.

Duquesnoy, R. J., 1975, Approach to a molecular model for HL-A antigenicity, in: *Histocompatibility Testing, 1975* (F. Kissmeyer-Nielsen, ed.), pp. 747–752, Munksgaard, Copenhagen.

Duquesnoy, R. J., Testin, J., and Aster, R. H., 1977, Variable expression of w4 and w6 on platelets: possible relevance to platelet transfusion therapy of alloimmunized thrombocytopenic patients, *Transpl. Proc.* **9:**1829–1831.

Eguro, S. Y., Dorf, M. E., and Amos, D. B., 1973, Cross-reactions of HL-A antibodies. VI. Dissection of a complex serum, *Tissue Antigens* **3:**195–203.

Eijsvoogel, V. P., Schellekens, P. T. A., Breur-Vriesendorp, B., van Leeuwen, A., Koch, C., and van Rood, J. J., 1970, HL-A identity and one-allelic differences in families with unrelated individuals, in: *Histocompatibility Testing, 1970* (P. I. Terasaki, ed.), pp. 523–529, Munksgaard, Copenhagen.

Eijsvoogel, V. P., van Rood, J. J., Du Toit, E. D., and Schellekens, P. Th. A., 1972, Position of a locus determining mixed lymphocyte reactions distinct from the known HL-A loci, *Eur. J. Immunol.* **2:**413–418.

Eijsvoogel, V. P., du Bois, R., Melief, C. J. M., Zeylemaker, W. P., Roat-Koning, L., and de Groot-Kooy, L., 1973, Lymphocyte activation and destruction *in vitro* in relation to MLC and HL-A, *Transplant. Proc.* **5:**1301–1307.

Eisen, H. N., and Siskind, G. W., 1964, Variations in affinities of antibodies during the immune response, *Biochemistry* **3:**996–1008.

Faulk, W. P., and Temple, A., 1976, Distribution of $\beta_2$-microglobulin and HLA in chorionic villi of human placentae, *Nature (London)* **262:**799–802.

Faulk, W. P., Sanderson, A. R., and Temple, A., 1977, Distribution of MHC antigens in human placental chorionic villi, *Transplant. Proc.* **9:**1379–1384.

Fellous, M., Colle, A., and Tonnell, C., 1976, The expression of human beta$_2$-microglobulin on human spermatozoa, *Eur. J. Immunol.* **6:**21–24.

Fellous, M., Günther, E., Kembler, R., Wiels, J., Berger, R., Guenet, J. L., Jakob, H., and Jacob, F., 1978, Association of the H-Y male antigen with $\beta_2$-microglobulin on human lymphoid and differentiated mouse teratocarcinoma cell lines, *J. Exp. Med.* **148:**58–70.

Ferrara, G. B. (ed.), 1977, *HLA—New Aspects*, 170 pp., Elsevier/North-Holland Biomedical Press.

Ferrara, G. B., Tosi, R., Longo, A., Castellani, A., Viviani, C., and Carminati, G., 1978a, A safe blood transfusion producedure for immunization against MHC determinants in man, *Transplantation* **26:**150–152.

Ferrara, G., Tosi, R., Longo, A., Castellani, A., Viviani, C., and Carminati, G., 1978b, Silent alleles at the HLA-C locus, *J. Immunol.* **121:**731–735.

Ferrone, S., Belvedere, M., and Pellegrino, M. A., 1978, Structural relationship between w4/w6 antigens and the other surface markers on cultured human lymphoid cells as determined by the "lysostrip" method, *Immuno-genetics* **6:**161–169.

Festenstein, H., 1976, The Mls system, *Transplant. Proc.* **8:**339–342.

Festenstein, H., and Halim, K., 1977, HLA-D-locus determinants detected by sperm-lymphocyte culture, *Transpl. Proc.* **9:**1239–1241.

Flaherty, L., and Zimmerman, D., 1979, Further study of the surface mapping of mouse thymocytes, *Proc. Nat. Acad. Sci. USA* **76:**1990–1993.

Fradelizi, D., and Dausset, J., 1975, Mixed lymphocyte reactivity of human lymphocytes primed *in vitro*. I. Secondary response to allogeneic lymphocytes, *Eur. J. Immunol.* **5:**295–301.

Fradelizi, D., Charmot, D., Mawas, C., Sasportes, M., 1976, Secondary response of *in vitro* primed human lymphocytes to allogeneic cells. III. Specificity for the mixed lymphocyte reaction stimulating determinant of the secondary proliferative response, *Immunogenetics* **3:**29–40.

Fu, S. M., Chiorazzi, N., Wang, C. Y., Montazeri, G., Kunkel, H. G., Ko, H. S., and Gottlieb, A. B., 1978, Ia-bearing T lymphocytes in man, *J. Exp. Med.* **148:**1423–1428.

Fuller, T. C., Einarson, M., Pinto, C., Ahern, A., and Yunis, E. J., 1978, Genetic evidence that HLA-DR (Ia) specificities include multiple HLA-D determinants on a single haplotype, *Transplant. Proc.* **10:**781–784.

Gally, J. A., and Edelman, G. M., 1972, The genetic control of immunoglobin synthesis, *Ann. Rev. Genet.* **6:**1–46.

Gatti, R. A., and Leibold, W., 1979, HLA-D typing with lymphoblastoid cell lines. Allelic relationships, *Tissue Antigens* **13:**35–44.

Gedde-Dahl, T., Jr., Teisberg, P., and Thorsby, E., 1974, C3 polymorphism: genetic linkage relations, *Clin. Genet.* **6:**66–72.

Geha, R. S., Malakian, A., Geha, O., and Yunis, E., 1977, Genetics of cell-mediated lympholysis in man, *J. Immunol.* **118:**1286–1291.

Gibofsky, A., Jaffe, E. A., Fotino, M., and Becker, C. G., 1975, The identification of HL-A antigens on fresh and cultured human endothelial cells, *J. Immunol.* **115:**730–733.

Giles, C. M., Gedde-Dahl, T., Jr., Robson, E. B., Thorsby, E., Olaisen, B., Arnason, A., Kissmeyer-Nielsen, F., and Schreuder, I., 1976, Rgᵃ (Rogers) and the HLA region: linkage and associations, *Tissue Antigens* **8:**143–149.

Giphart, M. J., Doyer, E., Wisse, E., and Bruning, J. W., 1975, Quantitative aspects of HL-A2 antigenic surface determinants studies with radio-labelled antibodies, in: *Histocompatibility Testing, 1975* (F. Kissmeyer-Nielsen, ed.), pp. 739–746, Munksgaard, Copenhagen.

Giraldo, G., Degos, L., Beth, E., Sasportes, M., Marcelli, A., Gharbi, R., and Day, N. K., 1977, C8 deficiency in a family with xeroderma pigmentosum. Lack of linkage to the HLA region, *Clin. Imm. and Immunopath.* **8:**377–384.

Goodfellow, P. N., Jones, E. A., Heyningen, V. V., Solomon, S., Bobrow, M., Miggiano, V., and Bodmer, W. F., 1975, The β₂m gene is on chromosome 15 and not in the *HL-A* region, *Nature* **254:**267–269.

Gorer, P. A., and O'Gorman, P., 1956, The cytotoxic activity of isoantibodies in mice, *Transplant. Bull.* **3:**142–143.

Götze, D. (ed.), 1977, *The Major Histocompatibility System in Man and Animals*, 404 pp., Springer-Verlag, New York.

Goulmy, E., Termijtelen, A., Bradley, B., and van Rood, J., 1976, HLA restriction of non-HLA-A, -B, -C, and -D cell mediated lympholysis (CML), *Tissue Antigens* **8:**317–326.

Goulmy, E., Termijtelen, A., Bradley, B. A., and van Rood, J. J., 1977, Y antigen killing by T cells of women is restricted by HLA, *Nature (London)* **266:**544–545.

Greenberg, L. J., Gray, E. D., and Yunis, E. J., 1975, Association of HL-A 5 and immune responsiveness *in vitro* to streptococcal antigens, *J. Exp. Med.* **141:**935–943.

Grier, J. O., Abelson, L. A., Mann, D. L., Amos, D. B., and Johnson, A. H., 1977, Enrichment of B lymphocytes using goat anti-human F(ab')₂, *Tissue Antigens* **10:**236.

Grunnet, N., Kristensen, T., and Kissmeyer-Nielsen, F., 1976, Cell mediated lympholysis in man. The impact of HLA-C antigens, *Tissue Antigens* **7:**301–309.

Halim, A., Abbasi, K., and Festenstein, H., 1974, The expression of the HL-A antigens on human spermatozoa, *Tissue Antigens* **4:**1–6.

Halper, J., Fu, S. M., Wang, C. Y., Winchester, R., and Kunkel, H. G., 1978, Patterns of expression of human "Ia-like" antigens during the terminal stages of B cell development, *J. Immunol.* **120:**1480–1484.

Han, T., Dadey, B., and Minowada, J., 1977, Stimulating capacity of fresh and cultured human leukemic lymphoid and myeloid cells in "one-way" mixed lymphocyte culture reaction, *Immunol.* **33:**543–551.

Hanes, D., van Speybroeck, J., and Cockrum, K., 1978, The development of suppressor T cells in MLR. *Transplant. Proc.* **10:**895–899.

Hansen, H. E., Ryder, L. P., and Nielsen, L. S., 1975, Recombination between the second and third series of the HL-A stystem, *Tissue Antigens* **6:**275–277.

Hansen, J. A., Dupont, B., L'Esperance, P., and Good, R. A., 1977, Congenital neutropenia: abnormal neutrophil differentiation associated with HLA, *Immunogenetics* **4:**327–331.

Hartzman, R. J., Pappas, F., Romano, P. J., Johnson, A. H., Ward, F. E., and Amos, D. B., 1978, Dissociation of HLA-D and HLA-DR using primed LD typing, *Transplant. Proc.* **10:**809–812.

Hattler, B. G., Young, W. G., Amos, D. B., Hutchins, P., and McQueen, M., 1966, White blood cell antibodies. Occurrence in patients undergoing open heart surgery, *Arch. Surg.* **93:**741–746.

Hauptman, G., Tangio, M. M., Grosse-Wilde, H., and Mayer, S., 1977, Linkage between C2 defficiency and the HLA-A10,B18,Dw2,Bfs haplotype in a French family, *Immunogenetics* **4:**557–565.

Haverkorn, M. J., and Norrby, E., 1978, Measles antibodies and HLA, *J. Immunogenet.* **5:**129–134.

Heron, I., Hokland, M., and Berg, K., 1978, Enhanced expression of $\beta_2$-microglobulin and HLA antigens on human lymphoid cells by interferon, *Proc. Nat. Acad. Sci. USA* **75:**6215–6219.

Hirschberg, H., and Thorsby, E., 1975, Lymphocyte activating alloantigens on human epidermal cells, *Tissue Antigens* **6:**183–194.

Hirschberg, H., and Thorsby, E., 1977, Activation of human suppressor cells in mixed lymphocyte cultures, *Scand. J. Immunol.* **6:**809–815.

Hirschberg, H., Evensen, S. A., Henriksen, T., and Thorsby, E., 1974, Stimulation of human lymphocytes by allogeneic endothelial cells *in vitro, Tissue Antigens* **4:**257–261.

Hirschfeld, J., 1965, Serologic codes: Interpretation of immunogenetic systems, *Science* **148:**968–971.

Hirschhorn, K., Bach, F., Kolodny, R. L., Firschein, I. L., and Hashem, N., 1963, Immune response and mitosis of human peripheral blood lymphocytes *in vitro, Science* **142:**1185–1187.

Hobart, M. J., 1977, Complementary genetics, *Nature (London)* **266:**681–682.

Hobart, M. J., Cook, P. J. L., and Lachmann, P. J., 1977, Linkage studies with C6, *J. Immunogenet.* **4:**423–428.

Hsia, S., Howell, D. N., Amos, D. B., and Woodbury, M. A., 1977, Studies of viral antibody responses among Amish families, *J. Immunol.* **118:**1659–1663.

Hsu, S. H., Yates, K., Hopkins, K., and Bias, W. B., 1977, Evidence for a third lymphocyte-defined locus in the HLA region, *Transplant. Proc.* **9** (Suppl. 1):87–93.

Hunter, S. V., Benson, J. W., Bull, R. W., and Poulik, M. D., 1978, Use of turkey anti-human $\beta_2$-microglobulin antisera for identification of DR antibodies, *Transplant. Proc.* **10:**853–855.

Jackson, J. F., Currier, R. D., Terasaki, P. I., and Morton, N. E., 1977, Spinocerebellar ataxia and HLA linkage, *New Eng. J. Med.* **296:**1138–1141.

Janis, M., Hartzmann, R. J., and Bach, F. H., 1970, Lymphocyte reactivity *in vitro.* III. Soluble factors in histocompatibility matching, in: *Histocompatibility Testing, 1970* (P. I. Terasaki, ed.), pp. 517–521, Munksgaard, Copenhagen.

Jeannet, M., Schapira, M., Gervasoni, C., Metaxas-Buhler, M., Butler, R., and van Loghem, E., 1973, Study of the HL-A system and other polymorphisms in the Tibetan population, in: *Histocompatibility Testing, 1972* (J. Dausset and J. Colombani, eds.), pp. 241–250, Munksgaard, Copenhagen.

Jensen, E. B., Kristensen, T., Jorgensen, F., and Lamm, L. U., 1977, HLA-D typing by homozygous typing cells. A statistical analysis of experimental and biological variation, *Tissue Antigens* 10:83–98.

Jersild, C., Rubenstein, P., and Day, N. K., 1976, The HLA system and inherited deficiencies of the complement system, *Transplant. Rev.* 32:43–71.

Johnson, A. H., Rossen, R. D., and Butler, W. T., 1972, Detection of allo-antibodies using a sensitive antiglobulin microcytotoxicity test: identification of low levels of preformed antibodies in accelerated allograft rejection, *Tissue Antigens* 2:215–226.

Johnson, A. H., Amos, D. B., Noreen, H., and Yunis, E. J., 1975, Strong mixed lymphocyte reaction associated with the LA or first locus HL-A, *Transplantation* 20:291–295.

Johnson, A. H., Ward, F. E., and Amos, D. B., 1977, B-lymphocyte alloantigens, *Scand. J. Immunol.* 6:171–176.

Jongsma, A., Someren, H., Westerwald, A., Hagemeijer, A., and Pearson, P., 1973, Localization of genes of human chromosomes by studies of human-Chinese hamster somatic cell hybrids, *Humangenetik* 20:195–202.

Jørgensen, F., Lamm, L. U., and Kissmeyer-Nielsen, F., 1973, Mixed lymphocyte cultures with inbred individuals: An approach to MLC typing, *Tissue Antigens* 3:323–329.

Jørgensen, F., Lamm, L. U., and Kissmeyer-Nielsen, F., 1974, MLC typing and blastogenic factor, *Tissue Antigens* 4:404.

Kaakinen, A., and Hirschberg, H., 1977, Stimulation of human lymphocytes by allogeneic macrophages *in vitro, Tissue Antigens* 10:306–314.

Kachru, R. B., and Mittal, K. K., 1975, Serological detection of HL-A antigens in human mammary secretion, in: *Histocompatibility Testing, 1975* (F. Kissmeyer-Nielsen, ed.), pp. 404–413, Munksgaard, Copenhagen.

Käalén, B., Löw, B., and Nilsson, O., 1977, Confounding factors in HLA-Dw2 typing of human leucocytes, *Clin. Exp. Immunol.* 27:55–62.

Kamoun, M., Wiels, J., Lepage, V., Fellous, M., Chereau, C., Sasportes, M., and Dausset,-J., 1977, Presence of Ia equivalent on human spermatozoa detected by specific reagents, prepared by the absorption-elution technique on B cell lymphoid lines or PHA stimulated cells, *Tissue Antigens* 10:245.

Karush, F., 1962, Immunologic specificity and molecular structure, *Adv. Immunol.* 2:1–40.

Keuning, J. J., Termijtelen, A., Blusse van Oud Alblas, A., Gabb, B. W., D'Amaro, J., and van Rood, J. J., 1975, LD (MLC) population and family studies in a Dutch population, in: *Histocompatibility Testing, 1975* (F. Kissmeyer-Nielsen, ed.), pp. 533–543, Munksgaard, Copenhagen.

Kissmeyer-Nielsen, F. (ed.), 1975, *Histocompatibility Testing, 1975*, 1035 pp., Munksgaard, Copenhagen.

Kissmeyer-Nielsen, F., and Thorsby, E., 1970, Human transplantation antigens, *Transplant. Rev.* 4:1–175.

Klareskog, L., Sandberg-Trigardh, L., Rask, L., Lindblom, J. B., Curman, B., and Peterson, P. A., 1977a, Chemical properties of human Ia antigens, *Nature (London)* 265:248–251.

Klareskog, L., Tjernlund, U. M., Forsum, U., and Peterson, P. A., 1977b, Epidermal Langerhans cells express Ia antigens, *Nature (London)* 268:248–250.

Klareskog, L., Trägardh, L., Lindblom, J. B. and Peterson, P. A., 1978, Reactivity of a rabbit antiserum against highly purified HLA-DR antigens, *Scand. J. Immunol.* 7:199–208.

Klein, J. (ed.), 1975, *The Biology of the Mouse Histocompatibility-2 Complex*, 620 pp., Springer-Verlag, New York.

Klein, J., 1977, Evolution and function of the major histocompatibility system: Facts and Speculations, in: *The Major Histocompatibility System in Man and Animals* (D. Götze, ed.), pp. 339–378, Springer-Verlag, New York.

Klein, J., 1978, H-2 mutations: Their genetics and effect on immune functions, *Immunology* **26**:56–146.

Knowles, B. B., Mausner, R., and Aden, D. P., 1977, Preliminary characterization of human cell surface molecules controlled by human chromosomes 7 and 6, IVth International Workshop on Human Gene Mapping, August 14–18, Winnipeg, Canada.

Koch, G., and Shows, T. B., 1978, A gene on human chromosome 6 functions in assembly of tissue-specific adenosine deaminase isozymes, *Proc. Nat. Acad. Sci. USA* **75**:3876–3880.

Kostyu, D. D., Bernard, N. F., and Amos, D. B., 1979, Cross-reactions of HLA antibodies. VII. Rate of sensitization and serological specificity, *Tissue Antigens* **13**:298–306.

Kostyu, D. D., Cresswell, P., and Amos, D. B., 1980, A public HLA antigen associated with HLA-A9, Aw32 and Bw4, *Immunogenetics* (in press).

Kovithavongs, T., Shivji, S., and Dossetor, J. B., 1978, Human K cells do not have Ia antigens, *Transplant. Proc.* **10**:839–843.

Kristensen, T., 1978, Studies on the specificity of CML. Report from a CML workshop, *Tissue Antigens* **11**:330–349.

Kristensen, T., and Grunnet, N., 1975, Cell mediated lympholysis (CML) in man. Evidence of a separate locus within the major histocompatibility complex (MHC) and an approach to CML typing, in: *Histocompatibility Testing, 1975* (F. Kissmeyer-Nielsen, ed.), pp. 835–844, Munksgaard, Copenhagen.

Kristensen, T., and Jørgensen, F., 1978, False HLA-D assignments may be caused by cytotoxic responder lymphocytes, *Tissue Antigens* **11**:443–448.

Kuntz, M. M., Inness, J. B., and Weksler, M. E., 1976, Lymphocyte transformation induced by autologous cells. IV. Human T lymphocyte proliferation induced by autologous or allogeneic non-T lymphocytes, *J. Exp. Med.* **143**:1042–1054.

Lachmann, P. J., and Hobart, M. J., 1978, Complement genetics in relation to HLA, *Br. Med. Bull.* **34**:247–252.

Lamm, L. U., and Kristensen, T., 1977, Formal genetics of the HLA system, in: *HLA System—New Aspects* (G. B. Ferrara, ed.), pp. 1–20, Elsevier/North Holland Biomedical Press, New York.

Lamm, L. U., Kissmeyer-Nielsen, F., and Henningsen, K., 1970, Linkage and association studies of two phosphoglucomutase loci (*PGM₁* and *PGM₃*) to eighteen other markers, *Hum. Hered.* **20**:305–318.

Lamm, L. U., Friedrich, U., Petersen, G. B., Jørgensen, J., Nielsen, J., Therkelsen, A. J., and Kissmeyer-Nielsen, F., 1974, Assignment of the major histocompatibility complex to chromosome no. 6 in a family with a pericentric inversion, *Hum. Hered.* **24**:273–284.

Lamm, L. U. Thorsen, I.-L., Petersen, G. B., Jørgensen, J., Henningsen, K., Bech, B., and Kissmeyer-Nielsen, F., 1975, Data on the HL-A linkage group. *Ann. Hum. Genet.* **38**:383–390.

Lamm, L. U., Kristensen, T., Kissmeyer-Nielsen, F., and Jørgensen, F., 1977, On the HLA-B, -D map distance, *Tissue Antigens* **10**:394–398.

Lamm, L. U., Cullen, P., Edwards, J. H., van Leeuwen, A., Larsen, B., Cann, H., Thompson, J., Albert, E., Monk, K., Richards, S., and Bodmer, W. F., 1978, Joint family analysis, in: *Histocompatibility Testing, 1977* (W. F. Bodmer, J. R. Batchelor, J. G. Bodmer, H. Festenstein, and P. J. Morris, eds.), pp. 279–293, Munksgaard, Copenhagen.

Landsteiner, K., 1942, *The Specificity of Serological Reactions*, 330 pp., Dover Publications, New York.

Legrand, L., and Dausset, J., 1973, Serological evidence of the existence of several antigenic determinants (or factors) on the *HL-A* gene products, in: *Histocompatibility Testing, 1972* (J. Dausset and J. Colombani, eds.), pp. 441–453, Munksgaard, Copenhagen.

Legrand, L., and Dausset, J., 1975a, The complexity of the *HL-A* gene product. II. Possible evidence for a "public" determinant common to the first and second HL-A series, *Transplantation* 19:177–180.

Legrand, L. and Dausset, J., 1975b, A second lymphocyte system (Ly-Li), in: *Histocompatibility Testing, 1975* (F. Kissmeyer-Nielsen, ed.), pp. 665–670, Munksgaard, Copenhagen.

Lemke, H., Hämmerling, G. J., Höhmann, C., and Rajewsky, K., 1978, Hybrid cell lines secreting monoclonal antibody specific for major histocompatibility antigens of the mouse, *Nature (London)* 271:249–251.

Lepage, V., Degos, L., and Dausset, J., 1976, A natural anti-HLA-A2 antibody reacting with homozygous cells, *Tissue Antigens* 8:139–142.

Levine, B. B., Stember, R. H., and Fotino, M., 1972, Ragweed hay fever: Genetic control and linkage to HL-A haplotypes, *Science* 178:1201–1202.

Liberi, H. E., 1978, Production of allospecific antibodies to human DR antigens in a chimpanzee, *Fed. Proc.* 37:1757, Abstr. 2666.

Little, J. R., and Eisen, H. N., 1969, Specificity of the immune response to the 2,4-dinitrophenyl and 2,4,6-trinitrophenyl groups. Ligand binding and fluorescence properties of cross-reacting antibodies, *J. Exp. Med.* 129:247–265.

Lohrmann, H. P., Novikovs, L., and Graw, R. L., Jr., 1974, Stimulatory capacity of human T and B lymphocytes in the mixed leukocyte culture, *Nature (London)* 250:144–146.

Loke, Y. N., Joysey, V. C., and Borland, R., 1971, HL-A antigens on human trophoblast cells, *Nature (London)* 232:403–405.

Long, M. A., Handwerger, B. S., Amos, D. B., and Yunis, E. J., 1976, The genetics of cell-mediated lympholysis, *J. Immunol.* 117:2092–2099.

MacQueen, J. M., Ottesen, E. A., Weller, P. F., Ottesen, C., Amos, D. B., and Ward, F. E., 1979, HLA histocompatibility antigens in a Polynesian population—Cook islanders of Mauke, *Tissue Antigens* 13:121–128.

McCune, J. M., Humphreys, R. E., Yocum, R. R., and Strominger, J. L., 1975, Enhanced representation of HL-A antigens on human lymphocytes after mitogenesis induced by phytohemagglutinin or Epstein-Barr virus, *Proc. Nat. Acad. Sci. USA* 72:3206–3209.

Mann, D. L., Abelson, L., Harris, S., and Amos, D. B., 1976a, Second genetic locus in the HLA region for human B-cell alloantigens, *Nature (London)* 259:145–146.

Mann, D. L., Katz, S. I., Nelson, D. L., Abelson, L. D., and Strober, W., 1976b, Specific B-cell antigens associated with gluten-sensitive enteropathy and dermatitis herpetiformis, *Lancet* i:pp. 110–111.

Mardiney, M. K. Jr., Bock, G. N., and Chess, L., 1972, The role of the human granulocyte as an antigen in the mixed lymphocyte reaction, *Transplantation* 14:274–278.

Marsh, D. G., and Bias, W. B., 1977, Basal serum IgE levels and HLA antigen frequencies in allergic subjects. II. Studies in people sensitive to rye grass group I and ragweed antigen E and of postulated immune response (*Ir*) loci in the HLA region, *Immunogenetics* 5:235–251.

Martel, J. L., Jaramillo, S., Allen, F. H. Jr., and Rubenstein, P., 1974, Serology for automated cytotoxicity assays. Contrast fluorescence test, *Vox Sang.* 27:13–20.

Mattiuz, P. L., Massobrio, M., and Richiardi, P., 1973, Espressione degli antigeni del sistema HL-A sulle cellule fetali, *Estratto Minerva Ginecol.* 25:8–13.

Mawas, C., Sasportes, M., Christen, Y., Bernard, A., Dausset, J., Alter, B. J., and Bach, M. L., 1973, Cell-mediated lympholysis (CML) in the absence of LD2 mixed lymphocyte reaction and CML in the presence of SD1-SD2 identity in two HLA-genotyped families, *Transplant. Proc.* **5**:1683–1689.

Mawas, C. E., Charmot, D., and Sasportes, M., 1975, Secondary response of *in vitro* primed human lymphocytes to allogeneic cells, *Immunogenetics* **2**:449–463.

Mayr, W. R., Pausch, V., and Schnedl, W., 1979, Human chimaera detectable only by investigation of her progeny, *Nature (London)* **277**:210–211.

McMichael, A. J., Morhenn, V., Payne, R., Sasazuki, T., and Farber, E. M., 1978, HLA C and D antigens associated with psoriasis, *Br. J. Dermatol.* **98**:287–292.

Mendell, N. R., Lee, K. L., Reinsmoen, N., Yunis, E., Amos, D. B., and Emme, L., 1977, Statistical methods for evaluating responses in HLA-D typing, *Transplant. Proc.* **9**:99–106.

Mendell, N. R., Guppy, D. Bodmer, W. F., and Festenstein, H., 1978, Data management and assignment of scores to MLC data, in: *Histocompatibility Testing, 1977* (W. F. Bodmer, J. R. Batchelor, J. G. Bodmer, H. Festenstein, and P. J. Morris, eds.), pp. 90–102, Munksgaard, Copenhagen.

Mendes, N. F., Tolnai, M. E. A., Silveira, N. P. A., Gilbertsen, R. B., and Metzgar, R. S., 1973, Technical aspects of the rosette tests used to detect human complement receptor (B) and sheep erythrocyte-binding (T) lymphocytes, *J. Immunol.* **111**:860–867.

Menozzi, P., Piazza, A., and Cavalli-Sforza, L., 1978, Synthetic maps of human gene frequencies in Europeans, *Science* **201**:786–792.

Meo, T., Atkinson, J., Bernoco, M., Bernoco, D., and Ceppellini, R., 1977, Structural heterogeneity of C2 complement protein and its genetic variants in man: A new polymorphism of the HLA region, *Proc. Nat. Acad. Sci. USA* **74**:1672–1675.

Merritt, A. D., Petersen, B. H., Biegel, A. A., Meyers, D. A., Brooks, G. F., and Hodes, M. E., 1976, Chromosome 6: Linkage of the eighth component of complement (C8) to the histocompatibility region (HLA), in: *Baltimore Conference (1975), Third International Workshop on Human Gene Mapping. Birth Defects: Original Article Series*, Vol. 12, No. 7, pp. 364–366, The National Foundation, New York.

Michaelson, J., Flaherty, L., Vitetta, E., and Poulik, M. D., 1977, Molecular similarities between the Qa-2 alloantigen and other gene products of the 17th chromosome of the mouse, *J. Exp. Med.* **145**:1066–1070.

Mickey, M. R., Opelz, G., and Terasaki, P. I., 1975, Comparison of MLC typing response indexes, in: *Histocompatibility Testing, 1975* (F. Kissmeyer-Nielsen, ed.), pp. 563–568, Munksgaard, Copenhagen.

Middleton, J., Crookston, M. C., Falk, J. A., Robson, E. B., Cook, P. J. L., Batchelor, J. R., Bodmer, J., Ferrara, G. B., Festenstein, H., Harris, R., Kissmeyer-Nielsen, F., Lawler, S. D., Sachs, J. A., and Wolf, E., 1974, Linkage of Chido and HL-A, *Tissue Antigens* **4**:366–373.

Milgrom, F., Kano, K., and Witebsky, E., 1965, The mixed agglutination test in studies in human transplantation, *J. Am. Med. Assoc.* **192**:845.

Mintz, B., 1971, Genetic mosaicism *in vivo*: Development and disease in allophenic mice, *Fed. Proc.* **30**:935–943.

Mittal, K. K., 1975, Human histocompatibility (HL-A) antigens in semen and their role in reproduction, *Fertil. Steril.* **26**:704–710.

Mittal, K. K., and Terasaki, P. I., 1972, Cross-reactivity in the HL-A system, *Tissue Antigens* **2**:94–104.

Mittal, K. K., Wolski, D. P., Lim, D., Gewurz, A., Gewurz, H., and Schmid, F. R., 1976,

Genetic independence between the HLA system and deficiency of the first and sixth components of complement, *Tissue Antigens* 7:97–104.

Moraes, J. R., and Stastny, P., 1975, Alloantibodies to endothelial cell antigens, in: *Histocompatibility Testing, 1975* (F. Kissmeyer-Nielsen, ed.), pp. 391–397, Munksgaard, Copenhagen.

Moraes, M. E., Sittler, S., and Stastny, P., 1975, Development of methods for study of human alloantibodies reacting with subpopulations of lymphocytes, in: *The First HLA Workshop of the Americas*, DHEW Pub. 76–1064, pp. 186–193.

Moraes, M. E., Moraes, J. R., and Stastny, P., 1977, Separate Ia-like determinants in human lymphocytes and macrophages, *Transplant. Proc.* 9:1211–1213.

Morton, J. A., Pickles, M. M., Sutton, L., and Skov, F., 1971, Identification of further antigens on red cells and lymphocytes: Association of Bg$^b$ with w17 (Te 57) and Bg$^c$ with w28 (Dal5, Ba*), *Vox Sang.* 21:141–153.

Mowas, C. E., Charmot, D., and Sasportes, M., 1976, Secondary response of *in vitro*-primed human lymphocytes to allogeneic cells. IV. Evidence for a cell-mediated lympholysis target-antigen locus linked to, but different from, the classical human major histocompatibility complex, *Immunogenetics* 3:41–51.

Muller-Eberhard, H. J., 1975, Complement, *Ann. Rev. Biochem.* 44:697–724.

Murphy, G. P. (ed.), 1977, *HLA and Malignancy*, 246 pp., Alan R. Liss, New York.

Nabholtz, M., and Miggiano, V. C., 1978, The biological significance of the mixed leukocyte reaction, in: *B and T Cells in Immune Recognition* (F. Loor and G. E. Roelants, ed.), pp. 261–289, John Wiley and Sons, Ltd., New York.

Naeim, F., Leibold, W., Gatti, R. A., Ferrara, G. B., Johns, S., and Walford, R. L., 1978, Ia-like segregant series probably distinct from HLA-DRw: a study of lymphoblastoid cell lines and leukemia cells with evidence for a class of cytotoxic antibodies requiring the presence of monocytes, *Transplant. Proc.* 10:815–821.

Nau, D. S., Markowsky, G., Woodbury, M. A., and Amos, D. B., 1978, A mathematical analysis of human leukocyte antigen serology, *Math. Biosc.* 40:243–270.

Netzel, B., Grosse-Wilde, H., Rittner, Ch., Pretorius, A. M. G., Scholz, S., and Albert, E. D., 1975, HL-A/MLC recombination frequency and LD typing in HL-A/MLC/Bf/PGM3 recombinant families, in: *Histocompatibility Testing, 1975* (F. Kissmeyer-Nielsen, ed.), pp. 955–959, Munksgaard, Copenhagen.

Nicolson, G. L., 1976, Transmembrane control of the receptors on normal and tumor cells. I. Cytoplasmic influence over cell surface components, *Biochim. Biophys. Acta* 457:57–108.

Nielsen, L. S., Ryder, L. P., and Svejgaard, A., 1975, The third (AJ) segregant series, in: *Histocompatibility Testing, 1975* (F. Kissmeyer-Nielsen, ed.), pp. 324–329, Munksgaard, Copenhagen.

Nordhagen, R., and Orjasaeter, H., 1974, Association between HL-A and red cell antigens. An autoanalyzer study, *Vox Sang.* 26:97–106.

Ochs, H. D., Rosenfeld, S. I., Thomas, E. D., Giblett, E. R., Alper, C. A., Dupont, B., Scholler, J. G., Gilliland, B. C., Hansen, J. A., and Wedgwood, R. J., 1977, Linkage between the gene (or genes) controlling the synthesis of the fourth component of complement and the major histocompatibility complex, *New Eng. J. Med.* 296:470–475.

Olaisen, B., Gedde-Dahl, Jr., T., and Thorsby, E., 1976, Localization of the human *GLO* gene locus, *Humangenetik* 32:301–304.

Oliver, R. T. D., and Festenstein, H., 1975, Second, third locus and 4a/4b antigen associations in Negroids and Caucasoids, *Tissue Antigens* 5:395–401.

Olving, J. H., Olaisen, B., Teisberg, P., Gedde-Dahl, Jr. T., and Thorsby, E., 1977, Non-linkage between C6 and chromosome 6 markers, *Hum. Genet.* 37:125–129.

O'Neill, G. H., Yang, S. Y., Tegoli, J., Berger, R., and Dupont, B., 1978a, Chido and Rodgers blood groups are distinct antigenic components of human complement C4, *Nature (London)* **273:**668–669.

O'Neill, G. J., Yang, S. Y., and Dupont, B., 1978b, Two HLA-linked loci controlling the fourth component of human complement, *Proc. Nat. Acad. Sci. USA* **75:**5165–5169.

Osofsky, S. G., Thompson, B. H., Gewurz, H., Schmid, F. R., and Mittal, K. K., 1977, Evidence for lack of linkage between HLA and C3 deficiency in man, *Immunogenetics* **4:**195–197.

Ostberg, L., Rask, L., Wigzell, H., and Peterson, P. A., 1975, Thymus leukaemia antigen contains $\beta_2$-microglobulin, *Nature (London)* **253:**735–737.

Papermaster, B. W., Papermaster, V. M., Reisfeld, R. A., Pellegrino, M. A., Ferrone, S., Kahan, B. D., Terasaki, P. I., Takasugi, M., and Albert, E. D., 1972, Characterization and isolation of HL-A antigens from continuous cultured human lymphocyte cell lines: A report of current progress, in: *Cellular Antigens* (A. Nowotny, ed.), pp. 186–199, Springer-Verlag, New York.

Parham, P., and Bodmer, W. F., 1978, Monoclonal antibody to a human histocompatibility alloantigen, HLA-A2, *Nature (London)* **276:**397–399.

Parham, P., Alpert, B. N., Orr, H. T., and Strominger, J. L., 1977, Carbohydrate moiety of HLA antigens: antigenic properties and amino acid sequences around the site of glycosylation, *J. Biol. Chem.* **252:**7555–7567.

Parish, C. R., Higgins, T. J., and McKenzie, I. F. C., 1978, Comparison of antigens recognized by xenogeneic and allogeneic anti-Ia antibodies: evidence for two classes of Ia antigens, *Immunogenetics* **6:**343–354.

Payne, R., and Hackel, E., 1961, Inheritance of human leukocyte antigens, *Amer. J. Hum. Genet.* **13:**306–319.

Payne, R., Amos, B., Kostyu, D., Engelfriet, C. P., van den Berg-Loonen, P. M., Curtoni, E. S., and Richiardi, P., 1978, Subdivisions of the HLA-B5 and Bw35 complex, *Tissue Antigens* **11:**302–314.

Pellegrino, M. A., Curry, R. A., Pellegrino, A. G., and Hock, J. A., 1975, Linkage between the B-cell specific receptor for monkey red blood cells and HL-A, *Immunogenetics* **2:**543–549.

Pellegrino, M. A., Ferrone, S., Pellegrino, A. D., Oh, S. K., and Reisfeld, R. A., 1974, Evaluation of two sources of soluble HL-A antigens: Platelets and serum, *Eur. J. Immunol.* **4:**250–255.

Peterson, P. A., Cunningham, B. A., Berggard, I., and Edelman, G. M., 1972, $\beta_2$-microglobulin—a free immunoglobulin domain, *Proc. Nat. Acad. Sci. USA* **69:**1671–1701.

Piazza, A., and Galfré, G., 1975, A new statistical approach for MLC typing: A clustering technique, in: *Histocompatibility Testing, 1975* (F. Kissmeyer-Nielsen, ed.), pp. 552–556, Munksgaard, Copenhagen.

Pious, D., Bodmer, J., and Bodmer, W., 1974, Antigenic expression and cross-reactions in HL-A variants of lymphoid cell lines, *Tissue Antigens* **4:**247–256.

Plate, J. M., Ward, F. E., and Amos, D. B., 1970, The mixed leukocyte culture response between HL-A identical siblings, in: *Histocompatibility Testing, 1970* (P. I. Terasaki, ed.), pp. 531–535, Munksgaard, Copenhagen.

Pober, J. S., Guild, B. C., and Strominger, J. L., 1978, Phosphorylation *in vivo* and *in vitro* of human histocompatibility antigens (HLA-A and HLA-B) in the carboxy-terminal intracellular domain, *Proc. Nat. Acad. Sci. USA* **75:**6002–6006.

Popp, D. M., 1978, Use of congenic mice to study the genetic basis of degenerative disease, in: *Genetic Effects of Aging* (D. Bergsma and D. H. Harrison, eds.), p. 261, Alan R. Liss, New York.

Poulik, M. D., Ferrone, S., Pellegrino, M. A., Sevier, D. E., Oh, S. K., and Reisfeld, R. A., 1974, Association of HL-A antigens and $\beta_2$-microglobulin: Concepts and questions, Transplant. Rev. 21:106–125.

Ragab, A. H., and Cowan, D. H., 1973, Separation of cells involved in the mixed leukocyte culture by velocity sedimentation, Cell. Immunol. 7:336–340.

Raum, D., Glass, D., Carpenter, C. B., and Schur, P. H., 1976, C6 deficiency—HLA association, Fed. Proc. 35:655.

Rapaport, F. T., Thomas, L., Converse, J. M., and Lawrence, H. S., 1960, The specificity of skin homograft rejection in man, Ann. N.Y., Acad. Sci. 87:217–220.

Rask, L., Österberg, L., Lindblom, B., Rernstedt, Y., and Peterson, P. A., 1974, The subunit structure of transplantation antigens, Transplant. Rev. 21:85–105.

Reis, A. P., dos, Betuel, H., Reisner, E. G., and Amos, D. B., 1972, The utilization of antiglobulin reagents in the cytotoxicity testing for HL-A, Transplantation 15:36–41.

Reisfeld, R. A., Pellegrino, M. A., and Ferrone, S., 1977, The immunologic and molecular profiles of HLA antigens isolated from urine, J. Immunol. 118:264–269.

Richiardi, P., Castagneto, M., D'Amaro, J., Schruder, I., Vassalli, P., and Curtoni, E. S., 1974, Four new HL-A allelic factors subtypic to HL-A 12 and w15. Their correlation with w4 and w6, J. Immunogenet. 1:323–325.

Rittner, C., 1976, Genetic loci of components of the classical and alternate pathway of complement activation: A new dimension of the immunogenetic linkage group (HLA) on chromosome 6 in man, Hum. Genet. 35:1–20.

Rittner, C., Opferkuch, W., Wellek, B., Grosse-Wilde, H., and Wernet, P., 1976, Lack of linkage between gene(s) controlling the synthesis of the seventh component of complement and the HLA region on chromosome no. 6 in man, Hum. Genet. 34:137–142.

Robb, R. J., Terhorst, C., and Strominger, J. L., 1978, Sequence of the COOH-terminal hydrophilic region of histocompatibility antigens HLA-A2 and HLA-B7, J. Biol. Chem. 253:5319–5324.

Robinson, M. A., Noreen, H. J., Amos, D. B., and Yunis, E. J., 1978, Target antigens of cell-mediated lympholysis. Discrimination of HLA subtypes by cytotoxic lymphocytes, J. Immunol. 121:1486–1490.

Rodey, G. E., Sturm, B., and Aster, R. H., 1973, Cross-reactive HL-A antibodies. Separation of multiple HL-A antibody specificities by platelet absorption and acid elution, Tissue Antigens, 3:63–69.

Rogentine, G. N., Jr., 1967, Detection of isoantigens on human lymphocytes and tissue culture cells by the $^{51}$Cr cytotoxicity technique, in: Histocompatibility Testing, 1967 (E. S. Curtoni, P. L. Mattiuz, and R. M. Tosi, eds.), pp. 371–379, Munksgaard, Copenhagen.

Rosenfeld, S. I., Weitkamp, L. R., and Ward, F. E., 1977, Hereditary deficiency of the fifth component of complement in man. IV. Genetic linkage studies, J. Immunol. 119:604–610.

Rotman, B., and Papermaster, B. W., 1966, Membrane properties of living mammalian cells as studied by enzymatic hydrolysis of fluorogenic esters, Proc. Nat. Acad. Sci. USA 55:134–141.

Russell, P. S., and Winn, H. J. (eds.), 1965, Histocompatibility Testing, Natl. Acad. Sci. USA Publ. 1229, Washington, D.C.

Ryder, L. P., and Svejgaard, A., 1977, Histocompatibility associated diseases, in: B and T Cells in Immune Recognition (F. Loor and G. E. Roelants, eds.), pp. 437–456, John Wiley and Sons, Ltd. New York.

Ryder, L. P., Thomsen, M., Platz, P., and Svejgaard, A., 1975, Data reduction in LD-typing, in: Histocompatibility Testing, 1975 (F. Kissmeyer-Nielsen, ed.), pp. 845–848, Munksgaard, Copenhagen.

Sanderson, A., and Batchelor, R., 1967, Lymphocytotoxic reactions of human isoantisera detected by the release of chromium-51 label or by dye exclusion, in: *Histocompatibility Testing, 1967* (E. S. Curtoni, P. L. Mattiuz, and R. M. Tosi, eds.), pp. 367–369, Munksgaard, Copenhagen.

Sanderson, A. R., and Welsh, K. I., 1974, Properties of histocompatibility (HL-A) determinants. I. Site density of antigens of the two segregant series on peripheral human lymphocytes, *Transplantation* 17:281–289.

Sasazuki, T., McMichael, A., Radvany, R., Payne, R., and McDevitt, H., 1976, Use of high dose x-irradiation to block back stimulation in the MLC reaction, *Tissue Antigens* 7:91–96.

Sasazuki, T., Kohno, Y., Iwamoto, I., Tanimura, M., and Naito, S., 1978, Association between an HLA haplotype and low responsiveness to tetanus toxoid in man, *Nature (London)* 272:359–361.

Sasportes, M., Nunez-Roldan, A., and Fradelizi, D., 1978, Analysis of products involved in primary and secondary allogeneic proliferation in man. II. Further evidence for products different from Ia-like, DRw antigens, activating secondary allogeneic proliferation in man, *Immunogenetics* 6:55–68.

Saunders, J. B. de C. M., 1972, A conceptual history of transplantation, in: *Transplantation* (J. S. Najarian and R. L. Simmons, eds.), pp. 3–25, Lea and Febiger, Philadelphia.

Schendel, D. J., Wank, R., and Dupont, B., 1978, Cell-mediated lympholysis: Examination of HLA genetic fine structure and complementation using cytotoxic lymphocytes, *Eur. J. Immunol.* 8:634–640.

Scher, I., Berning, A. K., Strong, D. M., and Green, I., 1975, The immune response to a synthetic amino acid terpolymer in man: Relationship to HLA type, *J. Immunol.* 115:36–40.

Schurmann, R. K. B., van Rood, J. J., Vossen, J. M., Schellekens, P. Th. A., Feltkamp-Vroom, Th. M., Doyer, E., Gmellig-Mayling, F., and Vissner, H. K. A., 1979, Failure of lymphocyte-membrane HLA-A and B expression in two siblings with combined immunodeficiency, *Clin. Immunol. Immunopath.* (in press).

Seaman, M. J., Bemson, R., Jones, M. N., Morton, J. A., and Pickles, M. M., 1967, The reactions of the Bennett-Goodspeed group of antibodies with the Auto-Analyzer, *Br. J. Haematol.* 13:464–473.

Seigler, H. F., and Metzgar, R. S., 1970, Embryonic development of human transplantation antigens, *Transplantation* 9:478–486.

Seigler, H. F., Ward, F. E., Amos, D. B., Phaup, M. B., and Stickel, D. L., 1971, The immunogenicity of human HL-A haplotypes as measured by skin graft survival times and mixed leukocyte reactions, *J. Exp. Med.* 133:411–423.

Shaw, S., and Biddison, W. E., 1979, HLA-linked genetic control of the specificity of human cytotoxic T cell responses to influenza virus, *J. Exp. Med.* 149:565–575.

Sheehy, M. J., and Bach, F. H., 1976, Primed LD typing (PLT)—Technical considerations, *Tissue Antigens* 8:157–171.

Shreffler, D. C., David, C. S., Passmore, H. C., and Klein, J., 1971, Genetic organization and evolution of the mouse H-2 region: A duplication model, *Transplant. Proc.* 3:176–179.

Singal, D. P., Berry, R., and Naipaul, N., 1971, HL-A inhibiting activity in human seminal plasma, *Nature New Biol.* 233:61–62.

Smith, M., and Hirschhorn, K., 1978, Location of genes for human heavy chain immunoglobulin to chromosome 6. *Proc. Nat. Acad. Sci. USA* 75:3367–3371.

Snary, D., Barnstable, C., Bodmer, W. F., Goodfellow, P., and Crumpton, M. J., 1976,

Human Ia antigens—purification and molecular structure, *Cold Spring Harbor Symp. Quant. Biol.* **41**:379–386.

Snary, D., Barnstable, C. J., Bodmer, W. F., and Crumpton, M. J., 1977a, Molecular structure of human histocompatibility antigens: The HLA-C series, *Eur. J. Immunol.* **8**:580–585.

Snary, D., Barnstable, C. J., Bodmer, W. F., Goodfellow, P. M., and Crumpton, M. J., 1977b, Cellular distribution, purification and molecular nature of human Ia antigens, *Scand. J. Immunol.* **6**:439–452.

Snell, G. D., Dausset, J., and Nathenson, S. (eds.), 1976, *Histocompatibility*, 401 pp., Academic Press, New York.

Solheim, B. G., Thorsby, E., and Moller, E., 1976, Inhibition of the Fc receptor of human lymphoid cells by antisera recognizing determinants of the HLA system, *J. Exp. Med.* **143**:1568–1574.

Someren, H. van, Westerveld, A., Hagemeijer, A., Mees, J. R., Meera Khan, P., and Zaalberg, O. B., 1974, Human antigen and enzyme markers in man-Chinese hamster somatic cell hybrids: Evidence for synteny between the HL-A, $PGM_3$, $ME_1$, and IPO-B loci, *Proc. Nat. Acad. Sci. USA* **71**:962–965.

Sondel, P., and Bach, F., 1975, Recognitive specificity of human cytotoxic T lymphocytes, *J. Exp. Med.* **142**:1339–1348.

Sondel, P. M., Chess, L., and Schlossman, S. F., 1975, Immunologic functions of isolated human lymphocyte subpopulations. IV. Stimulation of MLC and CML by human T cells, *Cell. Immunol.* **18**:351–359.

Sorensen, S. F., 1972, The mixed lymphocyte culture interaction—techniques and immunogenetics, *Acta Pathol. Microbiol. Scand. Sect. B Suppl.* **230**:11–82.

Spencer, M. J., Cherry, J. D., and Terasaki, P. I., 1976, HL-A antigens and antibody response after influenza A vaccination, *N. Eng. J. Med.* **294**:13–16.

Spencer, M. J., Cherry, J. D., Powell, K. R., Mickey, M. R., Terasaki, P. I., Marcy, S. M., and Sumaya, C. V., 1977, Antibody responses following rubella immunization analysed by HLA and ABO types, *Immunogenetics* **4**:365–372.

Springer, T. A., and Strominger, J. L., 1976, Detergent-soluble HLA antigens contain a hydrophilic region at the COOH-terminus and a penultimate hydrophobic region, *Proc. Nat. Acad. Sci. USA* **73**:2481–2485.

Springer, T. A., Strominger, J. L., and Mann, D. L., 1974, Partial purification of detergent soluble HL-A antigen and its cleavage by papain, *Proc. Nat. Acad. Sci. USA* **71**:1539–1543.

Springer, T. A., Kaufman, J. F., Terhorst, C., and Strominger, J. L., 1977a, Purification and structural characterisation of human HLA-linked B cell antigens, *Nature (London)* **268**:213–218.

Springer, T. A., Kaufman, J. F., Siddoway, L. A., Mann, D. L., and Strominger, J. L., 1977b, Purification of HLA-linked B lymphocyte alloantigens in immunologically active form by preparative SDS-gel electrophoresis and studies on their subunit association, *J. Biol. Chem.* **252**:6201–6207.

Stastny, P., 1974, HL-A antigens in mummified pre-Columbian tissues, *Science* **183**:864.

Strominger, J. L., Ferguson, W., Fuks, A., Giphart, M., Kaufman, J., Mann, D., Orr, H., Parham, P., Robb, R., and Terhorst, C., 1977, Isolation and structure of HLA antigens, in: *Progress in Immunology III* (T. E. Mandel, ed.), pp. 109–117, Elsevier/North-Holland, New York.

Suciu-Foca, N., and Dausset, J., 1975, Complex MLR family patterns, *Immunogenetics* **2**:389–391.

Suciu-Foca, N., Susinno, E., McKiernan, P., Rohowsky, C., Werner, J., and Rubenstein,

P., 1978a, DRw determinants on human T cells primed against allogeneic lymphocytes, *Transplant. Proc.* **10**:845–848.

Suciu-Foca, N., Werner, J., Rohowsky, C., McKiernan, P., Susinno, E., and Rubenstein, P., 1978b, Indications that Dw and DRw determinants are controlled by distinct (but closely linked) genes, *Transplant. Proc.* **10**:799–804.

Svejgaard, A., and Kissmeyer-Nielsen, F., 1968, Cross-reactive human HL-A isoantibodies, *Nature (London)* **219**:868–869.

Svejgaard, A., Kissmeyer-Nielsen, F., and Thorsby, E., 1970, HL-A typing of platelets, in: *Histocompatibility Testing, 1970* (P. I. Terasaki, ed.), pp. 153–164, Munksgaard, Copenhagen.

Svejgaard, A., Hauge, M., Jersild, C., Platz, P., Ryder, L. P., Staub-Nielsen, L., and Thompson, M., 1975, The HLA system—an introductory survey, *Monogr. Hum. Genet.* **7**:1–100.

Tanigaki, N., Nakamuro, K., Natori, T., Minowada, J., and Pressman, D., 1975, Structure of HL-A antigens. The structural components of papain-solubilized HL-A molecules, *Transplant, Proc.* **7**:195–199.

Teisberg, P., Olaisen, B., Jonassen, R., Gedde-Dahl, Jr., T., and Thorsby, E., 1977, The genetic polymorphism of the fourth component of human complement: Methodological aspects and a presentation of linkage and associated data relevant to its localization in the HLA region, *J. Exp. Med.* **146**:1380–1389.

Terasaki, P. I. (ed.), 1970, *Histocompatibility Testing, 1970* 653 pp., Munksgaard, Copenhagen.

Terasaki, P. I., and McClelland, J. D., 1964, Microdroplet assay of human serum cytotoxins, *Nature (London)* **204**:998–1000.

Terhorst, C., Parham, P., Mann, D. L., and Strominger, J. L., 1976, Structure of HLA antigens: Amino acid and carbohydrate composition and $NH_2$-terminal sequences of four antigen preparations, *Proc. Nat. Acad. Sci. USA* **73**:910–914.

Terhorst, C., Robb, R., Jones, C., and Strominger, J. L., 1977, Further structural studies of the heavy chain of HLA antigens and its similarity to immunoglobulins, *Proc. Nat. Acad. Sci. USA* **74**:4002–4006.

Termijtelen, A., Bradley, B. A., and van Rood, J. J., 1977, The TYN-PLOP phenomenon in HLA-D typing, in: *Proceedings of the 11th Leukocyte Culture Conference "Regulatory Mechanisms in Lymphocyte Activation"* (D. O. Lucas, ed.), p. 388, Academic Press, New York.

Thomsen, M., Morling, N., Platz, P., Ryder, L. P., Staub-Nielsen, L., and Svejgaard, A., 1976, Specific lack of responsiveness to certain HLA-D (MLC) determinants with notes on primed lymphocyte typing (PLT), *Transplant. Proc.* **8**:455–459.

Thomson, G., 1977, The effect of a selected locus on linked neutral loci, *Genetics* **85**:753–788.

Thorsby, E., 1969, HL-A antigens on human granulocytes studied with cytotoxic iso-antisera obtained by skin grafting, *Scand. J. Haematol.* **6**:119–127.

Thorsby, E., 1974, The human major histocompatibility system, *Transplant. Rev.* **18**:51–129.

Thorsby, E., Hirschberg, H., and Helgesen, A., 1973, A second locus determining human MLC response: separate lymphocyte populations recognize the products of each different MLC-locus allele in allogeneic combinations. *Transplant. Proc.* **5**:1523–1528.

Thorsby, E., Albrechtsen, D., Hirschberg, H., Kaakinen, A., and Solheim, B.G., 1977, MLC-activating HLA-D determinants: Identification, tissue distribution, and significance, *Transplant. Proc.* **9**:393–400.

Ting, A., Mickey, M. R., and Terasaki, P. I., 1976, B-lymphocyte alloantigens in Caucasians, *J. Exp. Med.* **143**:981–986.

Tosi, R. M., Ferrara, G. B., Antonelli, P., and Longo, A., 1975, Shift from HL-A antibodies active in C' dependent cytotoxicity to antibodies active only in ADCC, in: *Histocompatibility Testing, 1975* (F. Kissmeyer-Nielsen, ed.), pp. 915–922, Munksgaard, Copenhagen.

Tosi, R., Tanigaki, N., Centis, D., Ferrara, G. B., and Pressman, D., 1978, Immunological dissection of human Ia molecules, *J. Exp. Med.* **148:**1592–1611.

Tragardh, L., Wiman, K., Rask, L., and Peterson, P. A., 1978, Amino acid sequence homology between HLA-A, B, C antigens, $\beta_2$-microglobulin and immunoglobulins, *Scand. J. Immunol.* **8:**563–568.

Trucco, M. M., Stocker, J. W., and Ceppellini, R., 1978, Monoclonal antibodies against human lymphocyte antigens, *Nature (London)* **273:**666–668.

Turner, M. J., Cresswell, P., Parham, P., Strominger, J. L., Mann, D. L., and Sanderson, A. R., 1975, Purification of papain-solubilized histocompatibility antigens from a cultured human lymphoblastoid line RPMI 4265, *J. Biol. Chem.* **250:**4512–4519.

Vande-Stouwe, R. A., Kunkel, H. G., Halper, J. P., and Weksler, M. E., 1977, Autologous MLC reactions and generation of cytotoxic T cells, *J. Exp. Med.* **146:**1809–1814.

van den Berg Loonen, E. M., de Bruin, T., and Schellekens, P. T. A., 1977, The complex nature of human D-locus determinants: Heterogeneity within Dw3, *Immunogenetics* **5:**261–270.

van Leeuwen, A., Schuit, H. R. E., and van Rood, J. J., 1973, Typing for MLC (LD): II. The selection of nonstimulator cells by MLC Inhibition tests using SD-identical stimulator cells (Misis) and fluorescence antibody studies, *Transplant. Proc.* **5:**1539–1542.

van Leeuwen, A., Winchester, R. J., and van Rood, J. J., 1975, Serotyping for MLC. II. Technical aspects, *Ann. N.Y. Acad. Sci.* **254:**289–295.

van Rood, J. J., 1962, *Leucocyte Grouping*, Thesis, London.

van Rood, J. J., and van Leeuwen, A., 1963, Leukocyte grouping. A method and its application, *J. Clin. Invest.* **42:**1382–1390.

van Rood, J. J., and van Leeuwen, A., 1965, Defined leukocyte antigenic groups in man, in: *Histocompatibility Testing*, (P. S. Russell and H. J. Winn, eds.), pp. 21–37, Natl. Acad. Sci. USA Publ. 1229, Washington, D.C.

van Rood, J. J., van Leeuwen, A., Keuning, J. J., and van Oud Alblas, A. B., 1975a, The serological recognition of the human MLC determinants using a modified cytotoxicity technique, *Tissue Antigens* **5:**73–79.

van Rood, J. J., van Leeuwen, A., Parlevliet, J., Termijtelen, A., and Keuning, J. J., 1975b, LD typing serology. IV. Description of a new locus with three alleles, in: *Histocompatibility Testing, 1975* (F. Kissmeyer-Nielsen, ed.), pp. 629–636, Munksgaard, Copenhagen.

van Rood, J. J., van Leeuwen, A., and Ploem, J. S., 1976, A method to detect simultaneously two cell populations by 2 colour fluorescence, *Nature (London)* **262:**795–797.

van Rood, J. J., van Leeuwen, A., Keuning, J. J., and Termijtelen, A., 1977a, Evidence for two series of B cell antigens in man and their comparison with HLA-D, *Scand. J. Immunol.* **6:**373–384.

van Rood, J. J., de Vries, R. R. P., and Munro, A., 1977b, The biological meaning of transplantation antigens, in: *Progress in Immunology III* (T. E. Mandel, ed.), pp. 345–347, Elsevier/North-Holland, New York.

van den Tweel, J. G., van Oud Alblas, A. B., Keuning, J. J., Goulmy, E., Termijtelen, A., Bach, M. L., and van Rood, J. J., 1973, Typing for MLC (LD). I. Lymphocytes from cousin marriage offspring as typing cells, *Transplant. Proc.* **5:**1535–1538.

Vitetta, E. S., Artzt, K., Bennett, D., Boyse, E. A., and Jacob, F., 1975a, Structural similarities between a product of the T/t-locus isolated from sperm and teratoma cells, and H-2 antigens isolated from splenocytes, *Proc. Nat. Acad. Sci. USA* **72:**3215–3219.

Vitetta, E. S., Uhr, J. W., and Boyse, E. A., 1975b, Association of a $\beta_2$-microglobulin-like subunit with H-2 and TL alloantigens on murine thymocytes, J. Immunol. 114:252–254.

Vives, J., Gelabert, A., and Castillo, R., 1976, HLA antibodies and period of gestation: decline in frequency of positive sera during last trimester, Tissue Antigens 7:209–212.

de Vries, R. R. P., Nijenhuis, L. E., Lai A Fat, R. F. M., and van Rood, J. J., 1976, HLA-linked genetic control of host response to Mycobacterium leprae, Lancet ii:1328–1330.

de Vries, R. R. P., Kreeftenberg, H. G., Loggen, H. G., and van Rood, J. J., 1977, In vitro immune responsiveness to vaccinia virus and HLA, New Eng. J. Med. 297:692–696.

Walford, R., 1964, Serologic typing of human lymphocytes with immune serum obtained after homografting, Science 144:868–870.

Walford, R. L., 1977, Human B-cell alloantigenic systems: Their medical and biological significance, in: HLA System—New Aspects (G. B. Ferrara, ed.), pp. 105–127, Elsevier, New York.

Walford, R. L., Gossett, T., Smith, G. S., Zeller, E., and Wilkinson, J., 1975, A new alloantigenic system on human lymphocytes, Tissue Antigens 5:196–204.

Walford, R. L., Smith, G. S., Meredith, P. J., and Cheney, K. E., 1978, The immunogenetics of aging, in: Genetics of Aging (E. L. Schneider, ed.), pp. 383–402, Plenum Press, New York.

Walsh, F. S., and Crumpton, M. J., 1977, Orientation of cell-surface antigens with lipid bilayer of lymphocyte plasma membrane, Nature (London) 269:307–311.

Wank, R., Schendel, D. J., Hansen, J. A., Yunis, E. J., and Dupont, B., 1977, Two different HLA restimulating determinants separated by recombination and titration, Transplant. Proc. 9:1771–1775.

Ward, F. E., and Seigler, H. F., 1973, Mixed lymphocyte reactions and skin graft survival in an HL-A recombinant family, Transplant. Proc. 5:359–362.

Ward, F. E., Southworth, J. G., and Amos, D. B., 1969, Recombination and other chromosomal aberrations within the HL-A locus, Transplant. Proc. 1:352–356.

Ward, F. E., Levy, S. B., and Pinnell, S. R., 1977, Mixed lymphocyte responses in a four generation C2 deficiency family, Transplant. Proc. 9:1733–1735.

Ward, F. E., Mendell, N. R., Seigler, H. F., MacQueen, J. M., and Amos, D. B., 1978, Factors which have a significant effect on the survival of human skin grafts, Transplantation 26:194–198.

Waters, L., and Walford, R. L., 1972, Detection of non-linear serological subgroups within the specificity HL-A 9, Fed. Proc. 31:737.

Weitkamp, L. R., 1976, Linkage of GLO with HLA and Bf. Effect of population and sex on recombination frequency, Tissue Antigens 7:273–279.

Weitkamp, L. R., 1977, Further data concerning the linkage relationships of loci for urinary pepsinogen and HLA, IVth International Workshop on Human Gene Mapping, Aug. 14–18, 1977, Winnipeg, Canada.

Weitkamp, L. R., van Rood, J. J., Thorsby, E., Bias, W., Fotino, M., Lawler, S. D., Dausset, J., Mayr, W. R., Bodmer, J., Ward, F. E., Seignalet, J., Payne, R., Kissmeyer-Nielsen, F., Gatti, R., Sachs, J. A., and Lamm, L. U., 1973, The relation of parental sex and age to recombination to the HL-A system, Hum. Hered. 23:197–205.

Welsh, K. I., and Turner, M. J., 1976, Preparation of antisera specific for human B cells by immunization of rabbits with immune complexes, Tissue Antigens 8:197–205.

Welsh, K. I., Dorval, G., Nilsson, K., Clements, G. B., and Wigzell, H., 1977, Quantitation of $\beta_2$-microglobulin on the surface of human cells. II. In vitro cell lines and their hybrids, Scand. J. Immunol. 6:265–271.

Wernet, P., Jersild, C., Cunningham-Rundles, C., and Svejgaard, A., 1975, Dynamic and molecular characteristics of HL-A and HL-B (Ia-type) antigens on the surface of human lymphoid cell, in: *Histocompatibility Testing, 1975* (F. Kissmeyer-Nielsen, ed.), pp. 735–738, Munksgaard, Copenhagen.

Wilson, A. B., Haegert, D. G., and Coombs, R. R. A., 1975, Increased sensitivity of the rosette-forming reaction of human T lymphocytes with sheep erythrocytes afforded by papain treatment of the sheep cells, *Clin. Exp. Immunol.* **22:**177–182.

Winchester, R. J., Ross, G. D., Jarowski, C. I., Wong, C. Y., Halper, J., and Broxmeyer, H. E., 1977, Expression of Ia-like antigen molecules on human granulocytes during early phases of differentiation, *Proc. Nat. Acad. Sci. USA* **74:**4012–4019.

Winchester, R. J., Wang, C-Y., Gibofsky, A., Kunkel, H. G., Lloyd, K. O., and Old, L. J., 1978, Expression of Ia-like antigens on cultured human malignant melanoma cell lines, *Proc. Nat. Acad. Sci. USA* **75:**6235–6239.

Yamazaki, K., Boyse, E. A., Mike, V., Thaler, H. T., Mathieson, B. J., Abbot, J., Boyse, J., Zayas, Z. A., and Thomas, L., 1976, Control of mating preferences in mice by genes in the major histocompatibility complex, *J. Exp. Med.* **144:**1324–1335.

Yunis, E. J., and Amos, D. B., 1971, Three closely linked genetic systems relevant to transplantation, *Proc. Nat. Acad. Sci. USA* **68:**3031–3035.

Yunis, E. J., Ward, F. E., and Amos, D. B., 1970, Observations of the CNAP phenomenon, in: *Histocompatibility Testing, 1970* (P. I. Terasaki, ed.), pp. 351–356, Munksgaard, Copenhagen.

Yunis, E. J., Amos, D. B., Eguro, S. Y., and Dorf, M. E., 1972, Cross-reactions of HL-A antibodies. I. Characterization by absorption and elution, *Transplantation* **14:**474–479.

Yunis, E. J., Seigler, H. F., Simmons, R. L., and Amos, D. B., 1973, HL-A typing, mixed leukocyte reactivity, and skin graft survival in a family with a recombinant at the HL-1 chromosomal region (Major Transplantation Region), *Transplantation* **15:**435–440.

Zeuthen, J., Friedrich, U., Rosen, A., and Klein, E., 1977, Structural abnormalities in chromosome 15 in cell lines with reduced expression of $\beta_2$-microglobulin, *Immunogenetics* **4:**567–580.

Zmijewski, C. M., Kelly, M. A., and Dzida, L., 1977, The effect of "T"-cells on the serologic detection of "B"-cell alloantigens, *Tissue Antigens* **10:**237.

*Chapter 3*

# Linkage Analysis in Man

P. Michael Conneally
*Department of Medical Genetics*
*Indiana University School of Medicine*
*Indianapolis, Indiana 46223*

Marian L. Rivas
*Neurological Sciences Institute*
*Good Samaritan Hospital and*
*Medical Center*
*Portland, Oregon 97219*

The exploration of the human chromosomes now so feverishly active has something of the excitement of geographical cartography, and quite a lot of people deserve a doublet of velvet such as Columbus offered to the first man to see land.

—Race and Sanger (1975)

## INTRODUCTION

The mapping of human chromosomes, though much more complex, is related to cartography. To quote McKusick (1971), "We have a general picture of the various countries (the chromosomes) of the genetic world and have identified many of the municipalities (genes) on the basis of the specific traits to which they give rise. We are still largely in the dark, however, about the location of most of the municipalities even from the standpoint of deciding in what country they belong."

Though a decade has passed since McKusick's statement and the pace of gene mapping has increased substantially, the human gene map is still far from complete. For example, over 1000 Mendelian autosomal disorders are known with confidence in man, over 1000 others are prime can-

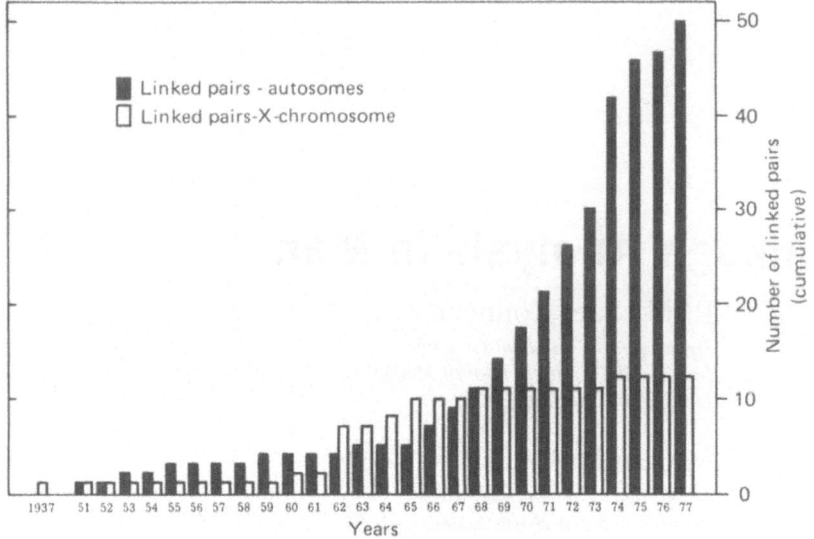

Fig. 1. Cumulative number (by year) of pairs of loci (autosomal and X-linked) shown to be linked by classical linkage methods.

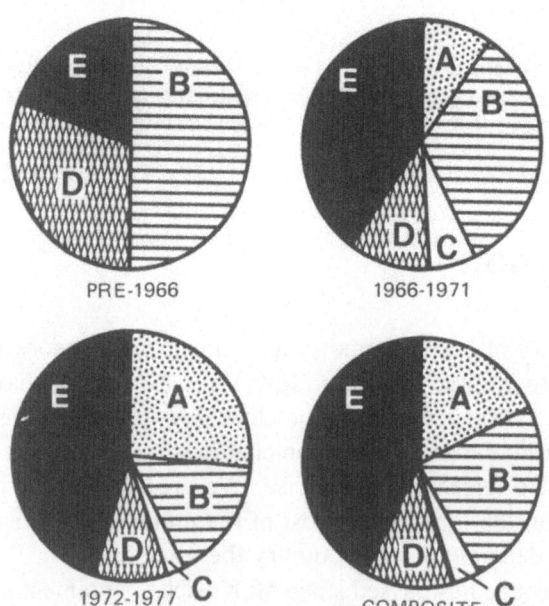

Fig. 2. Relative proportions of various types of genetic loci among all loci shown to be linked by classical linkage methods during the periods indicated. A, antigen locus; B, blood group locus; C, chromosome; D, disease locus; E, enzyme locus.

didates (McKusick and Ruddle, 1977), but less than one percent of these loci have been mapped.

Figure 1 illustrates the number of linked pairs of loci established through family studies since 1937, when the first linkage group was established. The exponential increase, noted since the late sixties, reflects recent developments in methodology including computer technology and the extension of genetic markers beyond the blood group antigens. As shown in Fig. 2, blood group loci comprised half of the established linked loci prior to 1966. After that, the relative involvement of blood group markers declined while enzyme (protein) polymorphisms and other antigenic markers (major histocompatibility complex) increased. In addition, the development of new cytogenetic techniques which permitted identification of chromosome polymorphisms, have made chromosomal and regional assignments possible.

# GENERAL CONSIDERATIONS

## Approaches to Gene Mapping

In essence, there are three approaches to gene mapping in man. The oldest is the family method, which is the main topic of this paper. The second approach is somatic cell hybridization, which has the advantage of allowing the mapping of proteins in which allelic intraspecies variation is not known. Both interspecies allelic variation and the constitutive expression of these genes in the hybrid fibroblast cells can be used to map the human gene. Furthermore, regional mapping, i.e., mapping of a human gene locus to a specific segment of a chromosome, can be accomplished using human cells with chromosomal rearrangements. A detailed review may be found in Ruddle (1977). The third method is *in situ* RNA hybridization. Theoretically, RNA that can be obtained in sufficient amount and made radioactive can be used for mapping multiple-copy DNA sequences. Using autoradiography, one can identify the specific genes and thus their location on the chromosome from which that RNA is normally transcribed. This method has been used to localize tRNA and ribosomal RNA loci; however, its usefulness for localization of single-copy genes is controversial. Recently, a technique for gene mapping using a combination of somatic cell and molecular hybridization has been developed by Deisseroth *et al.* (1977). This method promises to be sufficiently sensitive for localization of single-copy genes. Deisseroth *et al.* used it to localize the α-globin structural gene to chromosome 16.

## Linkage and Synteny

Loci on the same chromosome are said to be syntenic (Renwick, 1969*a*). Linkage may be defined as the occurrence of two loci sufficiently close together on a chromosome such that their assortment is recognized as being nonindependent. Thus linked loci are syntenic while the converse is not necessarily true.

## Crossing-Over, Recombination, and Genetic Map Distance

The map interval between two loci on the same chromosome is measured in terms of the average number of crossover events affecting a *single* strand between the loci. It also equals half the mean number of chiasmata occurring between the loci, since each strand is only one of four chromatids present at the crossing-over stage of meiosis and thus has only one-half chance of being involved in any one chiasma. The latter is usually given as the reason that the maximum frequency of recombination is 50 percent. The recombination fraction, which is defined as the proportion of strands that experience an odd number of crossover events between the loci, is the unit of measurement of map distance. Approximate formulae or mapping functions are used to define the relationship and will be discussed below. The unit of map distance, called a *Morgan*, is defined as the length of chromosomal segment which, on the average, experiences one exchange per strand. For short intervals the frequency of recombination will be directly proportional to the map interval since double crossovers will be negligible. For longer intervals the relationship is more complex; it is nonlinear for two reasons: the occurrence of multiple crossovers, and interference.

## Coincidence and Interference

Coincidence was defined by Muller in 1916 as a measure of the combined effects of chiasma and chromatid interference on recombination. Chromatid interference is the nonrandom selection of the pair of strands involved in the chiasma, i.e., if there is chromatid interference the frequency of one-, two-, and three-strand doubles will not be in the expected ratio of $1:2:1$. Chiasma interference is the tendency for an already established chiasma to suppress the formation of other chiasmata in nearby regions. The coefficient of coincidence ($c$) is defined as the ratio of the observed frequency of double recombinants to the expected frequency, the latter being the product of the recombination frequency for each of the two regions. In the absence of interference, $c$ takes the value 1, and if there is complete interference, $c = 0$, and no double recombinants will be found in that region.

## Linkage vs. Association

The first associations were between the ABO blood groups and diseases of the gastrointestinal tract (Clarke *et al.*, 1956). More recently the HLA system of antigens has been shown to be associated with numerous diseases. In general, the diseases found to be associated with ABO or HLA system antigens do not have a simple mode of inheritance; indeed, the majority have a small genetic component. Normally, association studies are performed on a populational rather than a familial basis. Linked loci will not show an association at a populational level unless there is linkage disequilibrium. Linkage, of course, will show an "association" within sibships; this, in fact, was the basis of Penrose's sib-pair method for detecting linkage, as described below.

## HISTORICAL PERSPECTIVE

With the active study of heredity following the rediscovery of Mendel's paper and the elucidation of the relationship between Mendelian factors and chromosomes by Sutton in 1903, it became apparent that the number of characters that individually followed Mendelian principles was greater than the number of chromosome pairs to which the differentiating genes could be assigned. In an earlier paper Sutton (1902) suggested that the association of paternal and maternal chromosomes in pairs and their subsequent separation during meiosis "may constitute the physical basis of the Mendelian law of heredity." His 1903 paper elaborated more fully on this hypothesis bringing together the fields of cytology and genetics.

## Linkage in Nonhumans

The first report of linkage was that of Correns (1905) in the stock plant *Matthiola*. He did not, however, recover any recombinants and thus thought in terms of complete linkage only. The first report of incomplete linkage (i.e., recombinants were recovered) was by Bateson and Punnet (1906) in the sweet pea; at this time the terms "coupling" and "repulsion" were coined. Reports of linkage in the next few years were scant and their interpretation was often incorrect. It remained for *Drosophila melanogaster* to be utilized in the new field of genetic analysis leading to the pioneering work of Morgan and his co-workers.

On the basis of studies with a number of X-linked mutants, Morgan (1911) suggested that genes are linked as a result of being carried on the same chromosome and that genes which were close together would be coupled more frequently than those more distant from one another. One of his co-workers, Sturtevant, argued in 1913 that if Morgan's explanation was correct it should be possible to map the genes in linear order using the frequency of recombination as an index of relative position on the chromosome. In fact, he was able to verify his hypothesis by the construction of a chromosome map of X-linked genes in *Drosophila melanogaster*.

Bridges and Morgan reported on the map of the second chromosome of *Drosophila* in 1919 and of the third chromosome in 1923. Thus, in a relatively short period a fairly sophisticated chromosome map of an organism was delineated. The cytological demonstration that recombination resulted from the physical exchange of chromosomal material was provided by Stern (1931) using *Drosophila*, and by Creighton and McClintock (1931) in maize. In 1933, Painter, using the giant chromosomes in larval salivary gland nuclei of *Drosophila*, assigned genes to specific areas on the X-chromosome. His method came to be widely used in what is now termed "regional mapping."

## Linkage in Man

Progress in human chromosome mapping was relatively slow. Due to limitations of family size and the lack of knowledge of phase in the informative parent (double heterozygote), it was not possible to analyze human linkage data in a mathematically simple manner. A number of mathematical approaches evolved; the more important of these will be discussed briefly.

## Y-Statistic (Bernstein)

The earliest approach to linkage analysis in man was by Bernstein in 1931, using data from two generations. His method may be illustrated using a double backcross, e.g., $AaBb \times aabb$. In the absence of linkage, the four gametes produced by the informative parent, $AB$, $Ab$, $aB$, and $ab$ will have equal expectations. However, if the loci are linked, either the $(AB,ab)$ or $(Ab,aB)$ set will be more common than the other, depending on the phase of the double heterozygote. Thus, if we obtain for each sibship the product $y$ of the sum of gametes $AB$ and $ab$ and the sum of gametes $Ab$ and $aB$ such that $y = (AB + ab) \times (Ab + aB)$, the expected value of $y$ is the same whether the informative parent is in coupling or repulsion. The value of $y$ is maximum if the loci assort independently and will decrease as the loci are closer together. The expected value of $y$ depends on the recombination fraction and sibship size and can be tabulated for various values of these parameters. The sum of the observed values of $y$ can be compared with the sum of the expected values to obtain an estimate of the recombination fraction ($\theta$). This method gives an approximate value of $\theta$ by comparing observed and expected values of $y$ but the significance of the estimate is difficult to determine.

## Sib-Pair Method (Penrose)

Penrose introduced his sib-pair method in 1935. The principle of this method is that if linkage exists between two conditions, examination of large numbers of pairs of siblings with respect to these conditions would show an excess of cases where the sibs are similar in both characters over those cases in which the sibs are similar for one character and dissimilar for the other. MacGregor (1953) reports on a number of linkages found using this method. However, these linkages often involved characteristics such as red hair and eye color which we now know are not inherited in simple Mendelian fashion. Finney (1942a) showed that this method extracts only a small fraction of the information on linkage compared to that obtained using maximum likelihood ($u$) scores. Also, sibships of size $n$ are partitioned into all $n(n - 1)/2$ possible pairs which are not independent, thus giving results which may be quite inexact.

## Maximum Likelihood Method—$u$ Scores (Fisher)

Fisher in 1935 developed a maximum-likelihood scoring procedure known as $u$ scores which is somewhat similar to Bernstein's $y$ scores but is more efficient for all linkage intensities and, in fact, is fully efficient in the limit for loose linkage. Finney (1940, 1941a,b, 1942a,b,c, 1943) extended the method of $u$ scores to cover a great variety of cases. This method has a number of disadvantages as pointed out by Smith (1953). The major ones are: (1) $u$ scores are fully efficient only in the limit for loose linkage which, in man, is not practical to detect; (2) it is not feasible to use three-generation data which greatly increase the amount of information on linkage; and (3) normality of the total score, which may be far from true in small or moderate samples is assumed. In fact, both Fisher's and Bernstein's methods are extremely inefficient for close linkage.

## Probability Ratio (Haldane and Smith)

Haldane and Smith (1947) developed a probability ratio test to extract information from families without making the assumption of normality that is required by the Fisher–Finney $u$-score method. This method is conceptually the simplest of all the methods and is the forerunner of the methods now in use. The ratio is the probability of the data given a specified value of the recombination frequency, $\theta$, divided by the probability of the data given independent assortment ($\theta = \frac{1}{2}$). If, for example, the probability of obtaining the observed distribution of two traits in a pedigree is higher when the genes are linked, then the odds are greater than 1; the converse is also true. In order to allow additivity of scores among families, the log of the probability ratio is used; hence the term *lod* (log odds) score, which was introduced by Barnard in 1949.

## Sequential Test (Morton)

Since information on linkage in man is obtained on a family basis it is normally accumulated as a succession of samples. Morton (1955) proposed that the best method of analysis was a sequential test. He combined the probability ratio test of Haldane and Smith with the method of sequential analysis devised by Wald (1947) in his now classic paper "Sequential tests for the detection of linkage."

The paper considered the properties of sequential linkage tests and the scoring types ($z$ scores) which arise when the parental genotypes are known and when there are only two alleles at each locus in two-generation data. In determining the criteria for a suitable sequential test, he suggested that the researcher should be "especially anxious to avoid the assertion that two genes are linked when they are not, since a misleading linkage map is worse than no map at all."

A sequential test would intuitively seem ideal for human linkage analysis. In nonsequential decision theory one rejects or accepts the null hypothesis. The sequential test allows a third decision, namely that evidence for acceptance or rejection is not decisive and judgment with the preassigned significance level and power must be suspended until more data can be collected. Two constants A and B, which are related to $\alpha$ and $\beta$ (the probabilities of type I and II errors, respectively), in the following approximation:

$$A = (1 - \beta)/\alpha$$

$$B = \beta/(1 - \alpha)$$

are used as a basis for the test of significance. The values of $\alpha$ and $\beta$ and thus $A$ and $B$ were determined by Morton (1955) based on the following argument.

Since there is a prior probability of linkage in man which Morton suggested might be approximately 0.05, in order that the posterior probability of a type I error be less than 0.05, $\alpha$ should be 0.02 if the average power of the test, i.e., the probability of detecting linkage, is 0.95. He also imposed a second condition on the power function of the test. If the test is to be useful it must have a power close to unity for values of $\theta$ near zero (close linkage).

Based on these considerations, Morton suggested the following criteria. After the lod scores (log of the probability ratio) are accumulated over families, if the total is 3 or greater, conclude that the frequency of recombination is significantly less than $\frac{1}{2}$; if the total is $-2$ or less conclude that the frequency of recombination is significantly greater than the value of $\theta$ for which the lods were calculated, i.e., linkage can be ruled out at that value of $\theta$ or less. If the total lod score lies between minus 2 and plus 3 suspend judgment about linkage until further data lead to a decision.

Morton (1955) gave tables of lod ($z$) scores for the various mating types for loci with two alleles and dominant, codominant, and recessive phenotypes. These tables, together with instructions for scoring, allowed researchers with minimal mathematical expertise to analyze two generation linkage data with known or unknown phase. Maynard-Smith *et al.* (1961) also published extensive tables of $z$ scores.

A second paper (Morton, 1956) obtained lod scores for multigeneration data on the Rh:elliptocytosis linkage. The likelihoods for these families were obtained by hand, a tedious process. The resulting lods were used to obtain likelihood ratio tests of genetic homogeneity and maximum likelihood estimates of linkage. The analysis revealed the first example in man of genetic heterogeneity based on linkage since the gene for elliptocytosis was found to be closely linked ($\theta = 3$ cM) to the Rh locus in four of seven large pedigrees while there was no evidence for linkage in the remaining three. A third paper (Steinberg and Morton, 1956) included application to multiple allelic test loci, e.g., *MNS*. A fourth and final paper (Morton, 1957) extended the lod scores to multiple alleles at both loci, pseudoalleles, and partial sex linkage.

Since human linkage data is usually obtained from extended families rather than nuclear families (a set of parents and their offspring) and Morton's $z$ scores are thus not directly applicable, methods to analyze extended families became available. Elston and Stewart (1971) described a method for computing the likelihood of a pedigree recursively beginning with the most recent generation and working back to the earliest known generation. This method will be discussed in more detail later.

Even with better mathematical techniques such as the sequential lod score method, the pace of mapping in humans was slow. With the discovery of many new polymorphic isozymes, better chromosome staining techniques, and the advent of somatic cell hybridization, rapid advances have occurred in the last ten years.

## APPROACH TO FAMILY STUDIES

### Framework of Family-Based Linkage Studies

A typical linkage study involves the following: (1) choosing the loci to be mapped; (2) determining the analytical method to be used; (3) selecting appropriate families for study; (4) phenotyping individuals; (5) analyzing the data; and (6) interpreting the results. The first three activities form the framework of the study; activity 4 generates data for analysis and is often the rate-limiting step; activity 5 generates the results on which conclusions (activity 6) are based.

## Mappable Loci

Not all of the 50,000 + loci in man are suitable for mapping by the family study method. Those which meet the following criteria can be used in linkage studies: (1) the mode of inheritance is known; (2) the phenotypic expression(s) of each genotype is well defined; (3) allelic frequencies are sufficiently high to ensure a "reasonable" level of heterozygosity in the population, and (4) phenotypic expression is detectable in tissues amenable to study.

Unfortunately, this set of criteria effectively eliminates most known loci from consideration at the present time. An increasing proportion of those loci which are not useful now, however, should be added to the repertoire of suitable loci as techniques become more refined, new techniques are applied to human gene products, and the genetic basis of human phenotypes is better defined.

Those loci which are mappable include disease loci (whose genotypes specifically give rise to clinical conditions); marker loci (whose genotypes give rise to apparently "neutral" or "benign" human variation), and chromosomal structural rearrangements (whose "loci" or break points represent physical points on a chromosome). The suitability of these loci for linkage studies will depend on the nature of the locus, the availability of families for study, the ease with which phenotypes are determined, and the availability of methods for analysis of data.

## Main vs. Test Locus

The *main* locus is the locus for which families are selected for study. Linkage relationship of the main locus is sought by studying its segregation with other or *test* loci. In order to provide information on linkage at best one parent must be doubly heterozygous; thus the loci to be studied should be chosen so as to maximize the occurrence of informative matings.

Double backcross matings such as $MmTt \times mmtt$, $MmT1T2 \times mmT1T1$ and $MmT1T2 \times mmT2T2$ ($M$ = main locus, $T$ = test locus) yield the most information on linkage since the parental contribution to each offspring can be clearly determined and all offspring are informative. Other matings, such as single backcrosses with dominance in the intercross factor ($MmTt \times mmTt$), and double intercrosses with no dominance in either factor ($M1M2T1T2 \times M1M2T1T2$), double intercrosses with dominance in one factor ($MmT1T2 \times MmT1T2$ and $M1M2Tt \times M1M2Tt$), and double intercrosses with dominance in both factors ($MmTt \times MmTt$), yield progressively less information.

Thus, loci with allelic frequencies which maximize the frequency of informative matings are most suitable for linkage analysis. Given that the locus of a rare dominant condition is chosen as the main locus, the following matings are potentially informative for linkage: $MmTt \times mmtt$, $MmTt \times mmTt$; similarly, matings $MmT1T2 \times mmT1T1$, $MmT1T2 \times MmT1T2$, and $MmT1T2 \times mmT2T2$ are informative for a codominant marker system with two alleles. The maximum frequency of these informative matings occurs when both alleles are equally frequent (codominant marker locus) and when the frequency of the recessive allele, $q$, is 0.61 (dominant marker locus) (Rivas and Conneally, 1977).

## Efficiency and Power in Linkage Studies

### Marker Loci

Marker loci include those determining blood groups, other antigenic systems such as HLA, enzymes and proteins such as $PGM_1$ and Hp, as well as all chromosome polymorphisms (even though they are not loci in the strict sense of the term). An example of a chromosome polymorphism is $lqh$. Though the amount of heterochromatin is a continuous variable, it can be scored within a family on a graded scale of, say, 1 to 10, provided that a discrete difference in the homologs of an individual (at least 2 on the scale of 1 to 10) is used to define heterozygotes. For example, one should not attempt to distinguish $lqh$ 4/5 individuals from $lqh$ 5/5; however, a 3/5 can be distinguished from a 5/5 but not from a 4/5. (Rivas et al., 1975).

Figure 3 demonstrates the use of the $lqh$ polymorphism in a linkage study with congenital cataract (Conneally et al., 1979). The gene for cataract is segregating with chromosome 1 having the smaller ("2") $lqh$ re-

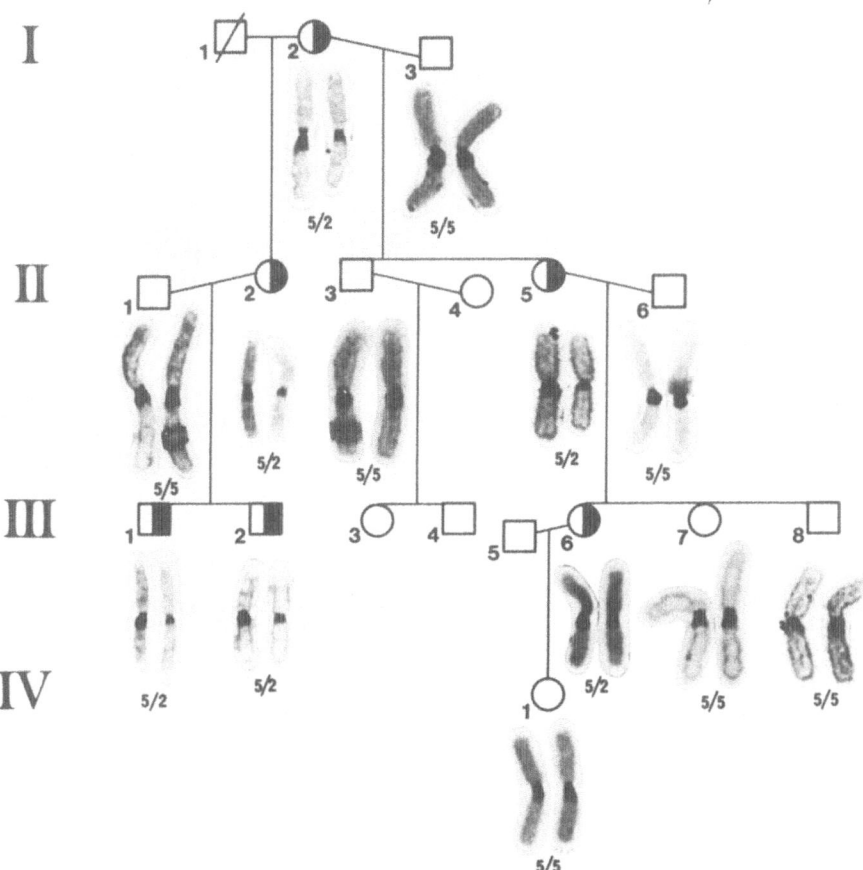

Fig. 3. Pedigree segregating for dominant congenital cataract showing linkage with *lqh*. Chromosome 1's from each individual are shown underneath. The homology having the smaller ("2") region is segregating with the gene for cataract. There are no crossovers between the cataract locus and the *lqh* region in this pedigree.

gion. Thus, for purposes of linkage analysis, the *lqh* region acts as a marker locus.

The mode of inheritance and phenotypic expression of most polymorphic loci are known. Suitability for linkage studies thus depends on allelic (and heterozygote) frequencies and the feasibility of phenotyping.

Table I lists allelic and heterozygote frequencies for some of the most commonly used genetic markers in man. It is readily apparent from the table that, as allelic frequencies approach 0.50 (for a two-allele system), the proportion of heterozygotes approaches the maximum value of 0.50.

**TABLE I. Human Marker Loci Suitable for Linkage Studies Based on Family Data**

| Genetic marker[a] | Tissue | Allelic frequencies[a] | Heterozygote frequency | Chromosomal assignment |
|---|---|---|---|---|
| **Blood group markers** | | | | |
| + ABO | rbc | $I^A = 0.27$; $I^B = 0.06$; $I^O = 0.67$ | 0.46 | 9 |
| Dombrock (Do) | rbc | $Do^a = 0.42$; $Do^b = 0.58$ | 0.49 | |
| + Duffy (Fy) | rbc | $Fy^a = 0.45$; $Fy^b = 0.55$ | 0.49 | 1 |
| + Kell (K) | rbc | $K = 0.05$; $k = 0.95$ | 0.10 | |
| + Kidd (Jk) | rbc | $Jk^a = 0.51$; $Jk^b = 0.49$ | 0.50 | |
| + Lewis (Le) | rbc | $Le^a = 0.15$; $Le^b = 0.85$ | 0.25 | |
| + Lutheran (Lu) | rbc | $Lu^a = 0.04$; $Lu^b = 0.96$ | 0.08 | |
| + MNSs | rbc | $M = 0.53$; $N = 0.47$ <br> $MS = 0.24$; $Ms \doteq 0.30$; $NS = 0.07$; $Ns = 0.39$ | 0.50 <br> 0.70 | 4 |
| + P | rbc | $P_1 = 0.46$; $P_2 = 0.54$ | 0.50 | |
| + Rhesus (Rh) | rbc | $R^1 = 0.42$; $R^2 = 0.15$; $R^0 = 0.03$; $r = 0.40$ | 0.64 | 1 |
| + Scianna (Sc) | rbc | $Sc^1 = 0.99$; $Sc^2 = 0.01$ | 0.02 | 1 |
| + Secretor (Se) | Saliva | $Se = 0.52$; $se = 0.48$ | 0.50 | |
| Xg | rbc | $Xg^a = 0.66$; $Xg = 0.34$ | 0.45 | X |
| **Antigenic markers (exclusive of blood groups)** | | | | |
| HLA-A | wbc | Highly polymorphic | >0.50 | 6 |
| HLA-B | wbc | Highly polymorphic | >0.50 | 6 |
| HLA-C | wbc | Highly polymorphic | | 6 |
| HLA-D | wbc | Highly polymorphic | | 6 |
| **Enzyme and protein markers** | | | | |
| Acidic protein (Pa) | Parotid saliva | $Pa^+ = 0.21$; $Pa^- = 0.79$ | 0.33 | |
| + Acid phosphatase-1 (ACP-1) | rbc | $ACP^A = 0.40$; $ACP^B = 0.55$; $ACP^C = 0.05$ | 0.55 | 2 |
| Aconitase (soluble) (ACON$_s$) | wbc | $ACON_s^1 = 0.85$*; $ACON_s^2 = 0.03$*; <br> $ACON_s^4 = 0.12$* | 0.25* | 9 |

| | | Alleles | | |
|---|---|---|---|---|
| \# Adenosine deaminase (ADA) | rbc | $ADA^1 = 0.95$; $ADA^2 = 0.05$ | 0.10 | 20 |
| + Adenylate kinase-1 (AK-1) | rbc | $AK_1^1 = 0.96$; $AK_1^2 = 0.04$ | 0.08 | 9 |
| \# Albumin (Alb) | Plasma | Several rare alleles = 0.13** | 0.25** | 4 |
| Amylase, salivary (AMY₁) | Saliva | Several rare alleles | 0.007 | 1 |
| + Amylase, pancreatic (AMY₂) | Urine | $Amy_2^A = 0.95$; $Amy_2^B = 0.05$ | 0.10 | 1 |
| | Serum | | | |
| α₁-Antitrypsin (Pi) | Plasma | $Pi^M = 0.95$; $Pi^Z = 0.01$; $Pi^S = 0.03$; $Pi^I = 0.01$ | 0.10 | |
| Carbonic anhydrase-2 (CA2) | rbc | $Ca_2^1 = 0.81*$; $Ca_2^2 = 0.19*$ | 0.31* | |
| Ceruloplasmin (CP) | Plasma | $Cp^A = 0.01***$; $Cp^B = 0.98***$; $Cp^C = 0.01***$ | 0.04*** | |
| \# Cholinesterase (E2) | Plasma | $E_2^+ = 0.05***$; $E_2^- = 0.95***$ | 0.10*** | |
| Complement | | | | |
| Second (C2) | Plasma | Σ Variants = 0.025 | 0.05 | 6 |
| Third (C3) | Plasma | $C_3^F = 0.77$; $C_3^S = 0.22$ | 0.35 | |
| Sixth (C6) | Plasma | $C_6^A = 0.61$; $C_6^B = 0.39$ | 0.48 | |
| Cytidine deaminase (CDA) | wbc | $CDA^1 = 0.65$; $CDA^2 = 0.35$ | 0.46 | |
| Diaphorase (NADPH-dependent) (DIA2) | rbc | Rare variants | 0.01 | |
| Double-band protein (DB) | Parotid saliva | $Db^+ = 0.16$; $Db^- = 0.84$ | 0.27 | |
| Esterase D (ESD) | rbc | $ESD^1 = 0.90$; $ESD^2 = 0.10$ | 0.18 | 13 |
| \# α-L-Fucosidase (α FUCA) | wbc | $\alpha\text{-}FUC^1 = 0.74$; $\alpha\text{-}FUC^2 = 0.26$ | 0.38 | 1 |
| \# Galactose-1-P-uridyl-transferase (GALT) | rbc | Duarte variant = 0.07; Los Angeles variant = 0.02 | 0.17 | 9 |
| \# Glucose-6-P-dehydrogenase (Gd) | rbc | $\Sigma Gd^A, Gd^{A-} = 0.20*$ | 0.32* | X |
| \# Acid α-glucosidase (GLUA) | wbc | $\alpha\text{-}GLU^1 = 0.97$; $\alpha\text{-}GLU^2 = 0.03$ | 0.06 | 17 |
| Glutamic-oxaloacetate transaminase (mitochondrial) (GOT_M) | wbc | $GOT_M^1 = 0.98$; $GOT_M^2 = 0.02$ | 0.04 | |
| | | $GOT_M^1 = 0.96*$; $GOT_M^2 = 0.01*$; $GOT_M^3 = 0.07*$ | 0.15* | |
| Glutamic-pyruvic transaminase (GPT1) | rbc | $GPT^1 = 0.52$; $GPT^2 = 0.48$ | 0.50 | |

*(Continued)*

**TABLE I. (Continued)**

| Genetic marker | Tissue | Allelic frequencies[a] | Heterozygote frequency | Chromosomal assignment |
|---|---|---|---|---|
| Enzyme and protein markers (cont.) | | | | |
| * Glutathione peroxidase (GPX1) | rbc | $\Sigma$ Several variants = 0.03* | 0.06* | |
| * Glutathione reductase (GSR) | rbc | $GSR^U = 0.87^*$; $GSR^V = 0.13^*$ | 0.23* | 8 |
| α-Acid glycoprotein (ORO) | Serum | $ORO^1 = 0.36$; $ORO^2 = 0.64$ | 0.46 | |
| Glyoxylase 1 (GLO1) | rbc | $GLO^1 = 0.40$; $GLO^2 = 0.60$ | 0.48 | 6 |
| + Haptoglobin (HPα) | Plasma | $Hp^1 = 0.40$; $Hp^2 = 0.60$ | 0.48 | 16 |
| Hexokinase-3 (HK3) | wbc | $HK_3^1 = 0.98$; $HK_3^2 = 0.02$ | 0.04 | |
| Immunoglobulin (Gm) | Serum | Highly polymorphic* | >0.50* | |
| Beta-lipoprotein (Ag) | Serum | $Ag^x = 0.23$; $Ag^y = 0.77$ | 0.35 | |
| Lipoprotein (Lp) | Serum | $Lp^a = 0.22$; $Lp = 0.78$ | 0.34 | |
| Malic enzyme (mitochondrial) ($ME_m$) | Skin | $MEM^1 = 0.69$; $MEM^2 = 0.31$ | 0.43 | |
| Pepsinogen (Pg) | Urine | $Pg^a = 0.62$; $Pg^b = 0.38$ | 0.47 | |
| Peptidase A (PEPA) | rbc | $PEPA^1 = 0.75$; $PEPA^2 = 0.25$ | 0.38 | 18 |
| Peptidase C (PEPC) | rbc | Several rare va riants | 0.01 | 1 |
| Peptidase D (PEPD) | rbc | $PEPD^1 = 0.96^*$; $PEPD^2 = 0.02^*$; $PEPD^3 = 0.02^*$ | 0.08* | 19 |
| + Phosphoglucomutase-1 (PGM1) | rbc | $PG\ M_1^1 = 0.75$; $PGM_1^2 = 0.25$ | 0.38 | 1 |
| Phosphoglucomutase-2 (PGM2) | rbc | $PGM_2^1 = 0.95^*$; $PGM_2^2 = 0.05^*$ | 0.10* | 4 |
| Phosphoglucomutase-3 (PGM3) | wbc | $PGM_3^1 = 0.75$; $PGM_3^2 = 0.25$ | 0.38 | 6 |
| + Phosphogluconate dehydrogenase (PGD) | rbc | $PGD^A = 0.95^*$; $PGD^C = 0.05^*$ | 0.10* | 1 |
| Phosphoglycolylate phosphatase (PGP) | rbc | $PGP^1 = 0.83$; $PGP^2 = 0.13$; $PGP^3 = 0.04$ | 0.30 | 16 |
| Proline-rich protein (Pr) | Parotid saliva | $Pr^1 = 0.68$; $Pr^2 = 0.32$ | 0.44 | |
| Properdin factor B (Bf) | Plasma | $Bf^1 = 0.71$; $Bf^2 = 0.28$; $Bf^s = 0.01$ | 0.41 | 6 |
| Transferrin (Tf) | Plasma | $Tf^c = 0.93^*$; $Tf^B = 0.01^*$; $Tf^D = 0.06^*$ | 0.13 | |

| | | | | |
|---|---|---|---|---|
| # Uridine monophosphate kinase (UMPK) | rbc | $UMPK^1 = 0.95$; $UMPK^2 = 0.05$ | 0.10 | 1 |
| + Vitamin D binding protein (Gc) | Plasma | $Gc^1 = 0.74$; $Gc^2 = 0.26$ | 0.38 | 4 |
| Chromosome heteromorphisms | | | | |
| 1qh | wbc | Variations in size and morphology of heterochromatic regions reported for different staining techniques. | Varying levels of heterozygosity depending on the specific variant(s), technique(s) used, and the population studied. | 1 |
| 9qh | wbc | | | 9 |
| 16qh | wbc | | | 16 |

a Symbols: *, African Blacks; **, North American Indians; ***, Asiatics; +, commonly used markers; #, site of one or more mutations that "cause" disease (McKusick, 1979).

Multiple-allelic systems ensure an even greater proportion ($1 - \Sigma p_i^2$, where $p_i$ is the frequency of $i$th allele) of heterozygous individuals.

Not all of the markers listed in Table I, however, are tested routinely. It is the rare laboratory indeed which has the means and the funding to use its entire repertoire of markers on *every* individual in *every* family in *every* linkage study. Considerations such as technical limitations (availability of antisera, substrates, and equipment), cost per test, difficulty in obtaining appropriate samples/tissues, degree of polymorphism, and established linkage relationships with other loci determine whether the marker system should be used for general linkage screening (i.e., one of many in a battery of markers) or should be reserved for more refined mapping of specific regions.

## Test Screening Panels

A greater degree of efficiency in the use of marker loci might be achieved if their chromosomal assignments are considered in choosing markers for routine screening. For example, an indirect test of linkage with the HLA complex could be done by routinely using the less expensive marker, *Bf*, whose locus is between *HLA-A* and *HLA-D*, i.e., within the *HLA* complex. If there is an indication of linkage with Bf or other loci on chromosome 6, HLA testing could be done on individuals in the most potentially informative sibships and/or kindreds. Similarly, the rather time consuming and expensive methods for determining chromosomal heteromorphisms or structural rearrangements could be limited to a subset of available families once linkage to a locus assigned to that chromosome is suspected.

The concept of developing a test panel of families or series of panels in order to increase efficiency in linkage studies is not new. Carter and Falconer (1951) discussed the rationale of using linkage testing stocks in mice, and suggested loci which they considered suitable for selection. The 21 loci which they selected and allocated to 5 stocks represented 11 linkage groups and 5 independent loci. They found that their set of stocks allowed the testing of a "new" locus against approximately 50% of the genome at the expense of raising 500 offspring. Using a set of 7 stocks containing 26 loci representing 16 linkage groups, Green (1963) showed that 70% of the mouse genome was covered at the cost of examining 700 offspring. Both studies indicate the increased power of test stocks over the traditional, rather opportunistic approaches in the detection of linkage. Although the theory of constructing test stocks has been applied to mouse and other organisms, in which breeding experiments are possible, the concept, with modifications, may be applicable to man.

The chromosomal assignments of loci listed in Table I illustrate the point that presently known marker loci are not randomly distributed among the chromosomes. Of the 35 autosomal marker loci listed for which chromosomal assignment is known, 10 (29%) are known to be on chromosome 1, 8 (23%) on chromosome 6, and 4 (11%) on chromosome 9. If one determines the swept radius of each locus, i.e., the length of chromosome on either side of a marker gene within which a new locus can be effectively excluded, the assigned autosomal marker loci in Table I collectively cover approximately 33% of the genome and represent 12 linkage groups. Limiting the battery of test loci to those 17 markers routinely used by the majority of linkage investigators (designated by a "+" sign in Table I), the test panel would contain 11 marker loci representing 5 known linkage groups (1, 2, 4, 9, and 16) and 6 nonassigned (presumably independent) loci; thus only 21% of the genome is covered. New, more efficient panels will develop as the number of marker loci increases and the "gaps" in the human map become filled. The function of these test panels is rapid screening for linkage; other test panels could conceivably be designed to map more precisely the location of a new locus. Thus it may be possible in the near future to rapidly screen for linkage using a limited number of loci whose phenotypes are quickly and inexpensively determined without sacrificing the power of detection.

## Power of a Linkage Study

Elston and Lange (1975) have examined the power of linkage studies. They considered the general problem of determining the prior probability that the main locus under study is within a certain distance of any one of a set of marker loci. They considered each locus to be a point on a line—the chromosome—and assumed the loci to be uniformly distributed across the genome. They arbitrarily used a cutoff point of $\theta = 0.40$, beyond which it would not be feasible to detect linkage, as previously suggested by Renwick (1969). They computed the *a priori* probabilities of detecting linkage for 1, 10, 20, 30, 50, and 100 random marker loci, the results of which are depicted in Fig. 4. For 20 marker loci, the *a priori*

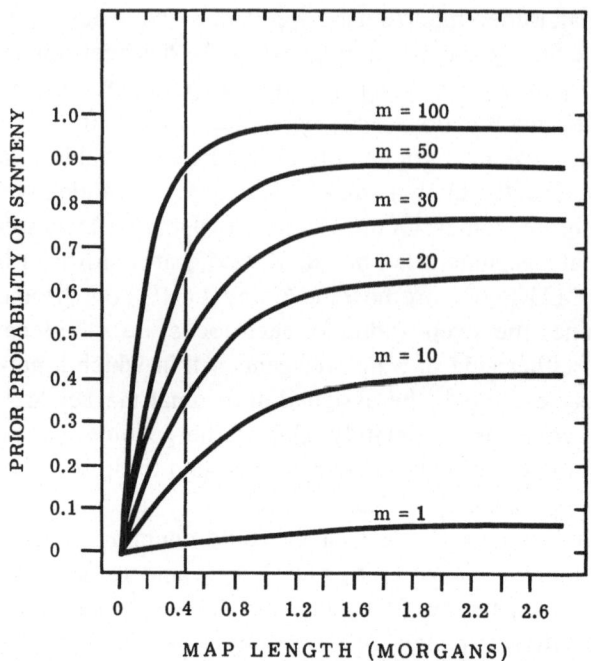

Fig. 4. Probability (ordinate) that a random locus is within a specific map distance (abcissa) of at least one of *m* random marker loci. The vertical line is at a distance of 44 cM which is usually taken as the limit for which linkage can be detected in man (modified from Elston and Lange, 1975).

probability of detecting linkage ($\theta \leq 0.40$) was 0.35; for 30 markers this probability rose to 0.50. Many laboratories now test for 30 or more marker loci; however, lest there be too much optimism, it should be stressed that the 50 percent probability is based on 30 *random* marker loci. Many of the marker loci now available are not independent (e.g., $PGM_1$-*UMPK*-*Rh-PGD* on *lp*). To the extent that they are not randomly distributed the probability of detecting linkage will be decreased.

# PREPARATION OF DATA PRIOR TO ANALYSIS

## Consistency Checking

Mistyping and nonpaternity are probably the more common reasons for an inconsistent pedigree though other factors such as unreported adoptions may also be responsible. Consistency checking may be done by inspection of the genotypes but this is by no means satisfactory since it may not detect allelic exclusion. An example of allelic exclusion would be an $A_1$ individual, the product of an $A_1 \times O$ mating who is married to an $O$ individual and produces an $A_2$ offspring. Inspection of nuclear sibships would not find this inconsistency. Thus, the optimal approach to consistency checking is to obtain the likelihood of the whole pedigree. This can be accomplished using, for example, the program LIPED (Ott, 1974) which is described later. In this case any genetic inconsistency will cause the likelihood to be zero.

## Segregation Analysis

For proper linkage analysis the segregation ratios for the loci being tested should not be disturbed by incomplete penetrance or differential viability. (If these factors exist, are known, and are taken into account in the linkage analysis, the above caveat does not hold.) In order to determine if the loci behave in simple Mendelian fashion, a segregation analysis of the data should be performed. If the segregation frequency is not significantly different from the expected, say $\frac{1}{2}$ or $\frac{1}{4}$, and if there is no evidence for sporadic cases due to new mutations or phenocopies, only then is linkage analysis feasible. In addition to testing genetic hypotheses, segregation analysis is useful in detecting mistyping errors, an important consideration especially if the typing system is new to the genotyping laboratory. Ott (1977) has shown that misclassification leads to a bias in the estimation of the recombination fraction. In particular, if the misclassification error is not taken into account at all in the analysis, the recombination fraction is overestimated.

## Age-Dependent Penetrance

A problem arises in linkage analysis when one of the traits followed is a disorder which is not fully penetrant. Among such disorders are those with late age of onset. Examples are Huntington disease (HD), myotonic dystrophy, and the hereditary ataxias. In this situation precise genotypic classification of at-risk individuals (those with an affected parent who show no signs of the disorder) is impossible. Using the standard lod score method, for example, only older individuals over, say, the 90th percentile for risk can be scored. This significantly decreases the amount of information available on a particular family and one has to select families with two or three living affected generations. Alternatively one could wait for at-risk family members to become affected or pass into the low-risk age group; however, the time span involved normally makes this approach impractical.

The development of a general algorithm for obtaining the likelihood of a pedigree by Elston and Stewart (1971) allows information on individuals at risk to be incorporated into the analysis. The computer program LIPED (Ott, 1974) based on the above algorithm, can be used to analyze all family members. As can be seen in the Appendix, the program requires, as one of its input parameters, $P(x|g_i)$, the probability of the phenotype x given a specific genotype $g_i$. In the case of at-risk individuals, this is the probability of being normal given that the individual has the abnormal allele.

The method can be illustrated using Huntington disease. In order to obtain the above mentioned conditional probability, i.e., the probability of the individual being normal given that he has inherited the Huntington gene, the cumulative age of onset distribution for HD is needed. Pericak-Vance *et al.* (1978) used the following approach for a linkage analysis of HD. Data on age of onset were obtained from their own sample of families as well as those from the literature. A function was determined, using asymptotic regression analysis, that best describes the cumulative age of onset curve. This function was $y = \exp(\alpha + \beta\rho^x)$, where $y$ is the cumulative relative frequency of being affected at age $x$. The least squares estimates of $\alpha$, $\beta$, and $\rho$ are 0.284, $-11.385$, and 0.947 respectively. The distribution is shown in Fig. 5. If one takes, for example, an individual age 46, who is at risk for HD (i.e., has an affected parent) the probability that he would be affected by that age, if he carries the HD gene, is 0.52. Thus the probability that such an individual is normal is the complement of this, or 0.48. The latter probabilities for the age range of at-risk individuals are used as input to LIPED.

This method, therefore, can add substantial information on linkage in late age of onset disorders. Normally in HD, even with this method, individuals under age 20 offer little information on linkage and thus, from an economic point view, probably should not be sampled.

Wilson *et al.* (1977) simulated a fully penetrant dominant disorder to behave as an *HD* locus and compared lod scores for different values of the recombination fraction before and after simulation. They concluded

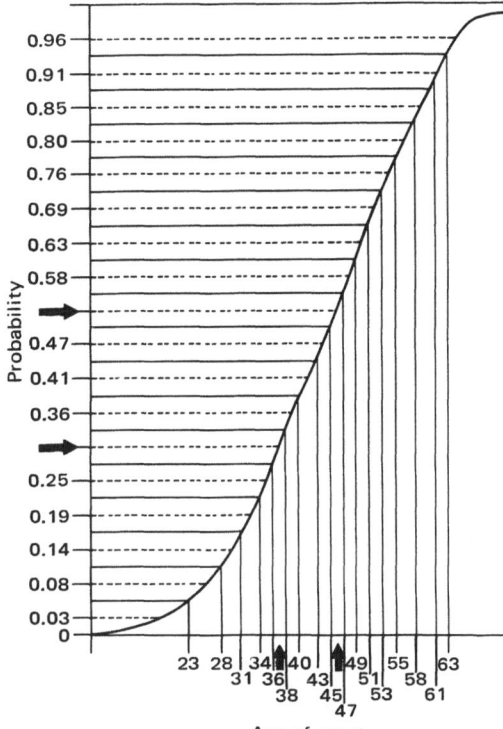

Fig. 5. Cumulative distribution of age of onset in Huntington Disease (HD). The ordinate gives the probability of being affected by a given age (abcissa) if one carries the *HD* gene. The information required by LIPED (i.e., the probability of being normal at a specific age given that one inherited the *HD* gene) is the complement of this probability. Two examples are shown by arrows; the probabilities for age 37 and 46 are 0.7 (1–0.3) and 0.48 (1–0.52) respectively.

that at least five times as much data are necessary to detect close linkage with the *HD* locus as compared to a fully penetrant disorder. This factor increases rapidly as the distance between the loci increases.

# ANALYSIS OF DATA

## Mendelian Traits

### Nuclear Family Units

In his 1955 paper, Morton used a computer to tabulate lod scores. These tables for nuclear families were used extensively during the next decade. However, they did not cover all mating types and furthermore, classification of the offspring had to be performed by hand. Some successful attempts were made to score nuclear families using the computer. Simpson (1958) wrote a program for linkage analysis of two generation family data and pointed out the possibility, by extending the program, of using it for large multigeneration families. Similar programs were written by Falk and Edwards (1970) and Gedde-Dahl *et al.* (1971). The likelihood for large pedigrees, however, could only be calculated by hand (Morton, 1956), a difficult task that required expertise in the calculation of likelihoods, as well as patience and considerable perseverance. Renwick and Schulze (1961) and Renwick and Bolling (1969) developed a program to calculate odds for large pedigrees. Their approach is difficult to assess since their algorithm was never published; it was also written in machine-dependent language and was not exportable. Friedhoff and Chase (1975) developed a program for analyzing multigeneration families; the input, however, was complex and the program has not been used to any extent.

## Multigeneration Family Units

When large families were encountered the usual method of analysis was to break down a large pedigree into subunits to which the lod score method could be applied. The lods were then summed to obtain the lods for the whole pedigree. Since the subunits are not independent of one another this procedure will not yield correct results. In fact it decreases the amount of information on $\theta$. An example is given in Fig. 6 for a main locus with two marker loci one of which is closely linked ($\theta = 0.05$) and the other independent ($\theta = 0.5$). Table II compares the lod scores using LIPED with those obtained if we assume four independent sibships and use Morton's $z$ scores. For the A:B linkage the maximum lod score is

TABLE II. Comparison of Lod Scores for Pedigree in Figure 6 Using Morton's $z$ Scores Separately for Each Sibship vs. LIPED

| Loci | Method | Recombination fraction ($\theta$) | | | | | |
|------|--------|------|------|------|------|------|------|
| | | 0.0 | 0.05 | 0.10 | 0.20 | 0.30 | 0.40 |
| A:B | z score | $-\infty$ | 1.143 | 1.171 | 0.908 | 0.521 | 0.160 |
| | LIPED | $-\infty$ | 3.118 | 3.019 | 2.451 | 1.648 | 0.689 |
| A:C | z score | $-\infty$ | $-2.627$ | $-1.560$ | $-0.642$ | $-0.238$ | $-.054$ |
| | LIPED | $-\infty$ | $-3.607$ | $-2.209$ | $-0.937$ | $-0.346$ | $-0.075$ |

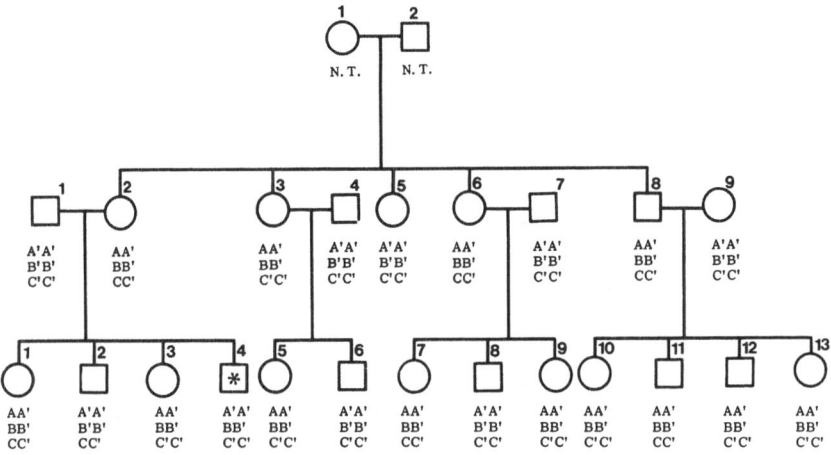

Fig. 6. Pedigree with three hypothetical loci, *A*, *B*, and *C* where *A* and *B* are closely linked and *A* and *C* are independent. The data for both pairs of loci were scored for linkage using LIPED, which gives a score for the whole pedigree, and also using $z$ scores for each sibship. The results, given in Table II, demonstrate the increase in efficiency of the former method. $A:B$ = 5 cM; $A:C$ = 50 cM; * = crossover between *A* and *B*; N.T. = not tested.

3.118 at $\theta$ = 0.05 while the score at $\theta$ = 0.05 using $z$ scores is only 1.143. For the A:C linkage, the scores were much more negative using LIPED. This latter is also important since, if loci are not linked the test should also be optimal in rejecting linkage.

Elston and Stewart (1971) developed a procedure for computing the likelihood recursively, starting with the most recent generation and working back from it. The results for a group of sibs can be computed first and the result attached to their parents; once attachment takes place these individuals are no longer needed in further computations.

Ott (1974) developed a general linkage program (LIPED) based on the algorithm of Elston and Stewart. The Elston-Stewart algorithm and Ott's program were restricted to simple pedigrees, i.e., those with no loops (consanguinity) and those in which parents of only one member of a pair of parents appeared in the pedigree. This deficiency was rectified by Lange and Elston in 1975 who presented an algorithm to calculate the likelihood of any pedigree including complex ones. Ott (1977) then incorporated their methods into his program producing a new version (LIPED 3). Thus, to quote Morton (1979), "the main problems in reducing raw data to a standard lod table have been solved."

The LIPED program requires the family structure, one record per individual as input. The record contains three unique numbers, one for the individual and one for each of his parents unless the individual is on the periphery of the pedigree (e.g., married in), in which case his parents' numbers will be recorded as unknown. It also must include the sex of the individual. This is sufficient to define a family pedigree.

In addition to the family structure and the phenotypes of the individuals, the program uses the following quantities which are intrinsically necessary for calculating the likelihood in a linkage analysis.

1. *Population gene frequencies for the loci being analyzed and the values of the recombination fraction for males and females.* Gene frequencies are necessary to obtain the likelihoods of individuals with unknown phenotypes and also to infer genotypes in dominant marker systems. Ott has suggested that small changes in gene frequency are not likely to affect the values of the lod scores very much. However, there is evidence, (Spence *et al.*, 1977) that large changes in gene frequency can substantially affect the lods. The magnitude of the effect will depend not only on the change in gene frequency but also on the number of individuals in the pedigree whose phenotype is unknown.

2. *A matrix which describes each locus.* The elements of the matrix give the probability of observing phenotype x given genotype $g$, $P(x|g)$. The number of rows in the matrix equals the number of genotypes, i.e., $k(k + 1)/2$, where $k$ is the number of alleles. Likewise the number of columns equals the number of observed phenotypes. Usually the matrix consists of zeros and ones but it may contain intermediate values as in the case of reduced penetrance. Calculations of the likelihood of a pedigree based on the Elston–Stewart algorithm are given in the appendix. Two examples are used. The first one involves, for simplicity, the likelihood for one locus while the second example involves two loci as is the case in linkage analysis.

## Quantitative Traits

Renwick (1971), in discussing quantitative linkage stated that, in his view, "the mapping of a locus in man through its influence on a 'metrical' trait will generally not be practical by statistical means." He felt that mapping would only be feasible after identifying the various genotypes "through properties more specific than metrical ones usually are." However, a number of contributions have been made in this area which may allay some of Renwick's pessimism.

Lowry and Shultz (1959), in a study of association of metric traits and marker genes in chickens, failed to show any association. They recognized that their analysis was limited in several ways. Only some of the genes responsible for the expression of the metric trait will be linked with the test locus, thus increasing the volume of data necessary to obtain statistical significance. Also part of the variation of the metric trait is environmental in nature. Thus the probability of obtaining evidence for linkage for a character with low heritability is slight, since it requires that an appreciable proportion of its variance be controlled by genes actually linked to the marker.

Jayakar (1970) described a method based on the ratio within families, of the between-marker-genotype variance to the within-marker-genotype variance. This $F$ ratio has an expected value of 1 in the absence of linkage. His method has a drawback in that it requires at least two members of one marker genotype and one of another in each sibship, a fairly serious restriction for human families. Furthermore, the method uses data from two generations only. He also did Monte Carlo simulation to test the efficiency of his method and, in general, found that large numbers of families (over 1000) would probably be required for his method to be feasible. Hill (1975) described in more detail an essentially similar method; she apparently was unaware of Jayakar's paper.

Smith (1975) described a nonparametric test for the detection of linkage between a quantitative and a Mendelian character. His method is based on within-family association of a marker phenotype with a higher or lower level of the quantitative trait.

Ott's program LIPED can be used for linkage analysis where one locus results in a continuously distributed phenotype. In this case $P(x|g)$, i.e., the probability of the phenotype x given genotype $g$, is taken to be the density of a normal distribution with mean $m$ and standard deviation $s$. Each row (corresponding to each genotype) of the matrix will contain the $m$ and $s$ for the given genotype. Thus the lod method may also be used to detect linkage when one of the loci has quantitative variation.

In order to test the efficiency of this method, Lange et al. (1976) did a simulation experiment. They used data from 61 informative families with 364 individuals on the established linkage between the $Amy_2$ and $Fy$ loci, added Gaussian noise to the $Amy_2$ phenotypes and then calculated lod scores for various values of the recombination fraction. They concluded that linkage could still be detected in their sample when the heritability is as low as 40 percent. They also found that by converting the original qualitative $Amy_2$ to a quantitative trait, the maximum likelihood estimates of the recombination fraction were biased towards lower values of θ.

Haseman and Elston (1972) developed parametric and nonparametric methods for estimating linkage between a qualitative locus with multiple alleles and a hypothesized two-allele locus that governs a quantitative trait. They gave both parametric and nonparametric methods. Their non-parametric method for detecting linkage is based on the premise that, if there is a major trait gene located near a marker locus there should be an inverse association between the sib pair difference for the trait and the proportion of genes identical by descent that they share in common. On the null hypothesis these should be independent. The method of rank correlations is then applied. This test procedure is easy to apply requiring only the calculation of the proportion of shared "identical by descent" genes and the sib-pair differences. A major disadvantage is that, being a nonparametric test, it is likely to require large samples in order to detect anything but close linkage.

Their parametric test involves maximum likelihood and unlike the previous method, which can only at best detect close linkage, the recombination fraction can be estimated.

Suarez et al. (1978) derived a general expression for the distribution of identity by descent scores at a marker locus for sib pairs given neither, one, or both sibs affected with a disorder determined by a linked-trait locus. They suggested that the affected sib-pair methodology is especially suited to traits determined by single loci with non-Mendelian transmission. Their method is similar to the approach of Haseman and Elston (1972) just described.

Thus, it would seem that linkage with a quantitative trait is feasible if a substantial proportion of the variance in the trait is due to alleles at one locus which is closely linked to one or more of the marker loci used. In view of the increasing number of marker loci that are becoming available in man these techniques should become more useful in the future.

# INTERPRETATION OF RESULTS

## Sex Differences in Recombination

In the majority of cases in man the estimate of the recombination fraction which gives the largest lod score is higher for females than for males. Haldane (1922) noted that in higher organisms, when a difference in recombination frequency occurs, it is lower in the heterogametic sex. Dunn and Bennett (1967) tabulated the recombination frequency for 53 linkage pairs in the mouse. Among 23 pairs for which a significant difference ($p < 0.05$) among the sexes existed, the lower estimate was for males in 18 cases and for females in 5. They found this difference to be region-specific. The five pairs for which the female recombination frequency was lower covered a distance (in terms of male recombination frequency) of approximately 43 cM in linkage groups VI and VII.

Thus it is important to obtain a separate estimate of $\theta$ for males and females. Likelihoods should be derived from the raw data for different pairs of values $\theta_m$ and $\theta_f$ and maximum likelihood estimates can then be obtained for each sex. Renwick (1968) coined the term *susceptibility ratio*, which he defined as the ratio of the female to male recombination fraction. Ott (1974) discussed the approximate factorization introduced by Falk and Edwards (1970):

$$z(\theta_m, \theta_f) \doteq z(\theta_m, \tfrac{1}{2}) + z(\tfrac{1}{2}, \theta_f)$$

which does not yield the joint maximum likelihood estimates $\hat{\theta}_m$ and $\hat{\theta}_f$. Morton (1979) has suggested a better, though still approximate, factorization:

$$z(\theta_m, \theta_f) \doteq \overset{*}{z}(\theta_m, \hat{\theta}_f) + \overset{*}{z}(\hat{\theta}_m, \theta_f)$$

where

$$\overset{*}{z}(\theta_m, \hat{\theta}_f) = \log\,[L(\theta_m, \hat{\theta}_f)/L(\tfrac{1}{2}, \hat{\theta}_f)] = z(\theta_m, \hat{\theta}_f) - z(\tfrac{1}{2}, \hat{\theta}_f)$$

Similarly,

$$\overset{*}{z}(\hat{\theta}_m, \theta_f) = z(\hat{\theta}_m, \theta_f) - z(\hat{\theta}_m, \tfrac{1}{2})$$

This has a maximum at $\hat{\theta}_m, \hat{\theta}_f$ and, as Morton points out, allows presentation of the data as a standard lod table for each sex separately although the lod surface is not precisely recovered.

For an exact factorization, a bivariate lod table for $\theta_m$ and $\theta_f$ simultaneously is required but this complicates presentation of data. A three dimensional bivariate surface for lod scores for males and females is shown in Fig. 7. A more useful representation is given in Fig. 8 using contour lines. It is hoped that eventually a standardized presentation of linkage data will be adopted.

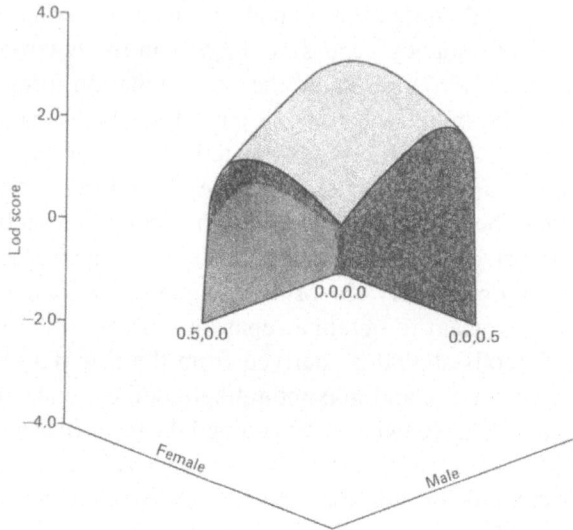

Fig. 7. Three dimensional surface of lod scores for male and female recombination fractions analyzed separately. Generation of this surface requires a large number of points $(\theta_m, \theta_f)$ and thus is normally not economical.

## *Acceptance and Significance of Linkage*

Morton (1955) suggested criteria for accepting or rejecting the null hypothesis. As mentioned earlier, in the sequential test for linkage, two constants A and B are used to determine one of three decision outcomes.

1. If $Z \geq \log A$ ($Z$ is the total lod score) there is significant evidence for linkage under the assumptions of the test.
2. If $Z \leq \log B$ the recombination fraction is significantly greater than the value for which the lod score was determined.
3. If $\log B < Z < \log A$ the evidence for linkage is not decisive and more data is required to make a decision.

As stated earlier the values of $A$ and $B$ are related to $\alpha$ and $\beta$, the probabilities of Type I and II errors respectively as follows:

$$A = (1 - \beta)/\alpha$$
$$B = \beta/(1 - \alpha)$$

Morton suggested that $\alpha$ be set at 0.001 and $\beta$ at 0.01 giving values of 3 and $-2$ for log $A$ and log $B$ respectively.

These criteria have been used up to now in linkage analysis and would appear from the recent data of Rao *et al.* (1978) to have been a good choice. Using the empirical distribution of lods from data since Morton's original paper led them to conclude that less than 2% of tests with total lod score greater than 3 were Type 1 errors.

It is important to realize that, though a lod score of 3 gives a probability ratio of 1000 to one in favor of linkage at the specific value of $\theta$ vs. independent assortment, this does not indicate a probability of a Type I error as low as 0.001 but in fact, as we will show, it is very close to 0.05, the standard significance level used in statistics.

The reason that the Type I error probability ($\alpha$) is not a true value is due to the fact that there is a prior probability of linkage of approximately 1/46 (Renwick, 1970) where linkage is defined as a map distance $\leq$

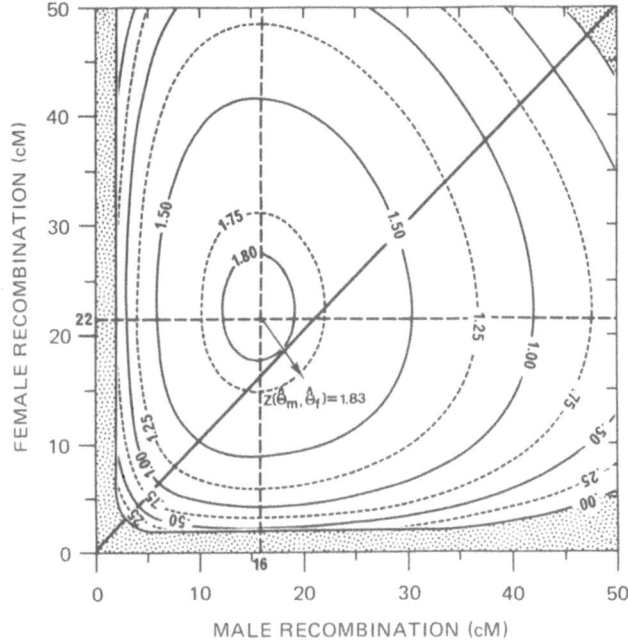

Fig. 8. Contour lines from a three dimensional distribution similar to Fig. 7. The diagonal line represents $z(\theta_m,\theta_f) = z(\theta_m, 1/2) + z(1/2, \theta_f)$. The horizontal dashed line represents $z(\theta_m,\hat{\theta}_f)$ and the vertical $z(\theta_m,\hat{\theta}_f)$. Their intersection is $z(\hat{\theta}_m,\hat{\theta}_f) = 1.83$ which is the peak or maximum lod score.

TABLE III. Posterior probability of a Type I Error When the
Probability of Linkage is 1/46 (0.022)

| State of nature | Linked ($\leq$44 cM) | Not linked |
|---|---|---|
| Prior probability | 0.022 | 0.978 |
| Apparent probabiity[a] | $0.95 = (1 - \beta)$ | $0.001 = (\alpha)$ |
| Joint probability | 0.021 | 0.00098 |
| Posterior probability | 0.96 | 0.04 |

[a] This is the conditional probability of rejecting the null hypothesis (stating that the loci are linked) given the state of nature.

44 cM. Thus the posterior probability of a Type I error is approximately 0.04 when the apparent $\alpha$ is 0.001. This is illustrated in Table III.

This point has been lost on many researchers who place emphasis on lods on the order of 1.3 (odds of 20:1) in the mistaken belief that they are significant. It should be emphasized that the posterior probability will vary with the prior probability which in turn is modified if more information is available on the location of one of the markers. The foregoing discussion assumes that only two loci are being tested. If multiple marker loci are utilized, as is usually the case, the apparent significance of a given lod score may be further inflated.

## Confidence Intervals

A number of procedures have been used to estimate limits for the recombination fraction. Where the likelihood function has a clear maximum in the 0.0–0.5 range its sampling variance can be estimated on the assumption that the likelihoods have a normal distribution such that the natural logs of the likelihoods have a parabolic distribution. Since lod scores differ from the natural log of the likelihoods only by two constants, (1) the denominator, i.e. the likelihood of the sample given that the two loci are independent, and (2) $\log_e 10$, they will also have the same distribution.

Edwards (1971) gives the following methods for obtaining the standard error of $\theta$. Consider the case of three serial values of the recombination fraction, $\theta$, with one unit separation, and lod scores $z_1$, $z_2$, and $z_3$. Then the lod function will be approximated by the parabolic function,

$$z = a\theta^2 + b\theta + c$$

where $a$, $b$, and $c$ are constants. Then

$$a = (z_1 - 2z_2 + z_3)/2$$

$$b = (z_3 - z_1)/2$$

$$c = z_2$$

with a peak at

$$b/2a = (z_3 - z_1)/2(z_1 - 2z_2 + z_3)$$

If $u$ is the distance between $\theta_1$ and $\theta_2$ and also between $\theta_2$ and $\theta_3$, then

$$\hat{\theta} = \theta_2 + u(z_3 - z_1)/(z_1 - 2z_2 + z_3)$$

with standard error

$$u/[(2.303)(z_1 - 2z_2 + z_3)]^{\frac{1}{2}}$$

where the factor 2.303 or $\log_e 10$ is necessary since lod scores are to the base 10. The large sample confidence interval for $\hat{\theta}$ is $(\hat{\theta} - t\sigma) < \theta < (\hat{\theta} + t\sigma)$ where $t$ is a standard normal deviate with confidence coefficient $1 - \alpha$. It should be stressed that these estimates of $\hat{\theta}$ and its standard error are only meaningful when the likelihoods have an approximately normal form. Morton (1956) has suggested that in small samples a suitable transformation of $z$ be made to make the likelihood distribution more nearly normal.

Renwick and Schulze (1964) suggest a graphical method to obtain an estimate and limits of the map interval. They avoid using the term "confidence interval." In their case they incorporate the prior probability of linkage with the relative likelihood (antilog of the lod scores) to obtain a final distribution of the map interval $w$. In this case $\theta$ is transformed to $w$ using a suitable mapping function [they used the Carter–Falconer (1951) transformation]. The narrowest limits, which Renwick and Schulze suggest are the most appropriate, are those which have the same relative probabilities (same ordinates) and which together exclude a proportion $\alpha$ of the area under the curve. The narrowest limits can be readily found by trial and error, using a planimeter.

Repeated sampling techniques can also be used to estimate the confidence limits for the recombination fraction. Although this approach is not applicable to real data due to generally small sample sizes, valuable insights can be provided using models based on computer simulation techniques. The construction of a simulation model incorporating two-generation double-backcross mating types provides means and variances. An estimate of true confidence limits, based on repeated sampling techniques, can be computed from these means and variances for any given recombination fraction and/or distribution of family size in the population. The major advantage of simulation modeling lies in the fact that very complex problems can be investigated, e.g., the model mentioned above can be extended to include multigeneration families with multiple loci (Wilson et al., 1978).

## Prior Probability of Linkage

Since man has 22 autosomes, there is a relatively high prior probability that two loci chosen at random are syntenic. For example, the probability that two loci are on chromosome 1 is $(1/11)^2$ or $1/121$ since that chromosome is approximately $1/11$ of the total autosomal length. If we assume that the positions of selected loci can be taken to be a random sample from a uniform distribution, the overall probability of synteny is

$$\sum_{i=1}^{22} 1/L_i^2$$

where $L_i$ is the relative length of the $i$th autosome. This figure is approximately $1/18.5$ (Renwick, 1969a).

Thus, in significance tests for linkage, it would seem reasonable that prior probabilities be included. By using Bayes' theorem, we can combine these prior probabilities with the relative likelihoods obtained from the data to obtain a posterior probability of linkage. Bayes' theorem has the advantage that, unlike any other method, it gives the probability of linkage rather than acceptance or rejection of the null hypothesis.

Renwick (1968, 1969a,b, 1971) has been the main proponent of Bayesian methodology in linkage analysis. He further refined the prior distribution to obtain the prior probability for particular lengths of map interval on any one of the 22 autosomes. The distribution of intervals for a given chromosome is triangular, the base being the relative length of the chromosome and its area related to the chance that the two loci are on the

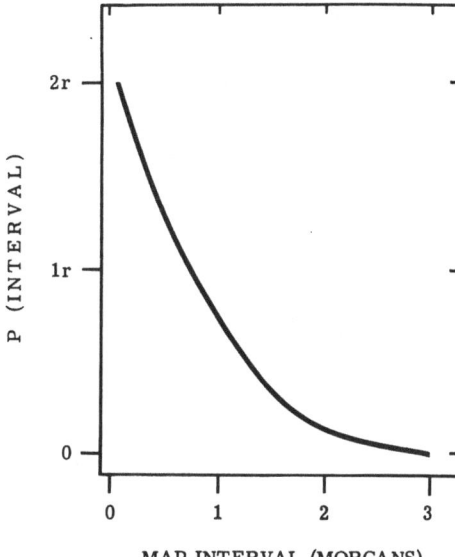

Fig. 9. Relative probability of synteny (loci on same chromosome) for intervals up to three Morgans which is assumed to be the length of the longest autosome, chromosome 1. The curve is obtained as the sum of 22 triangles, all of the same shape with the base of each triangle proportional to the relative length ($r$) of the corresponding autosome and its area proportional to the square of the length.

MAP INTERVAL (MORGANS)

chromosome. The distribution of intervals over all the autosomes is obtained as the summation of the individual prior probabilities as shown in Fig. 9.

The utility of the Bayesian method has been discussed in detail by Smith (1959). Unfortunately, it has fallen into disfavor mainly because the assumption of a random distribution of loci along the chromosomes may not be valid. Furthermore, if results are given only as posterior probabilities it is almost impossible to compare or combine them with other sets of data. Morton (1979) has made a plea that all linkage data be published in conventional form (i.e., lod scores for various recombination fractions) so that they can be used for combining with other data and for use in multipoint mapping.

## Linkage Heterogeneity

A major reason for linkage analysis is the detection of genetic heterogeneity resulting from the phenotype being caused by two or more loci. Recognition of genetic heterogeneity may help resolve biochemical and clinical heterogeneity. Morton (1956) used large sample theory for the following test of heterogeneity: $\chi^2 = 2 (\log_e 10) (\Sigma \hat{z}_i - \hat{z})$ with $n -$

1 degrees of freedom where $\hat{z}_i$ is the maximum lod score in the interval $0 \leq \theta \leq \frac{1}{2}$ for the $i$th family, $\hat{Z}$ is the maximum of $\Sigma\ z_i$ in the same interval, and the sum is over all families. Using this test, Morton (1956) has shown that in some families elliptocytosis appears to be closely linked with the Rh blood group while in other pedigrees there is no evidence for linkage, suggesting that there are at least two loci for elliptocytosis.

Since this test was based on large sample theory, Smith (1963) described a method for testing for heterogeneity that may be more appropriate in man for the small size of samples (pedigrees) that constitute the units being tested. The method is Bayesian and thus requires prior probabilities. It does, however, include an estimate of $\alpha$, the proportion of families in which the two loci are linked. The likelihood for the $r$th family may be expressed as $L_r(\theta, \alpha) = \alpha L_r(\theta = \theta_1) + (1 - \alpha)L_r(\theta = \frac{1}{2})$. The likelihood for the whole sample is the product of the likelihoods for specific families $L_S(\theta, \alpha) = \Pi\ L_i\ (\theta, \alpha)$. A likelihood which is the average of $L_S(\theta, \alpha)$ over all $\theta$ between 0 and $\frac{1}{2}$ and over all $\alpha$ between 0 and 1 is then obtained. This likelihood and the two alternate likelihoods, $L_S(\theta = 0; \alpha = 0)$ and $L_S(\theta; \alpha = 0)$, the latter averaged over all values of $\theta$ between 0 and $\frac{1}{2}$, are then modified by multiplying by their prior probabilities. If the modified relative likelihood for the hypothesis $\alpha > 0; \theta < \frac{1}{2}$, is much greater than the other two, there is evidence for heterogeneity.

The values of $\theta$ and $\alpha$ which maximize $L_S(\theta, \alpha)$ can be found, thus simultaneously obtaining estimates of the recombination fraction $\theta$ and the proportion of families showing linkage with the marker locus ($\alpha$). While this latter is the obvious advantage of the method it does have the disadvantage, as do other Bayesian approaches in linkage, of requiring prior probabilities.

## Age and Recombination

As early as 1915, Bridges showed a nonlinear effect of age on recombination in Drosophila, which followed a W-shaped curve with a low at 11–13 days and another low at 30 days. The effect appeared to be more marked for regions near the centromere.

In the case of mammals, Fisher (1949) noted a decrease in recombination with maternal age in mice. This was substantiated by Reid and Parsons (1963) whose data suggested that with increasing age there is decreasing recombination in female and increasing recombination in male mice.

In man, Renwick and Schulze (1965) compared the regression of re-combination fractions on mean parental age in the Lutheran : Secretor and ABO : nail patella linkages. They found only small differences in maternal ages; the differences in paternal ages were greater but nonsignificant. Weitkamp *et al.* (1973) performed a similar analysis for the closely linked *HLA-A* and *HLA-B* loci and again found no significant age effect for either sex. When they scored families on the basis of whether recombination occurs in the first or second half of the sibship their results were also nonsignificant. However, when Weitkamp (1973) used this latter method for the Lutheran : Secretor and Lutheran : myotonic dystrophy linkages he found a significant excess of paternal recombinants in the second half of the sibships. He also found a significant excess of maternal recombi-nants in the first half of sibships for the Rh : 6-PGD linkage.

Elston *et al.* (1976) incorporated paternal age into the Elston–Stewart (1971) algorithm. Using the likelihood ratio test and maximum likelihood estimates of parental age parameters they were unable to detect a sig-nificant age effect on recombination frequency for the ABO : nail patella linkage data.

Another approach to the study of age effects on the frequency of recombination is the relationship between chiasma frequencies and age. Henderson and Edwards (1968) and Luthardt *et al.* (1973) found a sig-nificant decrease in chiasmata with increasing age in female mice.

In man, data on chiasma frequencies in females are scant and thus no conclusions on their correlation with age can be drawn. In males, however, a much larger body of data is available. Lange *et al.* (1975) subjected data from 183 males to analysis of covariance. There appeared to be little or no linear trend in chiasma frequency with age. They did, however, find significant differences in mean chiasma frequencies among the eight investigators from which the data were obtained. Mayo (1974) suggested a curvilinear relationship between age and chiasma frequency but the numbers were not high enough for convincing statistical tests.

## Mapping Functions

A mapping function is a mathematical expression relating the fre-quency of recombination ($\theta$) to the map distance ($w$).

The first mapping function was derived by Haldane in 1919, and was based on the assumption of no interference, i.e., all chiasmata were dis-tributed uniformly along the chromosome, independently of one another.

He proposed the differential equation $d\theta/dw = 1 - 2c\theta$, where $c$ is the coincidence over a finite interval with an infinitesimally small adjacent interval, and from it derived the mapping function $\theta = \frac{1}{2}(1 - e^{2w})$. He then fit an empirical curve using data from the X chromosome of *Drosophila* and noted that the function, chosen to give as good a fit as possible, probably had no theoretical significance.

Kosambi in 1944 suggested that $c = 2\theta$ is more realistic than the estimate of Haldane, giving the differential equation $d\theta/dw = 1 - 4\theta^2$. On integration he obtained the formula $\theta = \frac{1}{2} \tanh (2w)$ or $w = \frac{1}{4} \log [(1 - 2\theta)/(1 + 2\theta)]$. This formula gave a good fit to *Drosophila* data. It did not however, give a satisfactory fit to mouse data for large recombination fractions. Carter and Falconer (1951) chose $c$ to be $(2\theta)^3$ and by integration obtained the formula $w = \frac{1}{4}(\tanh^{-1} 2\theta + \tan^{-1} 2\theta)$ which gave a better fit for mouse data. This mapping function has been the one generally used in man; a table of values of the function is given in Robinson (1972).

The first general mapping function was developed by Barratt *et al.* (1954), using a parameter $k$ which is a measure of interference. When $k = 1$ (complete interference) their formula reduced to that of Haldane and when $k = 0$ (no interference) it reduces to a straight line with $\theta = w$. When there is no interference, exchanges are distributed at random among bivalents following a Poisson distribution whose mean depends on the map length of the segment. Since positive interference decreases the proportion of multiple exchange tetrads relative to singles, these investigators approximated the new proportion of tetrads with $r$ exchanges by multiplying the Poisson term by $k^{n-1}$ and used the resultant family of functions to construct a genetic map in *Neurospora crassa*.

Recently, Rao *et al.* (1977) used the data of Hulten (1974) on male meiosis to determine a general mapping function for man,

$$w = \{p(2p - 1) (1 - 4p)ln(1 - 2\theta) + 16p(p - 1) (2p - 1)\tan^{-1}(2\theta)$$

$$+ 2p(1 - p) (8p + 2) \tanh^{-1}(2\theta) + 6(1 - p) (1 - 2p) (1 - 4p)\theta\}/6$$

where $p$ is a measure of coincidence. As in the case of the functions of Barratt *et al.* (1954), when $p = 1$ the formula reduces to that of Haldane and when $p = 0$, $w = \theta$. When $p = \frac{1}{2}$ it reduces to Kosambi's function and finally when $p = \frac{1}{4}$ it becomes the Carter–Falconer formula. They ignored terminal chiasmata and obtained an estimate of $p$ for each chromosome. Their mean value of $p$ was $0.351 \pm 0.007$. They found no significant variation of $p$ among chromosome groups within the metacentric and acrocentric classes, but acrocentrics showed significantly more interference than metacentrics ($\chi_1^2 = 27.7$) as was previously suggested by Carter and Falconer (1951) for the mouse.

Sturt (1976) proposed a new mapping function that provides for positive interference within chromosome arms but no interference across the centromere. The function was derived by assuming that all chromosome arms except the short arms of acrocentrics have an obligatory chiasma. Morton (1979), however, has suggested that "the effect of an obligate terminal chiasma may be negligible for all loci except those very close to the telomere which are not genetically mappable."

Figure 10 shows a number of these mapping functions. In summary, while the Carter–Falconer formula has been the most often used in man, the function proposed by Rao *et al.* (1977) is the first for man where human chiasma data were used in its determination. The latter also has

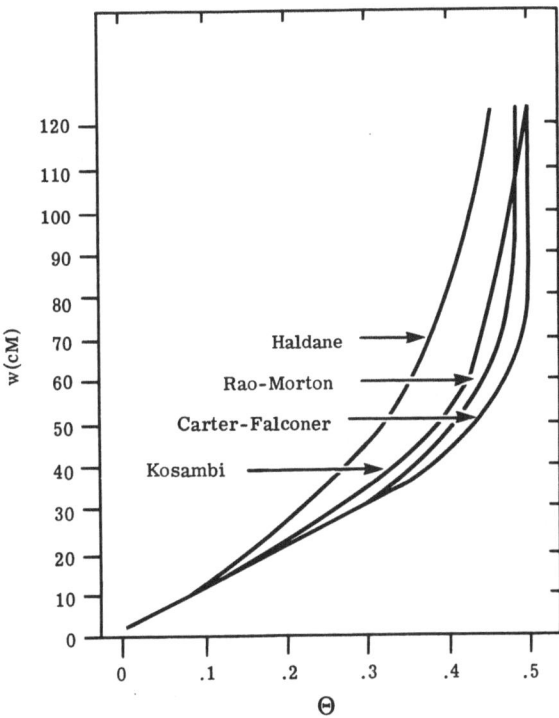

Fig. 10. Relationship between the recombination fraction, $\theta$ and the map interval $w$ in cM using various mapping functions, whose formulae are given in the text.

the advantage that it can be used for individual chromosomes assuming that a good estimate of coincidence is available for that chromosome.

## MULTIPOINT MAPPING

As the number of two-point linkages grew it was only a matter of time for triple and higher-order linkages to be discovered. The first autosomal linkage triplet, between ABO, nail-patella syndrome, and adenylate kinase, was described independently by Rapley *et al.* (1968) and Schleutermann *et al.* (1969). Many other multiple-point linkage groups have been described since.

Bolling (1970) and Renwick and Bolling (1971) described the first multipoint mapping approach for human data. The input to their program was the lod scores for each pair of linked loci for the various values of the recombination fraction ($\theta$). In order to obtain the relative odds of the different orders of the loci, the recombination fractions at which the lods were calculated had to be converted to map distances. This required the use of a mapping function; they used the Carter–Falconer function.

Since their approach was Bayesian, it required a prior distribution of the map distances. The prior probability was obtained using a density function derived by Irwin (1955) on the assumption that the loci are randomly situated along a fixed interval. For three loci with two intervals, $w_1$ and $w_2$, and a specific autosome length, $L$, the function is

$$f(w_1, w_2 | L) = \frac{6(L - w_1 - w_2)}{L^3} \qquad 0 \leqslant w_1 + w_2 \leqslant L$$

If more than one autosome is being considered, the function is summed over all of them. The likelihood of $w_1$ and $w_2$ given the lod scores from the two two-point analyses $\lambda(w_1 w_2 | S)$ is then multiplied by the prior probability to obtain a joint density function:

$$g(w_1, w_2 | S) = f(w_1 w_2 | L) \cdot \lambda(w_1 w_2 | S)$$

Through partial integration, the marginal function for each map interval and its most likely estimate is obtained. The unnormed marginal density function of $w_1$, $g(w_1 | S)$ is obtained by integrating $g(w_1, w_2 | S)$ over the interval $w_2$. Similarly, $g(w_1 w_2 | S)$ integrated over $w_1$ gives $g(w_2 | S)$, the unnormed marginal density function of $w_2$.

The unnormed probability of *synteny* is obtained by double integration. The probability

$$\int\int g(w_1, w_2 | S) dw_1 dw_2$$

is calculated for each order of loci; the most probable ordering of the loci will have the largest probability of synteny. An estimate of the odds by which one ordering is more likely than another is obtained by taking the ratio of the probabilities of the two orders.

If it is not known whether the three loci are syntenic, the relative frequency of 3-synteny, 2-synteny/1-asynteny, and 3-asynteny is obtained as follows. The probability of each order is summed and multiplied by the prior probability of 3-synteny to give joint odds. The joint odds of 2-synteny/1-asynteny are obtained by combining the likelihoods of the syntenic pair with the prior distribution of map intervals and multiplying by the prior probability of 2-synteny/1-asynteny. The joint odds for 3-asynteny are equal to the prior odds of 3-asynteny. The prior odds are as follows (where $L_i$ is the length of the $i$th autosome):

(1)  $\Sigma L_i^3$  for 3-synteny

(2)  $\Sigma L_i^2 (1 - L_i)$  for 2-synteny/1-asynteny

(3)  $1 - (i) - (ii)$  for 3-asynteny

Sturt (1975) used a similar approach and increased the number of loci to five. She then analyzed five loci, $PGM_1$, $Rh$, $PGD$, $Pep\ C$, and $Fy$, all known to be on chromosome 1. She assumed the total length of chromosome 1 to be 3 M. Her analysis did not allow a firm conclusion of their order since the probabilities for a number of orders were of similar magnitude.

The major problems with the methods of Renwick and Bolling (1971) and Sturt (1975) is their use of Bayesian methodology which requires prior probabilities. Moreover, data from triple- or higher-order heterozygotes cannot be incorporated into the calculations, nor can an estimate of interference be obtained.

Meyers *et al.* (1976, 1979) used a parametric non-Bayesian approach to obtain a multipoint map of chromosome 1. The method does not require the conversion of recombination fractions to map units. It uses data from triply and quadruply heterozygous crosses together with independent two-point data from nuclear families with known and unknown phase. This approach also allows for estimation of interference.

To explain the latter method, consider three loci, $A$, $B$, and $C$ in the order $A$-$B$-$C$.

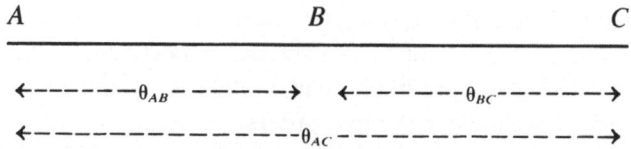

There are four classes of informative families, those segregating for the loci (1) $A$ and $B$; (2) $B$ and $C$; (3) $A$ and $C$ and (4) $A$, $B$, and $C$. Likelihood equations for two-point linkage are obtained in the usual manner and likelihood equations for triply heterozygous families are written and evaluated. Offspring of phase-known triple heterozygotes are classified into four groups.

For example, in the order $A$-$B$-$C$ there are single recombinants $r_{AB}$ and $r_{BC}$, double recombinants $r_{ABC}$, and nonrecombinants $r_{NR}$. The equation has three parameters, $\theta_{AB}$ and $\theta_{BC}$ (recombination fractions between $A$ and $B$, and $B$ and $C$, respectively) and the coefficient of coincidence, $c$. The likelihood ratio of linkage vs. nonlinkage for phase-known sibships is as follows:

$$\frac{L(H_1 : \theta_{AB}, \theta_{BC}, \theta_{AC})}{L(H_0 : \theta_{AB} = \theta_{BC} = \theta_{AC} = 0.5)} =$$

$$\frac{[\theta_{AB}(1 - c\theta_{BC})]^{r_{AB}}[\theta_{BC}(1 - c\theta_{AB})]^{r_{BC}}[c\theta_{AB}\theta_{BC}]^{r_{ABC}}\theta[1 - \theta_{AB} - \theta_{BC} + c\theta_{AB}\theta_{BC}]^{r_{NR}}}{(\frac{1}{4})^{r_{AB}}(\frac{1}{4})^{r_{BC}}(\frac{1}{4})^{r_{ABC}}(\frac{1}{4})^{r_{NR}}}$$

For phase-unknown sibships, the children are classified into four classes. A likelihood is obtained for each of the four possible phases which (under conditions of gametic phase equilibrium) are equally likely. The likelihood is proportional to

$$\tfrac{1}{4}L_{CC} + \tfrac{1}{4}L_{CR} + \tfrac{1}{4}L_{RC} + \tfrac{1}{4}L_{RR}$$

where, for example, $L_{CR}$ is the likelihood of the family with loci $A$ and $B$ in coupling and $B$ and $C$ in repulsion. The likelihood ratios obtained from each class of families are analyzed separately and, since they are independent, are combined. The maximum estimates from the likelihood surface for the three parameters $\theta_{AB}$, $\theta_{BC}$, and $c$ are obtained with the corresponding lod score. The parameter $\theta_{AC}$ is estimated through the relationship

$$\theta_{AC} = \theta_{AB} + \theta_{BC} - 2c\theta_{AB}\theta_{AC}$$

The analysis is repeated for each of the three possible orders of the loci. The lod scores for each order are compared to obtain an estimate of the most likely order and the relative odds for each order. This method has been programmed by Meyers (1976); the program is designated COM (crossover method).

Recently Keats *et al.* (1978) have used a maximum likelihood method for mapping human chromosomes. Details on their methodology have not yet been published.

## SIGNIFICANCE OF LINKAGE

There is a certain satisfaction in knowning where a piece of a puzzle fits and what its relationship is to neighboring pieces. So it is with the "puzzle" of how the vast amount of genetic information is packaged and distributed throughout the genome. To date, relatively small segments of the genome have been characterized, and interesting questions are beginning to surface: What relationship, if any, does linear order have with genetic regulation? with gene interaction? with position effect? How much redundancy is there in genetic information? How much genetic information has arisen through gene duplication? What effect, if any, do heterochromatic regions have on genetic material in euchromatic segments? Is there evidence of position effects in man? What is the significance of finding sex differences in recombination in specific chromosomal regions? What is the relationship between the genetic and physical map? Are there major gene effects in the expression of multifactorial disorders? What is the nature and extent of species differences in the packaging of genetic material? What role does selection play in the formation and population distribution of linked genes?

In helping to answer these questions, the human gene map will further our understanding of human biology and man's place in the natural order.

Attainment of a complete genetic map, however, is not in itself a prerequisite for the practical application of linkage data. The importance of the clinical applicability of linkage information was recognized long before the current growth spurt in human gene mapping. Haldane and Smith (1947) pointed out its value in counseling situations involving X-linked disorders. A decade later, Edwards (1956) extended this notion to prenatal diagnosis of disorders for which direct diagnosis *in utero* was not yet possible. More recently others have alluded to the applicability of linkage information in determining the parental origin of a new mutant allele (Renwick, 1969c) and in improving risk estimates for individuals at risk for genetic disorders (Edwards, 1969; Mayo, 1970; Lindstrom *et al.*, 1973; Murphy and Chase, 1975; Finley and Finley, 1976; Rivas and Conneally, 1977; Jackson *et al.*, 1977; Chakravarti and Nei, 1978).

It has been argued that linkage is of more theoretical than practical importance since its current clinical applications are rather limited and many hundreds of testable marker loci will be needed for the routine use of linkage data in prenatal diagnosis (Mayo, 1970; Edwards, 1956). It is true that linkage information has inherent limitations of precision and applicability (Rivas and Conneally, 1977). However, in spite of these drawbacks, its diagnostic value has been demonstrated in the indirect diagnosis of myotonic dystrophy (Schrott *et al.*, 1973) and of congenital adrenal hyperplasia due to 21-hydroxylase deficiency (Pollack *et al.*, 1979). There are indications that refinement of risk estimates, on the basis of linkage data, will be extended to other genetic disorders in the near future (Rivas and Conneally, 1977).

Increased efforts in establishing new linkage groups will not only allow more precision and applicability in counseling situations but will also demonstrate genetic heterogeneity in a number of clinical disorders. As Morton (1956) noted, detection of heterogeneity is the primary purpose of human linkage studies. The possibility that many dominant traits are genetically heterogeneous can best be resolved by linkage. A recent example of this is found in the class of disorders of congenital cataracts. Renwick and Lawler (1963) demonstrated close linkage in a large kindred of zonular pulverulent cataract with the Duffy (*Fy*) blood group locus, later assigned to chromosome 1 (Donahue *et al.*, 1968). In 1970, using data from two pedigrees, Renwick suggested that perhaps another form of nuclear cataract was linked to the *Fy* locus.

Recently, Conneally *et al.* (1979) described seven families with dominant forms of congenital cataract. Linkage to the *lqh* region was found in two of these families whereas linkage to this marker could be discounted in another family. The remaining four families were inconclusive.

The splitting out of distinct entities from a heterogeneous group of disorders is the first in a series of steps leading to complete clinical and biochemical characterization of genetic disorders. A more defined clinical population is essential if the biochemist is to identify the metabolic pathway involved, the specific defective protein, and finally the nature of the defect at the molecular level.

## APPENDIX

The following are two examples of the Elston–Stewart algorithm as used in the program LIPED. The first example (Pedigree A, Fig. 11) gives the likelihood of the pedigree for one autosomal locus while the second (Pedigree B) gives the likelihood for two autosomal loci with recombination frequency $\theta$.

The likelihood is computed recursively, starting with the most recent generation and working back to the most remote. The advantage of the method is that the likelihood for an individual can be calculated first and the result attached as a factor to the appropriate term for his parent. The individual is then no longer needed in further computations. The overall computation scheme is shown in Fig. 12. The likelihoods for the spouses and children of individuals 3, 5, and 7 are calculated and attached to them (the asterisk attached to their individual numbers indicates this). Thus, for example, $L_3*$ denotes the likelihood of individuals 3, 4, 9, 10, and 11. This procedure is then repeated attaching individuals 3*, 5*, 7*, and 2 to individual 1.

In general let $L$ denote the likelihood of the pedigree with $m$ individuals. This can be expressed as

$$L = \sum_{g_1} \dots \sum_{g_m} \prod_{i=1}^{m} P(X_i|g_i) P(g_i|\dots)$$

where $X_i$ denotes the phenotype and $g_i$ the genotype of individual $i$ and $P(g_i|\dots)$ denotes the probability of genotype $g_i$ for individual $i$ given his parents' genotypes or, if unknown, the population genotype frequency. The above expression is the basis for the calculations used in the two examples. The following are defined for both examples.

$L_i$ is the likelihood for individual $i$ and is the probability of observing his phenotype considering all information in the pedigree. $P(BB|AA)$ for

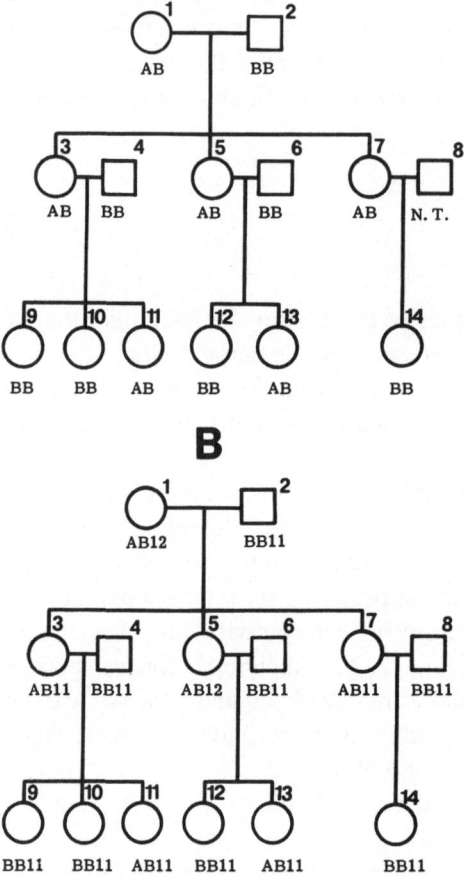

Fig. 11. Hypothetical pedigrees used in illustrations of algorithm for obtaining likelihood of pedigree. Pedigree A shows phenotypes for a codominant locus with two alleles $A$ and $B$. (N.T., not tested). Pedigree B shows phenotypes of two codominant loci each with two alleles, $A$ and $B$, and 1 and 2 respectively.

example, denotes the probability of phenotype BB given genotype $AA$. In both examples there is a one to one correspondence between phenotype and genotype (codominance) except in example 2 with two loci where two phases exist for the phenotype $AB12$. Thus, $P(BB|AA)$ is zero and $P(BB|BB)$ is unity.

$P(g_i|\ldots)$ denotes the probability of genotype $g_i$ given parental matings or population gene frequency. For example $P(AA|\text{Par} = AB \times AB) = \frac{1}{4}$ and $P(AA)$ with unknown parents $= p^2$.

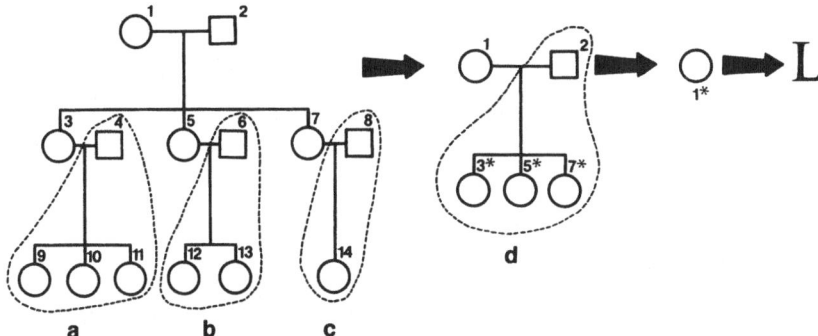

Fig. 12. Illustration of the recursive method as used in the Elston–Stewart algorithm for obtaining the likelihood of a pedigree. Details of the method are given in text.

In example 1, $p$ = gene frequency of $A = f(A)$; $q = f(B)$. In example 2,

$$p_1 = f(A); p_2 = f(B)$$

$$q_1 = f(1)\ q_2 = f(2)$$

## *Computation for Example 1—Pedigree A*

Indiv. #9:

$$L_9 = \sum_{g_i} P(X_9|g_i)P(g_i|\ldots)$$

$$L_9 = P(BB|AA)P(AA|\text{Par} = AB \times BB) + P(BB|AB)P(AB|\text{Par}$$

$$= AB \times BB) + P(BB|BB)P(BB|\text{Par} = AB \times BB)$$

where Par $= AB \times BB$ signifies that parental mating is $AB \times BB$

$$L_9 = (0 \times 0) + (0 \times \tfrac{1}{2}) + (1 \times \tfrac{1}{2}) = \tfrac{1}{2}.$$

Indiv. #10:

$$L_{10} = \tfrac{1}{2} \text{ (same as } L_9)$$

Indiv. #11:

$$L_{11} = P(AB|AA)P(AA|\text{Par} = AB \times BB) + P(AB|AB)P(AB|\text{Par}$$

$$= AB \times BB) + P(AB|BB)P(BB|\text{Par} = AB \times BB)$$

$$= (0 \times 0) + (1 \times \tfrac{1}{2}) + (0 \times \tfrac{1}{2}) = \tfrac{1}{2}$$

Indiv. #4:

$$L_4 = P(BB|AA)P(AA|f(AA)) + P(BB|AB)P(AB|f(AB))$$

$$+ P(BB|BB)P(BB|f(BB))$$

where $f(BB)$ = population frequency of $BB$

$$L_4 = (0 \times p^2) + (0 \times 2pq) + (1 \times q^2) = q^2$$

The likelihoods for Individuals 4, 9, 10, and 11 are now combined to give one likelihood $L_a$.

$$L_a = L_4 \times L_9 \times L_{10} \times L_{11} = \tfrac{1}{2} \times \tfrac{1}{2} \times \tfrac{1}{2} \times q^2 = \tfrac{1}{8}q^2$$

Follow the same procedure for individuals #12, #13, and #6 to obtain

$$L_b = L_6 \times L_{12} \times L_{13} = \tfrac{1}{2} \times \tfrac{1}{2} \times q^2 = \tfrac{1}{4}q^2$$

Consider individuals #14 and #8:
Indiv. #14:

$$L_{14} = P(BB|AA)P(AA|\;\text{Par} = AB \times AA) + P(BB|AA)P(AA|\;\text{Par} =$$

$$AB \times AB) + P(BB|AA)P(AA|\text{Par} = AB \times BB) + P(BB|$$

$$AB)P(AB|\text{Par} = AB \times AA) + P(BB|AB)P(AB|\text{Par} = AB \times$$

$$AB) + P(BB|AB)P(AB|\text{Par} = AB \times BB) + P(BB|BB)P(BB|\text{Par}$$

$$= AB \times AA) + P(BB|BB)P(BB|\text{Par} = AB \times AB) + P(BB|$$

$$BB)P(BB|\text{Par} = AB \times BB)$$

$$= (0 \times \tfrac{1}{2}p^2) + (0 \times \tfrac{1}{4}(2pq)) + (0 \times \tfrac{1}{2}q^2) + (0 \times \tfrac{1}{2}p^2) + (0 \times$$

$$\tfrac{1}{4}(2pq)) + (0 \times \tfrac{1}{2}q^2) + (1 \times 0p^2) + (1 \times \tfrac{1}{4}(2pq)) + (1 \times \tfrac{1}{2}q^2)$$

$$= \tfrac{1}{2}pq + \tfrac{1}{2}q^2 = \tfrac{1}{2}q(p + q) = \tfrac{1}{2}q$$

(Population frequencies are for unknown parent, Indiv. #8.)
Indiv. #8:

$$L_8 = P(x_8|\ldots) = 1$$

since his phenotype is unknown.

$$L_c = L_8 \times L_{14} = 1 \times \tfrac{1}{2}q = \tfrac{1}{2}q$$

To calculate $L_d$ the likelihoods for 3*, 5*, and 7* are obtained and combined with $L_2$.

$$L_3^* = 2 \text{ zero terms} + P(AB|AB)P(AB^*|\text{Par} = AB \times BB),$$

where * includes information on 4, 9, 10, and 11

$$L_3^* = 1 \times L_a \times \tfrac{1}{2} = \tfrac{1}{8}q^2 \times \tfrac{1}{2} = \tfrac{1}{16}q^2$$

Similarly,

$$L_5^* = 1 \times L_b \times \tfrac{1}{2} = \tfrac{1}{4}q^2 \times \tfrac{1}{2} = \tfrac{1}{8}q^2$$

and

$$L_7^* = 1 \times L_c \times \tfrac{1}{2} = \tfrac{1}{2}q \times \tfrac{1}{2} = \tfrac{1}{4}q$$

Indiv. #2: Similar to the computation of $L_4$,

$$L_2 = 2 \text{ zero terms} + P(BB|BB)P(BB|f(BB)) = 1 \times q^2$$

Then

$$L_d = L_3^* \times L_5^* \times L_7^* \times L_2$$

$$= \tfrac{1}{16}q^2 \times \tfrac{1}{8}q^2 \times \tfrac{1}{4}q \times q^2 = (\tfrac{1}{2})^9 q^7$$

Finally,

$$L = L_1^* = 2 \text{ zero terms} + P(AB|AB)P(AB^*|f(AB))$$

$$= 1 \times L_d \times 2pq$$

$$= (\tfrac{1}{2})^9 q^7 \times 2pq = (\tfrac{1}{2})^8 pq^8$$

When $p = q = 0.5$, $L = 7.6294 \times 10^{-6}$

## Computation for Example 2—Pedigree B

Indiv. #9:

$$L_9 = P(BB11|AA11)P(AA11|\text{Par} = AB11 \times BB11) + 7 \text{ more zero terms}$$

$$+ P(BB11|BB11)P(BB11|\text{Par} = AB11 \times BB11) = 1 \times \tfrac{1}{2} = \tfrac{1}{2}$$

(Zero terms are due to phenotype being inconsistent with genotype, or genotype inconsistent with parents' genotypes, or both.)

Similarly,

$$L_{10} = \tfrac{1}{2} \quad \text{and} \quad L_{11} = \tfrac{1}{2}$$

For $L_4$, population frequencies are used to obtain

$$L_4 = \Sigma \text{ zero terms} + P(BB11|BB11)P(BB11|f(BB11))$$

$$= 1 \times q_1^2 p_2^2$$

$$L_a = L_4 \times L_9 \times L_{10} \times L_{11} = q_1^2 p_2^2 \times \tfrac{1}{2} \times \tfrac{1}{2} \times \tfrac{1}{2}$$

$$= (\tfrac{1}{2})^3 q_1^2 p_2^2$$

$$L_{14} = \tfrac{1}{2} \quad \text{and} \quad L_8 = q_1^2 p_2^2 \quad \ldots \quad L_c = \tfrac{1}{2} q_1^2 p_2^2$$

In the case of Individuals 1 and 5 the genotypes may be in coupling or repulsion phase and the likelihood must be calculated for each phase. Let

$$C = \text{coupling} = \frac{A1}{B2} \quad \text{and} \quad R = \text{repulsion} = \frac{A2}{B1}$$

$$L_b{}^*_C = L_6 \times L_{12C} \times L_{13C} = q_1^2 p_2^2 \times \frac{\theta}{2} \times \frac{1 - \theta}{2}$$

$$L_b{}^*_R = L_6 \times L_{12R} \times L_{13R} = q_1^2 p_2^2 \times \frac{1 - \theta}{2} \times \frac{\theta}{2}$$

To calculate $L_d$:

$$L_3{}^* = 8 \text{ zero terms} + P(AB11|AB11)P(AB11^*|\text{Par} = AB12 \times BB11)$$

However, $L_3{}^*$ depends on the phase of #1

$$L_3{}^*_C = 8 \text{ zero terms} + P(AB11|AB11)P\left(AB11^*|\text{Par} = \frac{A1}{B2} \times BB11\right)$$

$$L_3{}^*_R = 8 \text{ zero terms} + P(AB11|AB11)P\left(AB11^*|\text{Par} = \frac{A2}{B1} \times BB11\right)$$

$$L_3{}^*_C = 1 \times (\tfrac{1}{2})^3 q_1^2 p_2^2 \times \frac{1 - \theta}{2}$$

$$L_3{}^*_R = 1 \times (\tfrac{1}{2})^3 q_1^2 p_2^2 \times \frac{\theta}{2}$$

Similarly

$$L_7{}^*{}_C = 1 \times \tfrac{1}{2}q_1{}^2p_2{}^2 \times \frac{1 - \theta}{2}$$

$$L_7{}^*{}_R = 1 \times \tfrac{1}{2}q_1{}^2p_2{}^2 \times \frac{\theta}{2}$$

$$L_5{}^*{}_C = 16 \text{ zero terms} + 1 \times L_b{}^*{}_C \times P\left(\frac{A1}{B2}\middle| \text{Par} = \frac{A1}{B2} \times BB11\right)$$

$$+ 1 \times L_b{}^*{}_R \times P\left(\frac{A2}{B1}\middle| \text{Par} = \frac{A1}{B2} \times BB11\right)$$

$$= (1 \times L_b{}^*{}_C \times 0) + \left(1 \times q_1{}^2p_2{}^2 \times \frac{1 - \theta}{2} \times \frac{\theta}{2}\right) \times \frac{\theta}{2}$$

$$L_5{}^*{}_R = 16 \text{ zero terms} + 1 \times L_b{}^*{}_C \times P\left(\frac{A1}{B2}\middle| \text{Par} = \frac{A2}{B1} \times BB11\right)$$

$$+ 1 \times L_b{}^*{}_R \times P\left(\frac{A2}{B1}\middle| \text{Par} = \frac{A2}{B1} \times BB11\right)$$

$$= (1 \times L_b{}^*{}_C \times 0) + \left(1 \times q_1{}^2p_2{}^2 \times \frac{1 - \theta}{2} \times \frac{\theta}{2}\right) \times \frac{1 - \theta}{2}$$

$$L_2 = 8 \text{ zero terms} + P(BB11|BB11)P(BB11|f(BB11))$$

$$= 1 \times q_1{}^2p_2{}^2$$

Now,

$$L_{dC} = L_2 \times L_3{}^*{}_C \times L_5{}^*{}_C \times L_7{}^*{}_C$$

$$= q_1{}^2p_2{}^2 \times \left[(\tfrac{1}{2})^3 q_1{}^2p_2{}^2 \times \frac{1 - \theta}{2}\right] \times \left[q_1{}^2p_2{}^2 \times \frac{1 - \theta}{2} \times\right.$$

$$\left.\left(\frac{\theta}{2}\right)^2\right] \times \left[\tfrac{1}{2}q_1{}^2p_2{}^2 \times \frac{1 - \theta}{2}\right] = (\tfrac{1}{2})^4 q_1{}^8p_2{}^8 \left(\frac{\theta}{2}\right)^2 \left(\frac{1 - \theta}{2}\right)^3$$

and

$$L_{dR} = L_2 \times L_3{}^*{}_R \times L_5{}^*{}_R \times L_7{}^*{}_R$$

$$= q_1{}^2 p_2{}^2 \times (\tfrac{1}{2})^3 q_1{}^2 p_2{}^2 \times \frac{\theta}{2} \times q_1{}^2 p_2{}^2$$

$$\times \left(\frac{1-\theta}{2}\right)^2 \times \frac{\theta}{2} \times \tfrac{1}{2} q_1{}^2 p_2{}^2 \times \frac{\theta}{2}$$

$$= (\tfrac{1}{2})^4 q_1{}^8 p_2{}^8 \left(\frac{\theta}{2}\right)^3 \left(\frac{1-\theta}{2}\right)^2$$

Finally,

$$L = L_1{}^* = 16 \text{ zero terms} + P\left(AB12 \,\middle|\, \frac{A1}{B2}\right) P\left(\frac{A1}{B2} * \middle| f\left(\frac{A1}{B2}\right)\right)$$

$$+ P\left(AB12 \,\middle|\, \frac{A2}{B1}\right) P\left(\frac{A2}{B1} * \middle| f\left(\frac{A2}{B1}\right)\right)$$

$$= 1 \times L_{dC} \times \tfrac{1}{2}(4p_1 p_2 q_1 q_2) + 1 \times L_{dR} \times \tfrac{1}{2}(4p_1 p_2 q_1 q_2)$$

$$= (\tfrac{1}{2})^3 p_1 p_2{}^9 q_1{}^9 q_2 \left(\frac{\theta}{2}\right)^2 \left(\frac{1-\theta}{2}\right)^3$$

$$+ (\tfrac{1}{2})^3 p_1 p_2{}^9 q_1{}^9 q_2 \left(\frac{\theta}{2}\right)^3 \left(\frac{1-\theta}{2}\right)^2$$

$$= (\tfrac{1}{2})^4 p_1 p_2{}^9 q_1{}^9 q_2 \left(\frac{\theta}{2}\right)^2 \left(\frac{1-\theta}{2}\right)^2$$

The following is a numerical example. Let

$$p_1 = q_1 = p_2 = q_2 = \tfrac{1}{2}$$

$$\theta = 0.5: \qquad L_{0.5} = 0.23283 \times 10^{-9}$$

$$\theta = 0.2: \qquad L_{0.2} = 0.95367 \times 10^{-10}$$

The $z$ score is simply the log of the ratio of two likelihoods.

$$z = \log_{10} \frac{L_{0.2}}{L_{0.5}} = \log_{10} (0.4096) = -0.38764$$

The above results can be verified using the program LIPED.

ACKNOWLEDGMENTS. This publication is No. 79-6 from the Department of Medical Genetics, Indiana University School of Medicine, and was supported in part by the Indiana University Human Genetics Center, USPHS GM 21054 and University of Oregon Grants USPHS HD 08237 and National Foundation CRBS 1-253. We wish to thank Drs. Margaret Pericak-Vance, Joe C. Christian, and Terry E. Reed and graduate students, Stephanie Sherman, Kathleen Stefanko, and Alexander Wilson for helpful comments on the manuscript. Computing services were contributed by the Indiana University Computing Network.

# REFERENCES

Barnard, G. A., 1949, Statistical inference, *J. Roy. Stat. Soc.* **B11**:115–135.

Barratt, R. W. A., Newmeyer, D. D., and Garnjobst, L., 1954, Map construction in Neurospora, *Adv. Gen.* **6**:1–93.

Bateson, W., and Punnett, R. C., 1906, Experimental studies in the physiology of heredity. Reports of the Evolution Committee, *Roy. Soc.* **3**:1–53.

Bernstein, F., 1931, Zur Grundlegung der Chromosomentheorie der Vererbung beim Menschen, *Zeitschr. Abst. Vererb.* **57**:113–138.

Bolling, D. R., 1970, Multipoint mapping of gene loci in man. M.S. Thesis, Johns Hopkins University, Baltimore, Maryland.

Bridges, C. B., 1915, A linkage variation in *Drosophila, J. Exp. Zool.* **15**:1–21.

Bridges, C. B., and Morgan, T. H., 1919, The second chromosome group of mutant characters of *Drosophila melanogaster,* Carnegie Inst. Washington Publ. **278**:123–304.

Bridges, C. B., and Morgan, T. H., 1923, The third chromosome group of mutant characters of *Drosophila melanogaster,* Carnegie Inst. Washington Publ. **327**.

Carter, T. C., and Falconer, D. S., 1951, Stocks for detecting linkage in the mouse and the theory of their design, *J. Genet.* **50**:307–323.

Chakravarti, A., and Nei, M., 1978, Utility of linked marker genes in genetic counseling with the Bayesian method, *Am. J. Hum. Genet.* **30**:122A.

Clarke, C. A., Edwards, J. W., Haddock, D. R. W., Howel-Evans, A. W., McConnell, R. B., and Sheppard, P. M., 1956, ABO blood groups and secretor character in duodenal ulcer. Population and sibship studies, *Br. Med. J.* **2**:725–736.

Conneally, P. M., Wilson, A. F., Merritt, A. D., Helveston, E. M., Palmer, C. G., and Wang, L. Y., 1979, Genetic heterogeneity in autosomal dominant forms of congenital cataract, in: *Winnipeg Conference (1977): Fourth international Workshop on Human Gene Mapping. Birth Defects: Original Article Series*, Vol. 14, No. 4, pp. 295–297, The National Foundation, New York.

Correns, C., 1905, Über Vererbungsgesetze, G. Bornträger, Berlin.

Creighton, H. B., and McClintock, B., 1931, A correlation of cytological and genetical crossing over in *Zea mays, Proc. Nat. Acad. Sci. USA* **17**:492–497.

Deisseroth, A., Nienhuis, A., Turner, P., Velez, R., French Anderson, W., Ruddle, F., Lawrence, J., Creagen, R., and Kucherlapati, R., 1977, Localization of human alpha-globulin structural gene to chromosome 16 in somatic cell hybrids by molecular hybridization assay, *Cell* **12**:205–218.

Donahue, R. P., Bias, W. B., Renwick, J. H., and McKusick, V. A., 1968, Probable assignment of the Duffy blood group locus to chromosome 1 in man, *Proc. Nat. Acad. Sci. USA* **61**:949–955.

Dunn, L. C., and Bennett, D., 1967, Sex differences in recombination of linked genes in animals, *Genet. Res.* **9**:211–220.

Edwards, J. H., 1956, Antenatal detection of hereditary disorders, *Lancet* **270**:579.

Edwards, J. H., 1969, The value of linkage in selective abortion. *Heredity* **25**(Abstr.):150.

Edwards, J. H., 1971, The analysis of X-linkage, *Ann. Hum. Genet.* **34**:229–250.

Elston, R. C., and Lange, K., 1975, The prior probability of autosomal linkage. *Ann. Hum. Genet.* **38**:341–350.

Elston, R. C., Lange, K., and Namboodiri, K. K., 1976, Age trends in human chiasma frequencies and recombination fractions. II. Method for analyzing recombination fractions and application to the ABO:nail patella linkage, *Am. J. Hum. Genet.* **28**:69–76.

Elston, R. C., Namboodiri, K. K., Lange, K., and Gedde-Dahl, T. Jr., 1976, Effect of age on the Gm-Pi linkage, in: *Baltimore Conference (1975). Third International Workshop on Human Gene Mapping. Birth Defects: Original Article Series*, Vol. 11, No. 3, pp. 298–301, The National Foundation, New York.

Elston, R. C., and Stewart, J., 1971, A general model for the analysis of pedigree data, *Hum. Hered.* **21**:523–542.

Falk, C. T., and Edwards, J. H., 1970, A computer approach to the analysis of family genetic data for detection of linkage, *Genetics* **64**(Abstr.):218.

Finley, W. H., and Finley, S. C., 1976, The diagnosis of genetic disorders before birth. *South. Med. J.* **69**:1486–1492.

Finney, D. J., 1940, The detection of linkage, *Ann. Eugen. (London)* **10**:171–214.

Finney, D. J., 1941a, The detection of linkage. II. Further mating types, scoring of Boyd's data, *Ann. Eugen. (London)* **11**:10–30.

Finney, D. J., 1941b, The detection of linkage. III. Incomplete parental testing. *Ann. Eugen. (London)* **11**:115–135.

Finney, D. J., 1942a, The detection of linkage. IV. Lack of parental records and the use of empirical estimates of information. *J. Hered.* **33**:157–160.

Finney, D. J., 1942b, The detection of linkage. V. Supplementary tables. *Ann. Eugen. (London)* **11**:224–232.

Finney, D. J., 1942c, The detection of linkage. VI. The loss of information from incompleteness of parental testing, *Ann. Eugen. (London)* **11**:233–242.

Finney, D. J., 1943, The detection of linkage. VII. Combination of data from matings of known and unknown phase, *Ann. Eugen. (London)* **12**:31–43.

Fisher, R. A., 1935, The detection of linkage, *Ann. Eugen.* **6**:187–201.

Fisher, R. A., 1949, A preliminary linkage test with agouti and undulated mice, *Heredity (London)* **3**:229–241.

Friedhoff, L. B., and Chase, G., 1975, A computer-oriented linkage analysis scheme, *Clin. Genet.* **7**:219–226.

Gedde-Dahl, T. Jr., Fagerhol, M. K. Cook, P. J. L. and Noades, J., 1942, Autosomal linkage between the *Gm* and *Pi* loci in man, *Ann. Hum. Genet.* **35**:393–399.

Green, M. C., 1963, Methods for testing linkage, in: *Methodology in Mammalian Genetics* (W. J. Burdette, ed.), pp. 56–82, Holden-Day, San Francisco.

Haldane, J. B. S., 1919, The combination of linkage values and calculation of distance between the loci of linked factors, *J. Genet.* **8**:299–309.

Haldane, J. B. S., 1922, Sex ratio and unisexual sterility in hybrid animals. *J. Genet.* **12**:101–109.

Haldane, J. B. S., and Smith, C. A. B., 1947, A new estimate of the linkage between the genes for colour-blindness and hemophilia in man, *Ann. Eugen.* **14**:10–31.

Haseman, J. K., and Elston, R. C., 1972, The investigation of linkage between a quantitative trait and a marker trait, *Behav. Genet.* **2**:3–19.

Henderson, S. A., and Edwards, R. C., 1968, Chiasma frequency and maternal age in mammals, *Nature (London)* **218**:22–28.

Hill, A. P., 1975, Quantitative linkage: a statistical procedure for its detection and estimation, *Ann. Hum. Genet.* **38**:439–449.

Hulten, M., 1974, Chiasma distribution at diakinesis in the normal human male, *Hereditas* **76**:55–78.

Irwin, J. O., 1955, A unified derivation of some well known frequency distributions of interest in biometry and statistics, *J. Roy. Stat. Soc. Series A.* **CXVII**:389–404.

Jackson, J. F., Currier, R. D., Terasaki, P. I., and Morton, N. E., 1977, Spinocerebellar ataxia and HLA linkage: Risk prediction by HLA typing, *New Engl. J. Med.* **296**:1138–1141.

Jayakar, S. D., 1970, On the detection and estimation of linkage between a locus influencing a quantitative character and a marker locus, *Biometrics* **26**:451–464.

Keats, B. J. B., Rao, D. C., and Morton, N. E., 1978, Maximum likelihood maps for human chromosomes, *Am. J. Hum. Genet.* **30**(Abstr.):84A.

Kosambi, D. D., 1944, The estimation of map distances from recombination values, *Ann. Eugen.* **12**:172–175.

Lange, K., and Elston, R. C., 1975, Extensions to pedigree analysis. I. Likelihood calculations for simple and complex pedigrees, *Hum. Hered.* **25**:95–105.

Lange, K., Page, B. M., and Elston, R. C., 1975, Age trends in human chiasma frequencies and recombination fractions. I. Chiasma frequencies, *Am. J. Hum. Genet.* **27**:41–418.

Lange, K., Spence, M. A., and Frank, M. B., 1976, Application of the lod method to the detection of linkage between a quantitative trait and a qualitative marker: a simulation experiment, *Am. J. Hum. Genet.* **28**:167–173.

Lindstrom, J. S., Bias, W. B., Schimke, R. N., Ziegler, D. K., Rivas, M. L., Chase, G. A., and McKusick, V. A., 1973, Genetic linkage in Huntington's Chorea, *Adv. Neurol.* **1**:203–208.

Lowry, D. C., and Schultz, F. T., 1959, Testing association of metric traits and marker genes, *Ann. Hum. Genet.* **23**:83–90.

Luthardt, F. W., Palmer, C. G., and Yu, P. L., 1973, Chiasma and univalent frequencies in ageing mice, *Cytogenet. Cell Genet.* **12**:68–79.

Maynard-Smith, S., Penrose, L. S., and Smith, C. A. B., 1961, *Mathematical Tables for Research Workers in Human Genetics*, 74 pp., Churchill, London.

Mayo, O., 1970, The use of linkage in genetic counseling, *Hum. Hered.* **20**:474–485.

Mayo, O., 1974, Effect of age on chiasma number in man, *Hum. Hered.* **24**:144–150.

McGregor, A. G., 1953, Evaluation of linkage, In: Clinical Genetics (A. Sorsby, ed.), pp. 65–73, C. V. Mosby, St. Louis.

McKusick, V. A., 1971, The mapping of human chromosomes, Sci. Am. 224:104–113.

McKusick, V. A., 1979, The Linkage Newsletter (Oct.), Johns Hopkins Hospital, Baltimore.

McKusick, V. A., and Ruddle, F. H., 1977, The status of the gene map of the human chromosomes, Science 196:390–405.

Meyers, D. A., Conneally, P. M., Lovrien, E. W., Magenis, R. E., Merritt, A. D., Norton, J. A., Palmer, C. G., Rivas, M. L., Wang, L., and Yu, P. L., 1976, Linkage group I: The simultaneous estimation of recombination and interference, in: Baltimore Conference (1975): Third International Workshop on Human Gene Mapping. Birth Defects: Original Article Series Vol. 11, No. 3, pp. 335–339, The National Foundation, New York.

Meyers, D. A., Merritt, A. D., Conneally, P. M., Norton, J. A., Rivas, M. L., Yu, P. L., and Palmer, C. G., 1979, Linage group I—a statistically significant locus order from family studies, in: Winnipeg Conference (1977): Fourth International Workshop on Human Gene Mapping. Birth Defects: Original Article Series, Vol. 14, No. 4, pp. 396–400, The National Foundation, New York.

Morgan, T. H., 1911, Random segregation versus coupling in Mendelian inheritance, Science 34:384.

Morton, N. E., 1955, Sequential tests for the detection of linkage, Am. J. Hum. Genet. 7:277–318.

Morton, N. E., 1956, The detection and estimation of linkage between the genes for elliptocytosis and the Rh blood type, Am. J. Hum. Genet. 8:80–96.

Morton, N. E., 1957, Further scoring types in sequential linkage tests with a critical review of autosomal and partial sex-linkage in man, Am. J. Hum. Genet. 9:55–75.

Morton, N. E., 1979, Analysis of crossing over in man, in: Winnipeg Conference (1977): Fourth International Workshop on Human Gene Mapping. Birth Defects: Original Article Series, Vol. 14, No. 2, pp. 15–36, The National Foundation, New York.

Muller, H. J., 1916, The mechanism of crossing over, Am. Nat. 50:193–221.

Murphy, E. A., and Chase, G. A., 1975, Principles of Genetic Counseling, 391 pp., Year Book Medical Publishers, Chicago.

Ott, J., 1974, Estimation of the recombination fraction in human pedigrees: efficient computation of the likelihood for human linkage studies, Am. J. Hum. Genet. 26:588–597.

Ott, J., 1977, Linkage analysis with misclassification at one locus, Clin. Genet. 12:119–124.

Painter, T.S., 1933, A new method for the study of chromosome rearrangements and plotting of chromosome maps, Science 78:585–586.

Penrose, L. S., 1935, The detection of autosomal linkage in data which consists of pairs of brothers and sisters of unspecified parentage, Ann. Eugen. 6:133–138.

Pericak-Vance, M. A., Conneally, P. M., Merritt, A. D., Roos, R., Norton, Jr., J. A., and Vance, J. M., 1979, Genetic linkage studies in Huntington Disease, in: Winnipeg Conference (1977), Fourth International Workshop on Human Gene Mapping. Birth Defects: Original Article Series, Vol. 14, No. 2, pp. 640–645, The National Foundation, New York.

Pollack, M. S., Levine, L. S., Pang, S., Owens, R. P., Nitowsky, H. M., Maurer, D., New, M. I., Duchon, M., Merkatz, I. R., Sachs, G., and Dupont, B., 1979, Prenatal diagnosis of congenital adrenal hyperplasia (21-hydroxylase deficiency) by HLA typing, Lancet 1:1107–1108.

Race, R. R., and Sanger, R., 1975, Blood Groups in Man, 665 pp., Blackwell, Oxford.

Rao, D. C., Morton, N. E., Lindsten, J., Hulten, M., and Yee, S., 1977, A mapping function for man, Hum. Hered. 27:99–104.

Rao, D. C., Keats, B. J. B., Morton, N. E., Yee, S., and Lew, R., 1978, Variability of human linkage data, *Am. J. Hum. Genet.* **30**:516–529.

Rapley, S., Robson, E. B., Harris, H., and Smith, S M., 1968, Data on the incidence, segregation and linkage relationships of the adenylate kinase (AK) polymorphism, *Ann. Hum. Genet.* **31**:237–242.

Reid, D. H., and Parsons, P. A., 1963, Sex of parent and variation of recombination with age in the mouse, *Heredity* **18**:107–108.

Renwick, J. H., 1968, Ratios of female to male recombination fractions in man, *Bull. Eur. Soc. Hum. Genet.* **2**:7–14.

Renwick, J. H., 1969*a*, Progress in mapping human autosomes, *Br. Med. Bull.* **25**:65–73.

Renwick, J. H., 1969*b*, Genetic linkage in man, in: *Computer Applications in Genetics* (N. E. Morton, ed.), pp. 103–116, University of Hawaii Press, Honolulu.

Renwick, J. H., 1969*c*, Widening the scope of antenatal diagnosis, *Lancet* **2**:386.

Renwick, J. H., 1970, Eyes on chromosomes, *J. Med. Genet.* **7**:239–243.

Renwick, J. H., 1971, Assignment and map-positioning of human loci using chromosomal variation, *Ann. Hum. Genet.* **35**:79–97.

Renwick, J. H., and Bolling, D. R., 1967, A program-complex for encoding, analyzing and storing human linkage data, *Am. J. Hum. Genet.* **19**:360–367.

Renwick, J. H., and Bolling, D. R., 1971, An analysis procedure illustrated on a triple linkage of use for prenatal diagnosis of myotonic dystrophy, *J. Med. Genet.* **4**:399–406.

Renwick, J. H., and Lawler, S. D., 1963, Probable linkage between a congenital cataract locus and the Duffy blood group locus, *Ann. Hum. Genet.* **27**:67–84.

Renwick, J. H., and Schulze, J., 1961, A computer program for the processing of linkage data from large pedigrees, *Excerpta Med. Int. Congr. Ser.* **32**:E145.

Renwick, J. H., and Schulze, J., 1964, An analysis of some data on the linkage between Xg and color-blindness in man, *Am. J. Hum. Genet.* **16**:410–418.

Renwick, J. H., and Schulze, J., 1965, Male and female recombination fractions for the nail-patella:ABO linkage in man, *Ann. Hum. Genet.* **28**:379–392.

Rivas, M. L., and Conneally, P. M., 1977, Application and significance of linkage in diagnosis and prevention of disease, in: *Genetic Counseling* (H. A. Lubs and Felix de la Cruz, eds.), pp. 447–475, Raven Press, New York.

Rivas, M. L., Conneally, P. M., Hecht, F., Lovrien, E. W., Magenis, E., Merritt, A. D., Meyers, D. A., Palmer, C. G., and Wang, L., 1975, Linkage relationships of 1qh to Amy, PGM₁, and Rh, in: *Rotterdam Conference (1974): Second International Workshop on Human Gene Mapping, Birth Defects: Original Article Series*, Vol. **11**, No. 3:274, The National Foundation, New York.

Robinson, R., 1972, *Gene Mapping in Laboratory Mammals*, Part B, 327 pp., Plenum Press, New York.

Ruddle, F. H., 1977, New approaches to human gene mapping by means of somatic cell genetics, in: *Human Genetics* (S. Armendares and R. Lisker, eds.), pp. 269–283, Excerpta Medica, Amsterdam.

Schleutermann, D. A., Bias, W. A., Murdoch J. L., and McKusick, V. A., 1969, Linkage of the loci for the nail-patella syndrome and adenylate kinase, *Am. J. Hum. Genet.* **21**:606–630.

Schrott, H. G., Karp, L., and Omenn, G. S., 1973, Prenatal prediction in myotonic dystrophy: Guidelines for genetic counseling, *Clin. Genet.* **4**:38–45.

Simpson, H. R., 1958, The estimation of linkage on an electronic computer, *Ann. Hum. Genet.* **22**:356–361.

Smith, C. A. B., 1953, The detection of linkage in human genetics, *J. Roy. Stat. Soc.* **15B**:153–192.

Smith, C. A. B., 1954, The separation of the sexes of parents in the detection of linkage in man, *Ann. Eugen.* (*London*) **18**:278–301.

Smith, C. A. B., 1959, Some comments on the statistical methods used in linkage investigations, *Am. J. Hum. Genet.* **11**:289–304.

Smith, C. A. B., 1963, Testing for heterogeneity of recombination fraction values in human genetics, *Ann. Hum. Genet.* **27**:175–182.

Smith, C. A. B., 1975, A non-parametric test for linkage with a quantitative character, *Ann. Hum. Genet.* **8**:451–460.

Spence, M. A., Sparkes, R. S., Heckenlively, J. R., Pearlman, J. T., Zedalis, D., Sparkes, M., Grist, M., and Tideman, S., 1977, Probable genetic linkage between autosomal dominant retinitis pigmentosa (RP) and amylase (Amy$_2$): Evidence of an RP locus on chromosome 1, *Am. J. Hum. Genet.* **29**:397–404; erratum, 592.

Steinberg, A. G., and Morton, N. E., 1956, Sequential test for linkage between cystic fibrosis of the pancreas and the MNS locus, *Am. J. Hum. Genet.* **8**:177–189.

Sturt, E., 1975, The use of lod scores for the determination of the order of loci on a chromosome, *Ann. Hum. Genet.* **39**:255–260.

Sturt, E., 1976, A mapping function for human chromosomes, *Ann. Hum. Genet.* **40**:147–164.

Stern, C., 131, Zytologisch-genetische Untersuchungen als Beweise für die Morganische Theorie des Faktorenaustausches, *Biol. Zentr.* **51**:547–587.

Sturtevant, A. H., 1913, The linear arrangement of six sex-linked factors in *Drosophila* as shown by their mode of association, *J. Exp. Zool.* **14**:43–59.

Suarez, B. K., Rice, J., and Reich, T. 1978, The generalized sib pair IBD distribution: its use in the detection of linkage, *Ann. Hum. Genet.* **42**:87–94.

Sutton, W. S., 1902, On the morphology of the chromosome group in *Brachystola magna*, *Biol. Bull.* **4**:24–39.

Sutton, W. S., 1903, The chromosomes in heredity, *Biol. Bull.* **4**:231–251.

Wald, A., 1947, *Sequential Analysis*, 212 pp., Wiley, New York.

Weitkamp, L. R., 1973, Human autosomal linkage groups, in: *Proceedings: Fourth International Congress of Human Genetics* (*Paris*), pp. 445–460, Excerpta Medica, Amsterdam.

Weitkamp, L. R., VanRood, J. J., Thorsby, E., Bias, W., Fotino, M., Lawler, S. D., Dausset, J., Mayr, W. R., Bodmer, J., Ward, F. E., Seignalet, J., Payne, R., Kissmeyer-Nielsen, F., Gatti, R. A., Sachs, J. A., and Lamm, L. U., 1973, The relation of parental sex and age to recombination in the HLA system, *Hum. Hered.* **23**:197–205.

Wilson, A. F., Bailey, J. E., Conneally, P. M., Yu, P. L. and Gersting, J. M., 1977, Genetic simulation: The relative efficiency of genetic linkage analysis in disorders with late age of onset, *Am. J. Hum. Genet.* **29**:115A.

Wilson, A. F., Conneally, P. M., Yu, P. L., Norton, J. A., and Gersting, J. M., 1978, An empiric distribution of the maximum likelihood of θ using complete simulation techniques, *Am. J. Hum. Genet.* **30**:129A.

*Chapter 4*

# Sister Chromatid Exchanges

Samuel A. Latt, Rhona R. Schreck,
Kenneth S. Loveday, Charlotte P. Dougherty, and
Charles F. Shuler
*Division of Genetics and Mental Retardation Center*
*Children's Hospital Medical Center and the Department of Pediatrics*
*Harvard Medical School*
*Boston, Massachusetts*

## INTRODUCTION

Sister chromatid exchanges (SCEs) represent the interchange of DNA replication products at apparently homologous loci. These exchanges presumably involve DNA breakage and reunion, although little is known about the molecular basis of sister chromatid exchange formation, and information about the biological significance of exchanges is largely circumstantial. In spite of these uncertainties, analysis of sister chromatid exchange formation in cytological systems has already provided information about chromosome structure and has been used to detect the effects of clastogens and to differentiate between chromosome fragility diseases.

Detection of SCEs in nonring chromosomes requires some means of differentially labeling sister chromatids. This was initially accomplished using tritiated thymidine, although most recent studies employ halogenated nucleosides. Sister chromatid exchanges were first described by J. Herbert Taylor and associates, who utilized autoradiography to detect differentially labeled sister chromatids in cells which had undergone one cycle of [³H]-dT incorporation followed by a replication cycle in nonradioactive medium.[301] Reciprocal alterations in labelling (SCEs) were detected along the chromatids of a number of metaphase chromosomes. In spite of its practical limitations, autoradiography permitted Taylor to characterize many basic features of SCEs, in which chromatid interchange followed constraints expected for individual DNA duplexes.[299] These results have been confirmed by more recent studies at higher resolution.

## BrdUrd METHODOLOGY FOR SCE DETECTION

The halogenated nucleosides BrdUrd and IdUrd have largely supplanted [³H]-dT for the purpose of differentially labeling sister chromatids. Initial observations of the effect of BrdUrd on differential chromosome staining (typically using Giemsa mixtures) were incidental to investigation of the effects of this nucleoside on chromosome integrity or condensation. For example, during the course of studies directed at evaluating the ability of agents, including BrdUrd, to affect rat chromosomes, Huang[117] noticed that metaphase chromosomes from cells harvested 2 cycles after initial BrdUrd exposure occasionally showed one dark and one light Giemsa-stained sister chromatid. Some causative role for BrdUrd was speculated, but this unexpected result was not pursued further. More recently, Huang's laboratory has utilized related BrdUrd–dye techniques to study SCE induction.[80,118,277]

Palmer[223] and Zakharov and Egolina[334] observed that exposure of cells to high concentrations of BrdUrd during the terminal segment of the DNA synthesis phase led to decondensation of late replicating chromosomal regions. Also, Zakharov and Egolina[335] showed that pulses of BrdUrd at the *end* of S of *two* successive cycles provided differential Giemsa staining of sister chromatids in late replicating regions. In contrast, exposure of cells to BrdUrd for an *entire* S phase had little effect on chromosome morphology.

In an attempt to find a fluorescent alternative to autoradiography for detecting DNA synthesis, our laboratory examined the ability of BrdUrd, in DNA or chromatin, to quench the fluorescence of DNA binding dyes.[169] The bisbenzimidazole dye, 33258 Hoechst, exhibits the greatest quenching,[169,172] while lesser reductions of fluorescence occurred with acridine orange and proflavine,[172] and at most very small effects on ethidium or quinacrine fluorescence were observed. Systematic analysis showed that quenching of 33258 Hoechst fluorescence reflected a reduction of dye fluorescence quantum yield, while dye binding affinity actually increased.[177] Consistent with the hypothesis prompting these studies, i.e., that BrdUrd might quench dye fluorescence by a heavy atom effect,[169] BrdUrd substitution into DNA leads to a reduction in the fluorescence lifetime of bound 33258 Hoechst.[173] Similarly, polymers containing IdUrd, instead of BrdUrd also quench 33258 Hoechst fluorescence.[172.173] Model system results on 33258 Hoechst fluorescence, as well as of yet unexplained abolition of BrdUrd-dependent quenching at pH 4,[172.177] were all applicable to the staining properties of cytological preparations, and 33258 Hoechst and structurally related derivatives[176] have proved useful for studying DNA synthesis both in fixed chromosome preparations and in unfixed cells.[16.176.178]

In addition to 33258 Hoechst, the dyes acridine orange[67.133] and 4',6-diamidinophenylindole (DAPI)[193.194] have been employed for fluorescent detection of BrdUrd incorporation and hence DNA synthesis. With acridine orange contrast due to dye fluorescence quantum yield reduction is enhanced by prolonged sample illumination. The mechanism of this "burning in" is unknown, but may involve BrdUrd-sensitized dye or DNA photodestruction. Evidence for a direct effect of BrdUrd on acridine orange fluorescence, in cytological systems, expected also because of its effect on dye phosphorescence,[81] can be found in recent flow cytometric studies using acridine orange to detect BrdUrd incorporation into proliferating lymphocytes.[58] DAPI fluorescence is insensitive to BrdUrd at neutral pH but is quenched by BrdUrd under highly alkaline conditions, e.g., pH 11.[194] Both with soluble dye–DNA complexes and in cytological preparations, DAPI–BrdUrd fluorescence effects mimic those of 33258 Hoechst but shifted several, i.e., 3–4, units to higher pH. One other fluorescent method for detecting BrdUrd, based on increased chromomycinone fluorescence (an effect presumably due to enhanced dye binding),[291.292] has not yet been found sensitive enough to provide sister chromatid differentiation necessary for SCE detection. Also, immunofluorescent techniques for detecting BrdUrd incorporation have found limited use for SCE detection.[99]

While useful for flow cytometric studies,[16,178] fluorescent methods for SCE detection do not provide permanent preparations, and rapid fading of stained specimens makes even initial photomicroscopy difficult. Giemsa methods, typically utilizing a BrdUrd-sensitive prestain for photosensitization, have thus largely replaced fluorescent techniques for routine SCE analysis (Fig. 1, 2). Soon after publication of fluorescent meth-

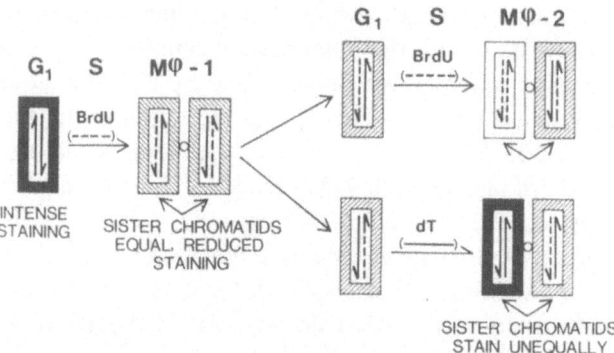

Fig. 1. Sister chromatid differentiation by BrdUrd–dye techniques. Cells are allowed to incorporate BrdUrd (- - -) for one cycle, followed by a second cycle of replication in which the presence of BrdUrd is optional. Sister chromatids in metaphase chromosomes from such second-division cells will exhibit unequal fluorescence, if stained, e.g., with 33258 Hoechst, or unequal intensity following Giemsa staining, reflecting different numbers of BrdUrd-substituted polynucleotide chains. Solid, hatched, and open areas surrounding each rectangle represent intense, intermediate, and pale staining, respectively.

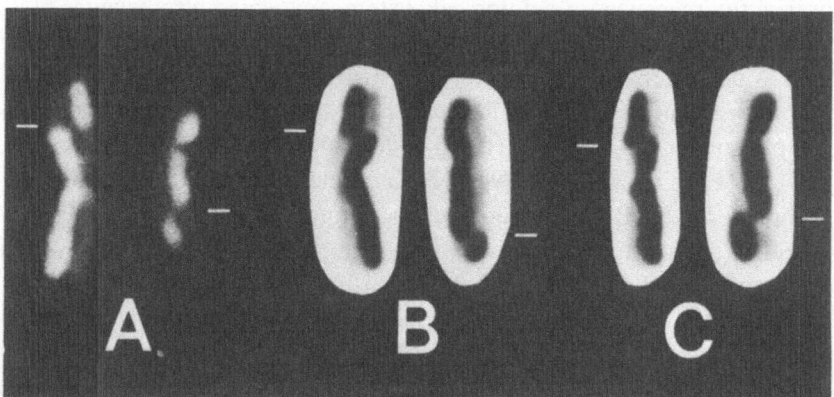

Fig. 2. Sister chromatid exchanges. The chromosomes in this figure are from human lymphocytes which replicated twice in medium containing $10^{-5}$ M BrdUrd, $6 \times 10^{-6}$ M U, and $4 \times 10^{-7}$ M FdUrd. Those in (A) were stained with 33258 Hoechst and photographed under conditions described for fluorescence microscopy. Chromosomes in (B) were previously photographed to record fluorescence, as in (A), and then washed with $H_2O$, incubated 15 min at 60–65° C in 2 × SSC, and stained with Giemsa. Chromosomes in (C) were exposed to fluorescent light while mounted in buffer containing $10^{-4}$ M 33258 Hoechst as described in Table 1, incubated in 2 × SSC and stained with Giemsa. Chromosomes shown were chosen to demonstrate relatively unambiguous sister chromatid exchanges (indicated by short, horizontal lines).[179]

odology for SCE detection, Ikushima and Wolff[124] described sister chromatid differentiation in Giemsa-stained preparations of Chinese hamster chromosomes from cells that had undergone two *complete* rounds of BrdUrd and IdUrd incorporation and were then exposed to preharvest pulses of light. However, the staining contrast achieved was minimal. Intense illumination of 33258 Hoechst-stained and BrdUrd-substituted slides during photomicroscopy[148] or extended moderate illumination with ambient light, followed by incubation in warm buffer,[234] greatly improved sister chromatid differentiation with Giemsa. This latter approach, with various modifications, has become the simplest and most popular method for SCE analysis. While the mechanism of this technique is still the subject of some debate,[321] Feulgen measurements of residual DNA content,[97,98] observations of electron dense material remaining after chromosome treatment,[44] and radioisotope measurements of DNA elution[183] indicate that nonfluorescent or poorly fluorescent dyes sensitize BrdUrd-substituted DNA to breakage, most likely creating single strand nicks, while warm saline incubation serves to elute the resultant small DNA fragments from the slides (Figs. 3, 4), rendering that chromatid less susceptible to Giemsa stain.

A variety of other modified Giemsa methods for SCE detection have also evolved. One, developed by Korenberg and Freedlender,[155] does not

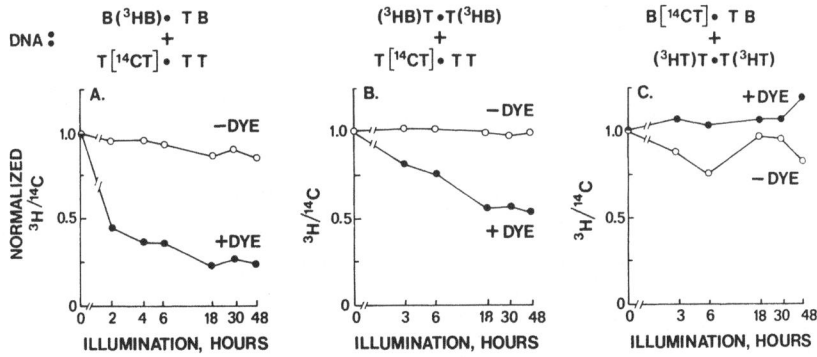

Fig. 3. DNA elution during a BrdUrd–dye–Giemsa procedure. Synchronized CHO cells were cultured to produce DNA substituted as shown at the top of each frame. Mixtures of colcemid-treated cells (average mitotic index approximately 40%) were applied to coverslips, mounted at pH 7 with or without prior staining with 33258 Hoechst, exposed 6 cm below a 20 watt cool white lamp, for time periods indicated in the graphs and subsequently incubated 15 min in 2 × SSC at 65°C. Relative elution of DNA species was estimated from the residual $^3$H/$^{14}$C ratio.[183]

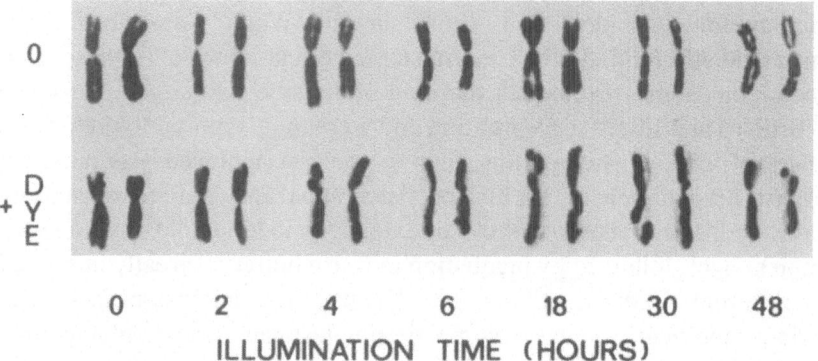

ILLUMINATION  TIME  (HOURS)

Fig. 4. Induction of sister chromatid differentiation in CHO chromosomes. The chromosomes shown are from synchronized CHO cells, that were allowed to incorporate [³H]-BrdUrd for one cycle followed by a cycle of nonradioactive BrdUrd. Slide treatment, including light exposure, was as described in the caption to Fig. 3, with or without 33258 Hoechst staining prior to light exposure. Photosensitization by 33258 Hoechst enhanced subsequent differential staining with Giemsa, and this increased with illumination time, up to 4–6 hr.

employ a dye for photosensitization, but utilizes incubation in 1 M pH 8.0 phosphate buffer at 88°C prior to Giemsa staining. This latter treatment should serve to elute even rather large fragments, which might be created in BrdUr-substituted DNA, e.g., by incidental light; evidence supporting this latter explanation has recently been published.[98] Other methods, employing acid pretreatment[296] or incubation in low pH buffers,[43,252,256] can produce a reverse staining pattern, in which BrdUrd-substitution correlates with *more* intense Giemsa staining. The mechanism of this latter effect, which can be reversed by exposure of slides to high pH (producing reduced staining in BrdUrd-substituted chromatids[43,256]), remains unknown. Data indicating that standard Giemsa sister chromatid differentiation (presumably due to breakage and elution of BrdUrd-substituted fragments) can be converted to an equally intense reverse staining pattern have not as yet been published.

BrdUrd-dependent sister chromatid differentiation can be achieved in most chromosomal regions by two related protocols. Both require one cycle of BrdUrd incorporation into chromosomal DNA; they differ in that only one involves the presence of BrdUrd during the second cycle (Fig. 1). (IdUrd can also produce sister chromatid differentiation, but it is more toxic to cells than is BrdUrd[63] and is thus seldom used.) *In vitro* studies typically employ two cycles of BrdUrd incorporation, primarily to avoid the difficulty of changing cell culture medium to remove the BrdUrd, at the appropriate time (between the first and second DNA synthesis periods). In contrast, *in vivo* studies usually involve BrdUrd incorporation for the first cycle only. BrdUrd is rapidly degraded in intact animals, and levels of BrdUrd drop rapidly as soon as external sources of BrdUrd are removed. A second cycle of BrdUrd incorporation has only a small effect on the baseline level of SCEs.[208] *In vitro* cultures must be protected from light (e.g., ≤ 313 nm) that can degrade BrdUrd-substituted DNA; such precautions do not appear to be necessary for most *in vivo* studies. For both protocols, cells are trapped at metaphase of the second cycle following initial exposure to BrdUrd, and cytological chromosome preparations are then made by standard techniques.

Exceptions to this discussion are chromosomal regions containing DNA with a markedly unequal distribution of thymine on complementary polynucleotide strands. In these regions, such as mouse centromeric heterochromatin,[195] the distal part of the long arm of the human Y,[182] the secondary constriction regions of human 1 and 16,[14,15,84] and in certain segments of human 6,[68] sister chromatid differentiation can be achieved after one cycle of BrdUrd incorporation. SCEs have been detected in first division metaphases in both mouse centromeric heterochromatic[193] and in the human Y.[94] After a second replication, SCEs formed during the first cycle appear as isolabeling, while second cycle SCEs appear as reciprocal interchanges.[94] This latter situation is analogous to patterns observed in most chromosomal regions after three, rather than two cycles of BrdUrd incorporation.[305]

Staining protocols used for BrdUrd detection have been described in detail and reviewed elsewhere.[169,172,179] The basic steps required in one fluorescent protocol, as well as in related Giemsa methods, are summarized in Table I. BrdUrd administration protocols can achieve greater than 80% substitution of BrdUrd for dT in one or both DNA strands.[11,178] BrdUrd detection under these circumstances presents little problem. The lower limit of BrdUrd incorporation which permits sister chromatid differentiation has not yet been determined.

Sister chromatid exchanges, which appear as reciprocal interchanges along differentially stained chromosomes, are easily scored on photographic prints obtained using any of the above methods (Fig. 2). Giemsa staining, which has the advantage of producing permanent chromosome preparations, allowing repeated examination by several observers, permits direct SCE scoring on microscope slides, and Giemsa stained slides lend themselves to automated analysis. Detection of an SCE, with es-

TABLE I. Staining Protocols for Detecting BrdUrd Incorporation into Metaphase
Chromosomes

*Fluorescence (33258 Hoechst)*[169,179]

1. Stain slides with 0.5 μg/ml dye in pH-7 phosphate buffer; mount at pH 7–7.5.
2. Excite fluorescence with near ultraviolet light, e.g., predominantly 365-nm Hg line, 400-nm dichroic mirror.
3. Observe fluorescence at or above 460 nm.
4. After fluorescence microscopy, slides can usually be incubated in 65°, 2× SSC buffer and overstained with Giemsa to obtain a permanent preparation reflecting sister chromatid differentiation.

*Fluorescence plus Giemsa*[179,234]

1. Stain slides with 33258 Hoechst or mount slides directly in excess dye (e.g., 50 μg/ml) in pH-7 phosphate buffer. Dilute dye into buffer from concentrated stock solution of dye in $H_2O$.
2. Expose slides, mounted in buffered dye solution, to light with appreciable intensity ≤ 400 nm, i.e., in a region absorbed by the dye. Exposure time is adjustable, typically a few hours if a standard 20 watt cool white fluorescent light is used.
3. Incubate slides 15–30 minutes in 65° 2× SSC buffer, rinse with $H_2O$.
4. Stain with Giemsa (e.g., 4% in 5 mM pH-6.8 phosphate buffer).

sentially redundant reciprocal information signaling exchange on sister chromatids, is probably simpler than automated recognition of banded chromosomes. Automated detection of SCEs can now be done at nearly the speed of manual studies, albeit with somewhat lower accuracy,[333] though this work is still at a fairly early stage. Some form of automation in SCE scoring may ultimately prove necessary, e.g., to screen hundreds of compounds or large numbers of individuals potentially exposed to clastogenic compounds.

# BASIC INFORMATION ABOUT SCEs

Newer techniques for sister chromatid differentiation have confirmed most of the conclusions about the overall features of SCE drawn from previous autoradiographic studies. For example, studies in third division cells,[305] and in cells with diplochromosomes,[323] indicated that sister chromatid exchange is constrained by the polarity of the DNA helix. Third division cell analysis showed that segregation at mitosis of sister chromatids into pairs of homologues in human lymphocytes is random (Figs. 5, 6);[55,187] and without marked bias in mouse spermatogonia (Fig. 7). How-

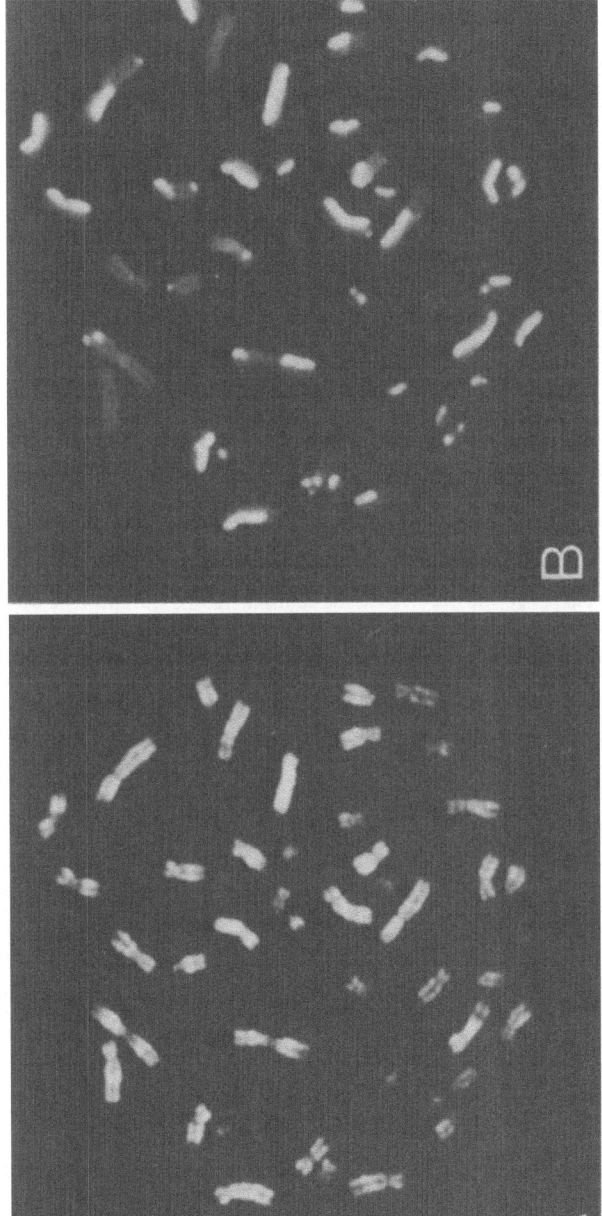

Fig. 5. Fluorescence of human metaphase chromosomes after three cycles of BrdUrd incorporation. Peripheral lymphocytes from a normal human female were cultured 3 days in medium containing $9 \times 10^{-5}$ M BrdUrd. $4 \times 10^{-7}$ M FdUrd. $6 \times 10^{-6}$ M U. Chromosomes from the cell shown were first stained with quinacrine. (A) photographed, destained in 3:1 methanol–acetic acid, stained with 33258 Hoechst, and (B) rephotographed.[187]

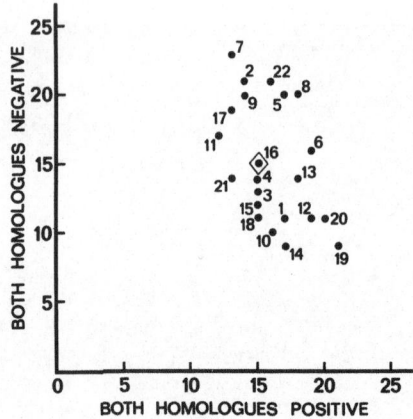

Fig. 6. Segregation of sister chromatids of homologous chromosomes during the third cycle of BrdUrd incorporation. Peripheral lymphocytes from normal humans were cultured 3 days in medium containing $1-9 \times 10^{-5}$ M BrdUrd, $4 \times 10^{-7}$ M FdUrd, $6 \times 10^{-6}$ M U, harvested, and stained sequentially with quinacrine and 33258 Hoechst as described in the legend to Fig. 5. A total of 60 cells which had replicated three times in this medium were scored. After this time, approximately one-fourth of the chromatids contain an unsubstituted polynucleotide chain and fluoresce very brightly. A chromosome was scored as positive if the centromere of one chromatid fluoresced brightly. Otherwise, it was scored as negative. If a sister chromatid exchange had occurred at the centromere, the chromosome was scored as positive if there was bright fluorescence in the long arm adjacent to the centromere. The results are shown for each pair of autosomes. If segregation of bright chromatids is random, there should be an average of 15 cells with both homologues positive, 15 cells with both homologues negative, and 30 cells with one of each. The results scatter around this average. Random segregation would result in this great a deviation from the expected average (evaluated by a $\chi^2$ test) 25% of the time.[187]

ever, other studies[238] suggest that segregation in certain specialized germ cells may be non-random. Analysis of endoreduplicated chromosomes indicates that apposition of newly synthesized polynucleotide chains is external to old chains with respect to centromeres (Fig. 8).[109,172,268,317,323] One study of SCE formation in ring chromosomes was interpreted as consistent with an occasional switch in DNA polarity along a chromosome,[327] but this conclusion has not yet been verified by an independent method, and it would be extraordinarily difficult to test by a direct chemical procedure.

The position of SCEs detected by fluorescence or Giemsa can be reasonably well localized relative to chromosome banding patterns. In human chromosomes, SCEs occur preferentially in Q-negative bands or at the junctions of Q-positive and Q-negative regions (Fig. 9).[57,170,210] Also,

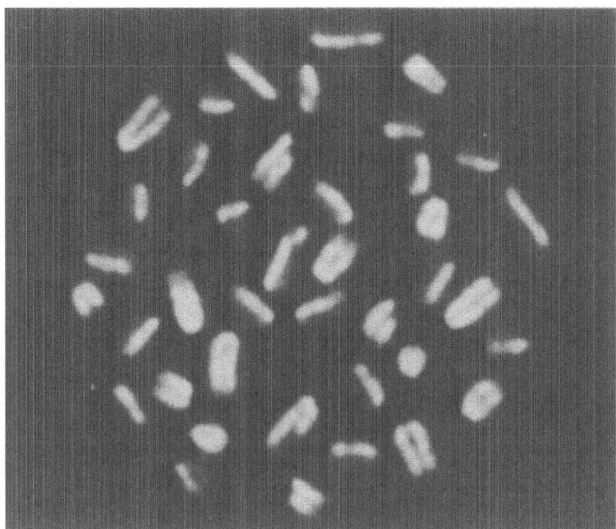

Fig. 7. Mouse spermatogonial cells at the third metaphase. This cell was harvested 72 hr subsequent to *in vivo* administration of BrdUrd. Third division cells stained with 33258 Hoechst reveal two types of chromosomes, those with sister chromatid differentiation and those with bright fluorescence in both chromatids.[8]

SCEs are very rare in homogeneously staining regions of human neuroblastoma cells.[20] Similar studies detected a clustering of SCE at junctions between heterochromatic and euchromatic regions in muntjac,[48] kangaroo rat,[36] microtus, and hamster chromosomes.[116] The significance of these "junctional" regions is as yet unknown. Although Dolfini[64] failed to observe SCE formation in heterochromatin of cultured drosophila lines, Gatti *et al.*[87] found a preponderance of SCEs in *Drosophila* cells (virtually all BrdUrd induced) at heterochromatin–euchromatin junctions but also found them to occur within heterochromatin. Lin and Alfi[193] observed, in one mouse marker chromosome, that both BrdUrd-induced and mitomycin C + BrdUrd-induced SCEs were *more* frequent in centric heterochromatin than in the chromosome arms. Similarly, Shubert *et al.*[265] found SCE hotspots near (though not necessarily within) heterochromatin in chromosomes from *Vicia* treated with alkylating agents, while Vosa[315] described the approximate location of SCEs in *Vicia* to be sparse in the vicinity of at least certain heterochromatic regions. Reexamination of the position of SCEs in highly extended chromosomes, prepared, e.g., as

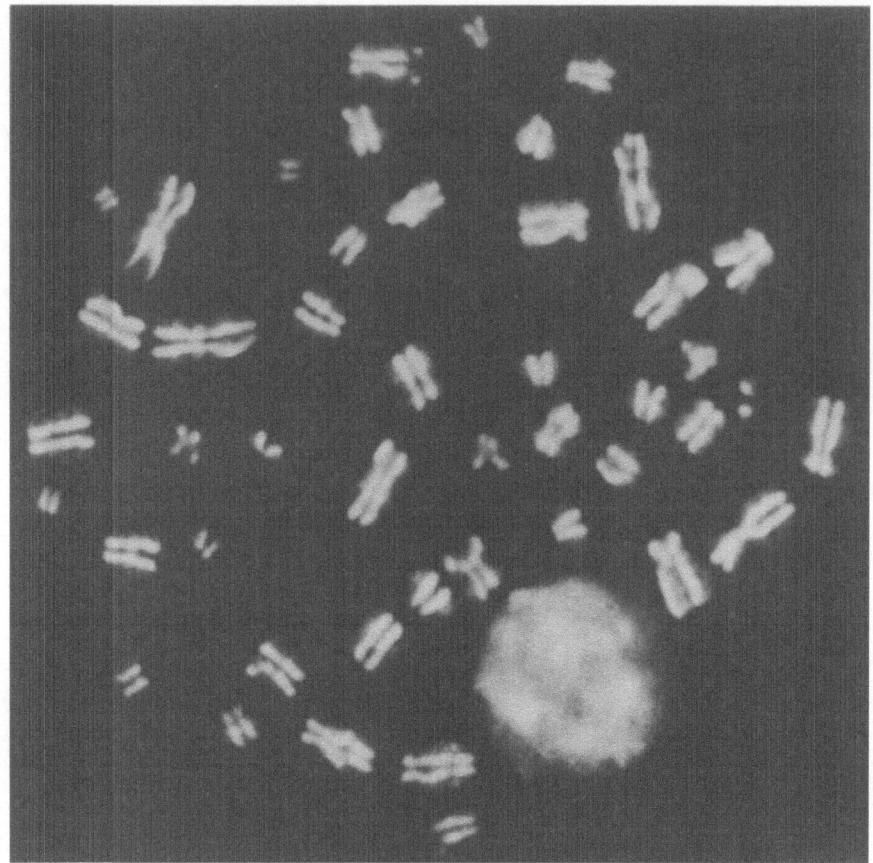

Fig. 8. 33258 Hoechst fluorescence of endoreduplication. The metaphase chromosomes shown are from a human lymphocyte which exhibited endoreduplication after 96 hr of growth in medium containing BrdUrd.[172]

described by Yunis,[331,332] or by premature chromosome condensation[189] should help elucidate systematic characteristics of SCE localization. It might prove especially interesting if the sites of SCE formation were somehow related to the DNA thought to be associated with the chromosome scaffolding structure,[4] since Razin *et al.*[241] have shown that this DNA contains moderately repetitious sequences which produce characteristic fragments following digestion with certain restriction endonucleases.

The greater effective resolution of BrdUrd dye techniques has facilitated the detection of multiple, closely spaced SCEs.[136,171,323] This ca-

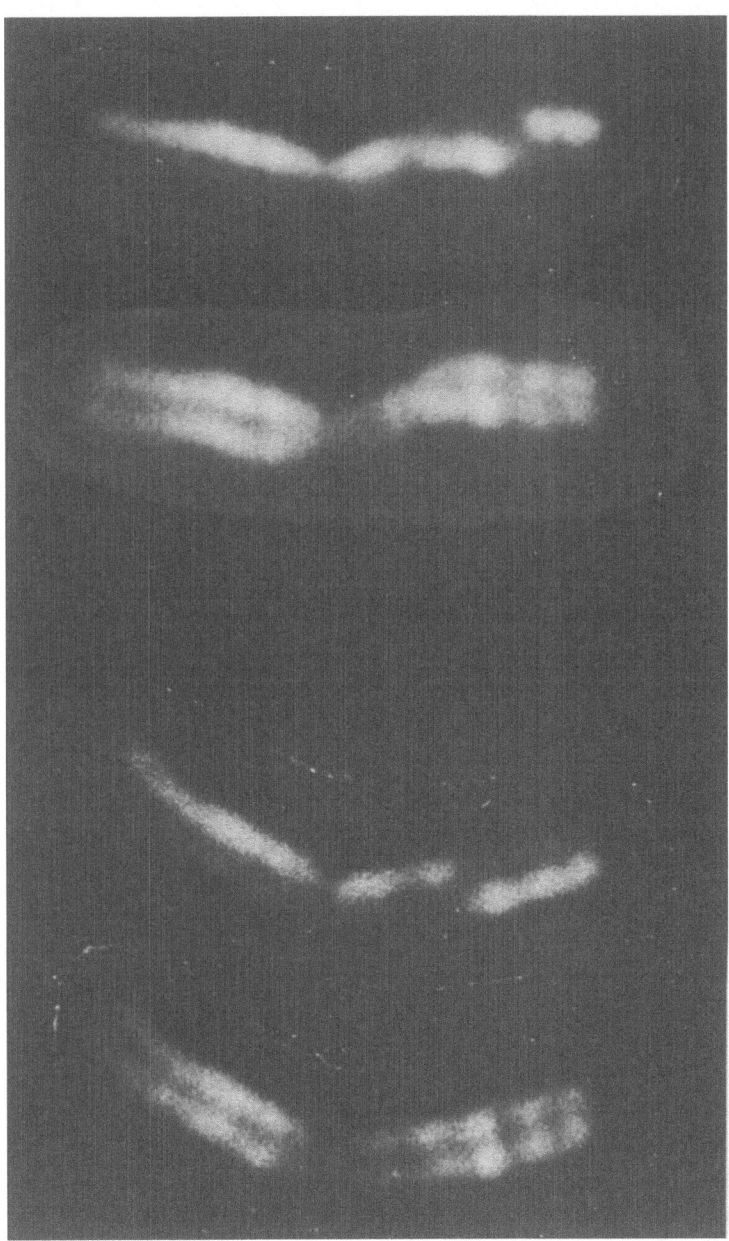

Fig. 9. Sister chromatid exchanges in human chromosome 1. Chromosomes were prepared from peripheral leukocytes obtained from normal human subjects and grown 70 to 72 hr in medium containing 0.01 or 0.02 mM BrdUrd. Chromosomes were stained with quinacrine (left-hand member of each pair), destained, and restained with 33258 Hoechst (right-hand member of each pair).[170] Sister chromatid exchanges are evident as abrupt reciprocal alternations in 33258 Hoechst fluorescence along chromatids.

pability has increased the accuracy and simplicity with which SCE induction by many clastogenic agents can be quantitated.[132,171,232] BrdUrd itself, like [3H]-dT,[39,95,202] induces SCEs,[87,133,164,171,206,322] and may be responsible for most of the baseline SCEs observed in the absence of additional clastogens. However, increments in SCEs can easily be scored, and the extent of SCE induction (at least by mitomycin C) does not seem to be very sensitive to BrdUrd levels to which cells are exposed.[126]

# INDUCTION OF SISTER CHROMATID EXCHANGE BY CLASTOGENS

Thus far, the most extensive use of SCE analysis has been to assess the impact of clastogens on chromosomes. Kato[132,134] had originally employed autoradiography to demonstrate SCE induction by alkylating agents and proflavine. However, quantitation of high SCE frequencies was difficult with this method. BrdUrd–dye methodology was used to show that low doses of alkylating agents such as mitomycin C (Fig. 10) or nitrogen mustard induced large numbers of SCEs at concentrations well below those causing significant numbers of chromosome breaks.[171] Numerous subsequent reports confirmed these observations and extended them to include other agents known to damage chromosomes either directly or after metabolic activation.

Dozens of mono- and bifunctional alkylating agents have been shown to induce SCEs (summarized in Table II, described in more detail elsewhere.[184,185,231,321] Since many of the agents initially used to induce SCEs are also well known mutagens and/or carcinogens, it was suggested that SCE analysis could be used as an assay for mutagens and carcinogens.[232] Comparison of SCE induction results with mutagenesis, carcinogenesis, and unscheduled DNA synthesis data[125,199,204] generally support this contention. SCE studies are still in a relatively early stage, and there are a number of agents for which information on SCE induction is conflicting, or for which induction is at most minimal (Table III), although these drugs are positive in other systems; additional tests on these compounds will be necessary. Importantly, a number of agents, which are known to cause genetic damage but which are relatively ineffective at inducing SCEs (X-irradiation, monomeric acrylamide, bleomycin) are able to induce chromosome breaks and/or rearrangements. The combination of SCEs *and*

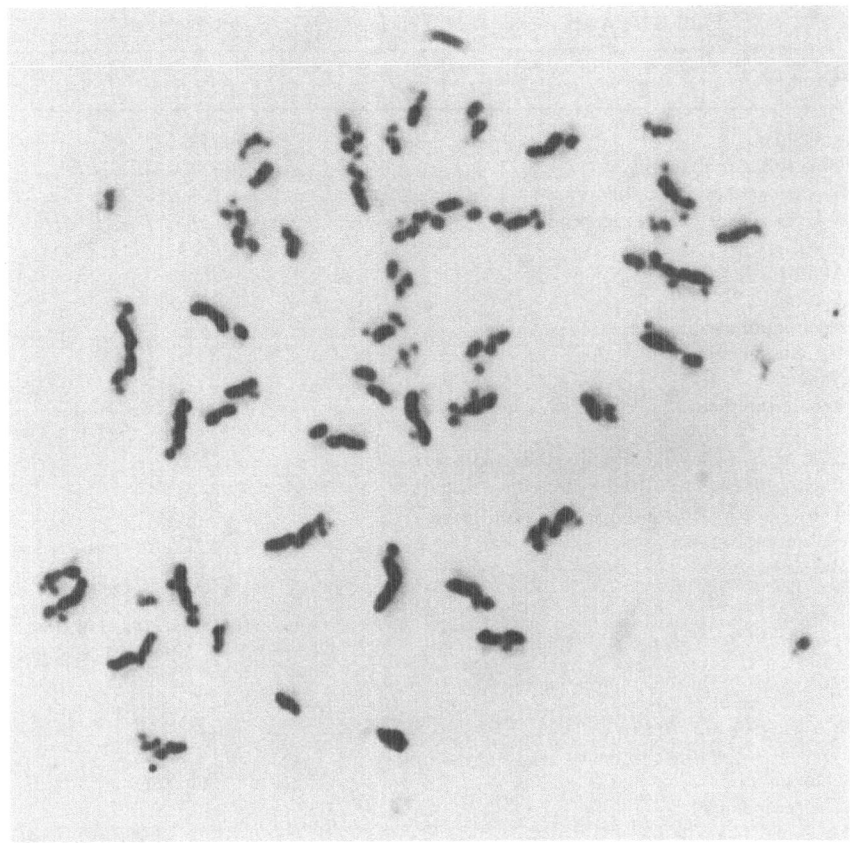

Fig. 10. Induction of sister chromatid exchanges in a human peripheral lymphocyte by mitomycin C. Mitomycin C (0.075 μg/ml) was present during the third and final day of cell culture. Slides of metaphase chromosomes were stained with 33258 Hoechst, exposed to light and 2 × SSC, and then stained with Giemsa. More than 50 SCEs can be detected in this cell; untreated cells exhibit approximately 15 SCEs.

chromosome aberrations thus appears to give very few "false negatives" when examining mutagen–carcinogens. Diethylstilbestrol is an example of a compound listed as negative in SCE induction in one system[2] but positive in another,[248a] and its action appears to be active as a mutagen[125] or inducer of unscheduled DNA synthesis[204]; it may require systems (e.g., hormone receptors, activating enzymes) which are inoperative in some cultured cells.

In a recent tabulation,[185] presumptive "false positives" were noted

TABLE II.  Agents Capable of Inducing SCEs (Strongly Positive)[a]

| Agent | Reference |
|---|---|
| Acetaldehyde | 219, 245 |
| N-Acetylaminofluorene | 237, 264, 297, 298 |
| N-Acetoxyacetylaminofluorene | 237, 260, 297 |
| N-Hydroxyacetylaminofluorene | 237, 297 |
| Adriamycin | 82, 157, 213, 232 |
| Aflatoxin B₁ | 297 |
| Alkeran | 239 |
| Aminofluorene | 239 |
| 4-Aminoquinoline-1-oxide | 3 |
| Aniline | 2 |
| Benzo(α)pyrene | 3, 26, 56, 221, 237, 248, 262, 277, 297 |
| *trans*-4,5-Dihydro-4,5-dihydroxybenz(α)pyrene | 221 |
| *trans*-9,10-Dihydro-9,10-dihydroxybenz(α)pyrene | 221 |
| *trans*-7,8-Dihydro-7,8-dihydroxybenz(α)pyrene | 221 |
| Betapropiolactone | 2, 232 |
| Busulfan | 239 |
| BrdUrd + light | 124, 135, 145, 316 |
| BrdUrd | 33, 66, 142, 150, 164, 169, 174, 208, 266, 283 |
| N-*n*-Butylurea | 3 |
| N-*n*-Butyl-N-nitrosourea | 3 |
| N-*n*-Butyl-N-nitrosourethane | 2 |
| Chlorambucil | 239, 279 |
| Chlorpropamide | 41 |
| Cyclophosphamide | 8, 9, 11, 24, 31, 59, 80, 118, 157, 232, 244, 264, 275, 276, 277, 285, 286, 304, 313 |
| N-Dibutylamine | 3 |
| Dibutylnitrosamine | 3 |
| Dibutylphthalate | 2 |
| Diethylnitrosamine | 24, 56, 212, 244, 277 |
| Diepoxybutane | 232 |
| Dimethylamine | 3 |
| 7,12-Dimethylbenzanthracene | 3, 26, 86, 275, 276, 277 |
| Dimethylnitrosamine | 3, 24, 25, 56, 212, 277, 304 |
| Dimethylphenyltriazine | 24 |
| Diphenyl | 2 |
| Ethylmethane sulfonate | 31, 46, 56, 82, 131, 136, 147, 186, 232, 260, 286 |

*(Continued)*

TABLE II. (*Continued*)

| Agent | Reference |
|---|---|
| Ethylnitrosourea | 46 |
| 33258 Hoechst | 232, 283 |
| 8-Methoxypsoralen + near UV light | 49, 88, 175, 211, 316 |
| 4,5,8-Trimethylpsoralen + near UV light | 88, 174 |
| Methylazoxymethanol acetate | 2, 70 |
| 7-Methylbenz($\alpha$)anthracene | 221 |
| *trans*-5,6-Dihydro-5,6-dihydroxy-7-methylbenz($\alpha$)anthracene | 221 |
| *trans*-1,2-Dihydro-1,2-dihydroxy-7-methylbenz($\alpha$)anthracene | 221 |
| *trans*-8,9-Dihydro-8,9-dihydroxy-7-methylbenz($\alpha$)anthracene | 221 |
| *trans*-3,4-Dihydro-3,4-dihydroxy-7-methylbenz($\alpha$)anthracene | 221 |
| 4-Methyl-*N'*-nitro-*N*-nitrosoguanidine | 24, 147, 232, 237 |
| Methylnitrosourea | 2 |
| 3-Methylcholanthrene | 3, 56, 237 |
| Methylmethane sulfonate | 31, 56, 147, 203, 232, 244, 286 |
| Mitomycin C | 7, 31, 45, 46, 82, 121, 126, 131, 134, 141, 147, 157, 164, 171, 186, 232, 239, 260 |
| Nitrogen mustard | 171, 232 |
| 2-Nitro-*O*-phenylenediamine | 233 |
| 4-Nitro-*O*-phenylenediamine | 233 |
| 4-Nitroquinoline-1-oxide | 3, 134, 232, 237 |
| *N*-Nitrosodiphenylamine | 2 |
| Procarbazine | 25, 244 |
| Proflavine | 46, 134, 237 |
| Propane sulfone | 2 |
| 1-(Pyridyl)-3,3-dimethyltriazine | 277 |
| Quinacrine mustard | 147, 232, 279 |
| Saccharin | 2, 324 |
| Sodium nitrite | 3 |
| Styrene | 60 |
| Styrene oxide | 60 |
| Thiotepa | 145 |
| Triaziquone | 24, 27, 89, 106, 314, 316 |
| Tris-(2,3-dibromopropyl)phosphate | 80 |
| Tritiated deoxythymidine | 95 |
| UV light (254 nm) | 132, 314, 326 |
| X-ray | 5, 82, 232, 279 |
| Virus (SV-40) | 214 |

*a* Details regarding conditions used for chemicals in Tables II–IV are given in reviews [184,185] dealing more specifically with testing details.

TABLE III. Agents Exhibiting Inconsistent or at Most Weak SCE Induction Behavior

| Agent | Reference |
|---|---|
| Acridine orange | 237 |
| Acrylamide | 270 |
| Anthracene | 3, 277 |
| Arsenic | 42 |
| Bleomycin | 89, 147, 232 |
| Butylbutanolamine | 3 |
| Butylhydroxyanisole | 2 |
| Caffeine | 23, 72, 127, 145, 147, 254, 314, 316 |
| Cytosine arabinoside | 239 |
| Deoxycytidine | 82, 186 |
| Deoxythymidine | 311 |
| Di-(2-ethylhexyl)-phthalate | 2 |
| Fluorescent brightner 24 (Kayaphor SN) | 2 |
| Fluorescent brightener 225 (Kayaphor LSK) | 2 |
| Maleic hydrazide | 147, 232, 285 |
| 2-Methyl-4-dimethylaminoazobenzene | 2 |
| Phenanthrene | 2, 26, 237 |
| Potassium metabisulfite | 2 |
| Potassium sorbate | 2 |
| Pyrene | 237, 277 |
| Pyridine | 2 |
| Sodium benzoate | 2 |
| Sunset yellow FCF (food yellow #5) | 2 |
| 4-*O*-Tolylazo-*O*-toluidine | 2 |
| Vincristine | 239, 289 |
| Virus (Vaccinia) | 153 |

in only two out of nearly fifty compounds (positive for SCE but negative in some other system). These two compounds, aniline and diphenyl, show no chromosome breakage or bacterial mutagenesis,[125,199] and neither of these compounds is an especially potent SCE inducer. Moreover, there does not yet appear to be any convincing example of an agent which is highly effective at inducing SCEs that is not also mutagenic or carcinogenic in at least some other system. Of equal importance, a large number of agents that are not thought to be mutagenic or carcinogenic appear incapable of inducing SCEs (Table IV).

A number of viruses have been observed to induce SCEs, although the extent of this induction is quite varied. For example, prior transfor-

TABLE IV. Agents Found Not to Induce SCEs[a]

| Agent | Reference |
|---|---|
| Acetone | 3, 31, 32 |
| Alcohols: | |
| Butanol | 31, 32, 219 |
| Ethanol | 3, 31, 32, 219 |
| Methanol | 219 |
| Propanol | 219 |
| Aminopyridine[b] | 2 |
| Arochlor 1254[c] | 277 |
| Bilirubin | 267 |
| N-n-Butylurethane | 2 |
| Dibutylhydroxytoluene | 2 |
| ε-Caprolactone | 2 |
| Cycloheximide | 254 |
| Dimethylsulfoxide | 24, 267, 277 |
| 8-Ethoxycaffeine | 143 |
| Ethylene glycol (50%) | 31, 32 |
| Fluorescent brightener (#260) | 2 |
| Fluorescent light[d] | 267 |
| Hydroxyurea | 237 |
| Lead acetate | 27 |
| 8-Methoxypsoralen | 49, 175, 211 |
| N-Methylurea | 2 |
| Near UV light | 49, 175, 211 |
| Ozone | 200 |
| Penicillin G | 31, 32 |
| Perylene | 237, 277 |
| Quinoline | 2 |
| S-9 | 28 |
| Salt solutions: | |
| Sodium acetate | 27 |
| Hanks balanced salt solution | 31 |
| 0.3 M NaCl + 0.03 M citrate | 31 |
| 0.2 M Phosphate + 0.1 M citrate | 31 |
| Sodium dehydroacetate | 2 |
| Streptomycin | 31 |
| Tetracycline | 32 |

[a] Negative results based only on a single test system, especially one that does not involve metabolic activation, should be viewed as tentative.
[b] This agent has been described as being mutagenic.[125]
[c] Arochlor 1254 is a potent inducer of monooxygenase activating enzymes,[13] in addition to any direct genetic effect it might have.
[d] Light of wavelength < 340 nm excluded by Plexiglas and neither phenol red nor tetracycline present. Irradiation of human fibroblasts with the 300- to 390-nm components of fluorescent light in medium containing phenol red, tetracycline, and riboflavin (or preirradiation of the medium itself) has been observed to induce SCEs.[208a]

mation by SV40 (although apparently not acute infection with SV40) more than triples SCE frequencies in some human diploid fibroblasts.[214] In other SV40 transformed human cells, the SCE frequencies are only slightly elevated above those in comparable untransformed cells.[326] Human lymphoblastoid cell lines, which are presumably transformed with Epstein–Barr virus,[215] show either normal SCE levels[260] or a very slight SCE elevation.[162] SCEs in mouse embryo fibroblasts are nearly doubled by infection with Rauscher leukemia virus, while SCEs in peripheral lymphocytes from recently vaccinated individuals, or individuals with other miscellaneous virus infections (e.g., herpes simplex, cold/flu, or hepatitis), show at most a modest SCE elevation.[153,162] However, herpes simplex virus, administered at the end of S, does not appreciably increase SCEs in human diploid fibroblasts.[139] This last result may be due, at least in part, to the insensitivity of cells[175] to SCE induction at the end of S; exposure of cells to virus at the start of S might produce a different response.


# EXTENSION OF SCE STUDIES FROM *IN VITRO* TO *IN VIVO* SYSTEMS

Bloom and Hsu[33] described the induction of SCEs *in ovo* in chick embryos exposed to BrdUrd. The chick embryo system has excellent potential for examining tissue-specific cytogenetic effects of mutagen-carcinogens during development.[31,32] Subsequent reports described the induction, by alkylating agents, of SCE formation in marrow cells or spermatogonia of mice which received repeated doses of BrdUrd,[7,8,313] and extension of *in vivo* SCE analysis to other rodent systems, as well as to the mud-minnow[150] has been accomplished. The host-mediated[13,190] aspects of *in vivo* systems, together with flexibility in choice of agent, exposure mode, and the tissue tested, make this approach unique for studying environmental mutagenesis.

In contrast to combined *in vivo–in vitro* studies, in which a microsomal system capable of activating some agents is added directly to *in vitro* cultures,[212,286] or in which cultured cells are enclosed in porous chambers and implanted in animals,[118,277] the *in vivo* systems permit examination of different processes in multiple tissues of a given organism. *In vivo* SCE analysis may prove particularly valuable, because recent data[30] suggest that the array of products produced by *in vivo* vs. *in vitro* activation of potential clastogens may be different. Also, *in vitro* "activating" conditions are capable of actually reducing the SCE inducibility of some agents, such as *N*-acetoxy-acetylaminofluorene,[297] and in at least one instance (styrene),[60] a microsomal activating system was effective only if accompanied by cyclohexene oxide, an epoxide hydrase inhibitor.

In our laboratory, SCE formation has been detected in a number of tissues, including mouse spermatogonia, bone marrow, thymus, and spleen cells.[7,8,9,10,11] Interestingly, spermatogonia have a lower baseline SCE level than the other tissues, and SCE induction by mitomycin C or cyclophosphamide is also lowest in spermatogonia. Very recently, a system for detecting SCE induction in regenerating mouse liver has been developed[11,264] (Fig. 11). Since the liver contains the highest level of mi-

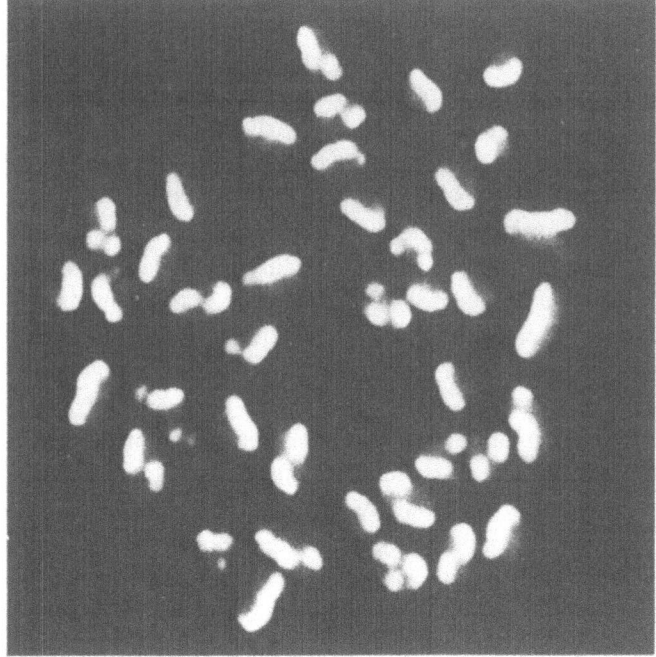

Fig. 11. Induction of SCEs in regenerating mouse liver cells by cyclophosphamide. Approximately 1 day after partial hepatectomy, a mouse received multiple BrdUrd injections; cyclophosphamide (5 mg/kg) was injected intraperitoneally one hour after the final BrdUrd injection. The animal was sacrificed and cells were harvested one day later. This cell exhibits more than 20 SCEs; cells not treated by the drug had, on the average, 5 SCEs per cell.[264]

crosomal activating activity,[35,100,108] chemical activation and SCE induction should be possible within the same cell. This system increases the sensitivity of detection of SCE induction by agents (e.g., acetylaminofluorene) which require activation but which have thus far appeared to be relatively ineffective at SCE induction,[264,297,298] perhaps because, once they are activated in the liver, they react without reaching more peripheral tissues. A liver system for SCE detection should also facilitate studies (Schreck, unpublished data) of the relative sensitivity of mice with different genetically determined basal and inducible liver arylhydrocarbon hydroxlase activity levels to clastogens requiring metabolic activation by associated enzyme complexes.

A major methodological difficulty with *in vivo* studies has been the requirement for multiple BrdUrd injections[7,8,313] or continuous BrdUrd infusion[229,257,261] because of rapid host catabolism of BrdUrd. The BrdUrd infusion method may prove especially valuable in studies in which sustained, known concentrations of clastogens must be administered to animals. We have introduced a simplified procedure, involving the use of BrdUrd in the form of a small tablet that can be implanted subcutaneously.[9] Tablets can be prepared with a small, commercially available pill press (e.g., Parr Co., Moline, Ill.). Nearly 100% unifilar replacement of dT by BrdUrd during a single cycle can thus be effected, and tablets with different release kinetics have been prepared.[11] The tablets will probably be more useful for large scale *in vivo* SCE studies in tissues such as bone marrow, the replication of which is apparently not seriously inhibited by the high BrdUrd levels provided by the tablets. However, relative to BrdUrd tablets, multiple BrdUrd injections give better results (e.g., a higher mitotic index) with regenerating liver cells and result in lower baseline SCE levels.[264*]

*In vivo* SCE analysis has now been performed on cells from Chinese hamster cheek pouch mucosa.[275,276] This tissue is accessible not only to systemic agents but to topically applied agents such as 7,12-dimethylbenzanthracene. In the latter situation, one cheek pouch can be exposed to clastogens, with the other serving as an internal control. This system should be especially useful for cytogenetic evaluation of putative topical carcinogens, and has recently been used to show SCE induction by a

---

* BrdUrd adsorbed to charcoal has also been used for depot BrdUrd administration.[10,130,251] Use of this method will require allowance for potential adsorption of exogenous test compounds (e.g., polycyclic aromatic hydrocarbons) to the charcoal.

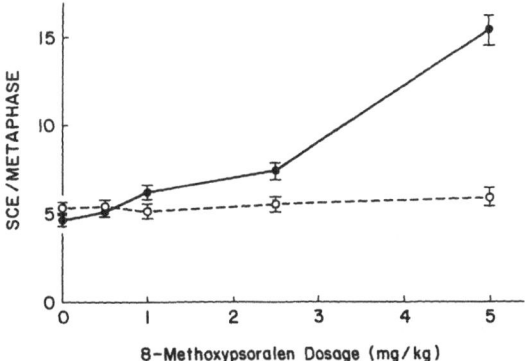

Fig. 12. Sister chromatid exchange induction by 8-methoxypsoralen and near UV light in Chinese hamster cheek pouch cells. One year old male Chinese hamsters were injected intraperitoneally with 8-methoxypsoralen at the doses shown. Forty-five minutes following the injection of 8-methoxypsoralen the left cheek pouches were everted and exposed to UV light (125 ergs/mm²/sec at 365 ± nm) for 5 minutes (●). The right cheek pouches were not exposed to UV light (○). Irradiated cells from animals given >1 mg/kg 8-methoxypsoralen exhibit more SCEs than do unirradiated cells.[270]

clastogen (8-methoxypsoralen) that is administered systemically but activated topically by near UV light (Fig. 12).[276]†

A different type of "*in vivo*" SCE analysis involves the use of SCE frequencies to assess the cytogenetic impact of clastogenic agents administered to patients, usually in the course of chemotherapy.[163,239] Peripheral lymphocytes withdrawn from patients exposed to various drugs are cultured for two cycles in medium containing BrdUrd prior to SCE analysis. Nevstad[213] utilized this approach to detail the time course of SCE elevation due to adriamycin, a compound previously stated to induce SCE in patients.[232] Perry[230] has continued this type of study. A similar type of SCE analysis of rabbit lymphocytes has shown that repeated exposure of an animal to an SCE inducer can result in a persistently elevated SCE level for as long as four months after drug exposure has been discontinued.[284] Widespread use of this procedure will require means to account for variations in the persistence of SCE elevation following treatment. This persistence depends on the drug used.[167] Such analyses will

---

† Consistent with these and previous SCE data, the combination of 8-methoxypsoralen plus near UV light, used to treat psoriasis, has been associated with a more than twofold increase in skin cancer.[282]

also be influenced by toxic effects of chemotherapy on cells; these effects compromise the yield of analyzable metaphases.

An alternative *in vivo* approach examines fetal cell exposure to agents administered to pregnant females. Thus far, cyclophosphamide has been found to be effective at SCE induction, *trans utero*, in mouse embryo and in maternal marrow.[156] This type of system may be useful for screening agents to which pregnant females may be exposed, and suggests that SCE analysis on blood samples from newborns may prove informative.

Recent observations of markedly elevated SCE frequencies in leukemic patients prior to therapy,[34,152,220] as the disease progresses[129] or following repeated therapy[34] may reflect the basic disease process, the result of extensive chemotherapy, and/or the response of the disease process to cumulative exposure to different agents known to damage DNA. The information obtained may prove of use in evaluating the status of patients with neoplasia, and it may assist interpretation of data emerging on SCE elevations in humans exposed to other environmental conditions (e.g., due to occupational conditions[79] or to cigarette-smoking habits.[61,113,165]) Such latter studies might also benefit from considerations of genetic differences in the ability of different individuals to activate polycyclic aromatic hydrocarbons.

## INTERPRETATION OF SCE INDUCTION TESTS

A number of potentially confounding variables and other limitations must be kept in mind, when interpreting the results of SCE tests. For example, exposure to BrdUrd must be high enough to permit good sister chromatid differentiation but not so high that it produces a variable and unacceptably high background level of SCEs. Also, while most early studies of SCEs were done with alkylating agents, chosen primarily to exemplify efficient SCE induction, it is desirable that future studies be capable of examining agents for which clastogenic activity is less certain. In these instances, at most a small increment in SCEs might be observed, and variables, such as effects due to the vehicles used to dissolve the agent, the time required for metabolic activation, or synergism between the test agent and BrdUrd may become important.

A major problem in arriving at a decision about the clastogenicity of a new compound is the upper limit of the concentration to be tested before negative results are to be accepted. Typically, this upper limit will be a treatment level that is sufficiently toxic to cells that proliferation necessary for SCE detection is inhibited. Such toxicity may become evident either in chromosome breakage or in alteration of specific cell kinetic parameters (and a reduced mitotic index). Also, especially when using high concentrations of agents, minor impurities might give spuriously positive results.

Finally, the limitations of the test system employed must be considered. Most frequently, one wishes to know whether an unknown agent will cause genetic damage to a variety of human tissues. If this agent is active without metabolic modification, a human peripheral lymphocyte test system (with at most very low monooxygenase activating capacity[101,102]), may be adequate, subject primarily to the possibility that different human tissues might have different repair capacities or drug metabolism rates. If metabolic activation of an agent is required, a rodent test system is most frequently used. However, DNA repair in rodents is known to differ both within rodent systems, e.g., as a function of age[71,228] and from that in humans,[192,308] and interpretation of results with rodent cells should consider this difference. If microsome preparations are used to activate the agent to be tested, differences between the modifications effected *in vivo* and those caused by isolated microsomes may prove important. Typically, most artifacts due to particular test systems will tend to produce false negative rather than false positive results. Because of the former possibility, utilization of multiple test systems is probably advisable. However, comparison of test data on different substances would be facilitated if the plethora of test systems currently utilized was reduced to a standard set, which, with limited but appropriate exceptions, was then applied to each compound.

It is possible that "positive" results might depend on the use of an unrealistically high treatment dosage. This problem is inherent in many short term tests, for which high level short term exposure is used to estimate the effect of low dose exposure over an interval of many years. Quantitative estimates of SCE induction efficiency per unit exposure will be important, both to characterize the potential hazard of an individual chemical and to estimate the possible additive effects of many different agents, each present in low amounts. Introduction of quantitative, rather than qualitative evaluations of chemicals may prove to be very important in large scale mutagen-carcinogen testing. SCE induction tests are very well suited for such a quantitative analysis.

# RELATIONSHIP OF SCE INDUCTION TO DNA DAMAGE, REPAIR, AND SYNTHESIS

A variety of chemical and physical agents, exhibiting diverse modes of interaction with DNA (Table II) as well as transformation of cells by SV40 virus,[214] are capable of inducing SCEs. Alkylating agents of many different types seem to be especially effective. SCEs can also be induced by irradiation of BrdUrd-substituted DNA,[124,135,137] a treatment causing predominantly (though not exclusively) single strand breaks.[120] Only fragmentary information exists, however, about the quantitative relationship between the number and types of alkylation products or DNA strand interruptions, the efficiency of their repair, and the number of SCEs produced.

Quantitation of DNA alkylation and removal can be accomplished by chemical analysis of reaction products or, if suitable isotopic derivatives can be obtained, by measurement of radioactivity in newly formed DNA adducts. We have obtained evidence that SCE may account for only a small fraction of DNA damage by 8-methoxypsoralen plus near UV light (Cassel and Latt, in press). The combination of 8-methoxypsoralen or trimethylpsoralen plus 365-nm light, but not either agent alone, is effective in inducing SCE in human and CHO chromosomes (Fig. 13).[49,88,174,175,179,180,181,211,316] The dependence of SCE on either light or 8-methoxypsoralen, keeping the other agent fixed, has been quantitated[175] and an assay for measuring the binding of tritiated 8-methoxypsoralen developed, so that the ratio between these two quantities can be compared (Figs. 14, 15). Data thus far indicate that one SCE is induced (in the two cycles following DNA damage) per approximately 200 8-methoxypsoralen-DNA adducts (Cassel and Latt, unpublished data). The majority of DNA adducts formed do not produce cross-links (under conditions used to score SCEs) but, with an SCE/adduct ratio of $\leq 0.01$, it cannot yet be exluded that the cross-links have a major role in SCE induction.

We have previously reported cytological evidence consistent with the persistence of alkylation by 8-methoxypsoralen during at least a few replication cycles. These data[175] consist of the observation of reciprocal interchanges of dark chromatids in third cycle metaphases, indicative of SCE formation after the second posttreatment cycle.[208,305] SCE formed during the first two cycles appear as isolated segments of darkly staining chromatids in third division metaphases (Fig. 13). Similar data implicating SCE induction during the third cycle following DNA damage have now

2ND DIV

3RD DIV

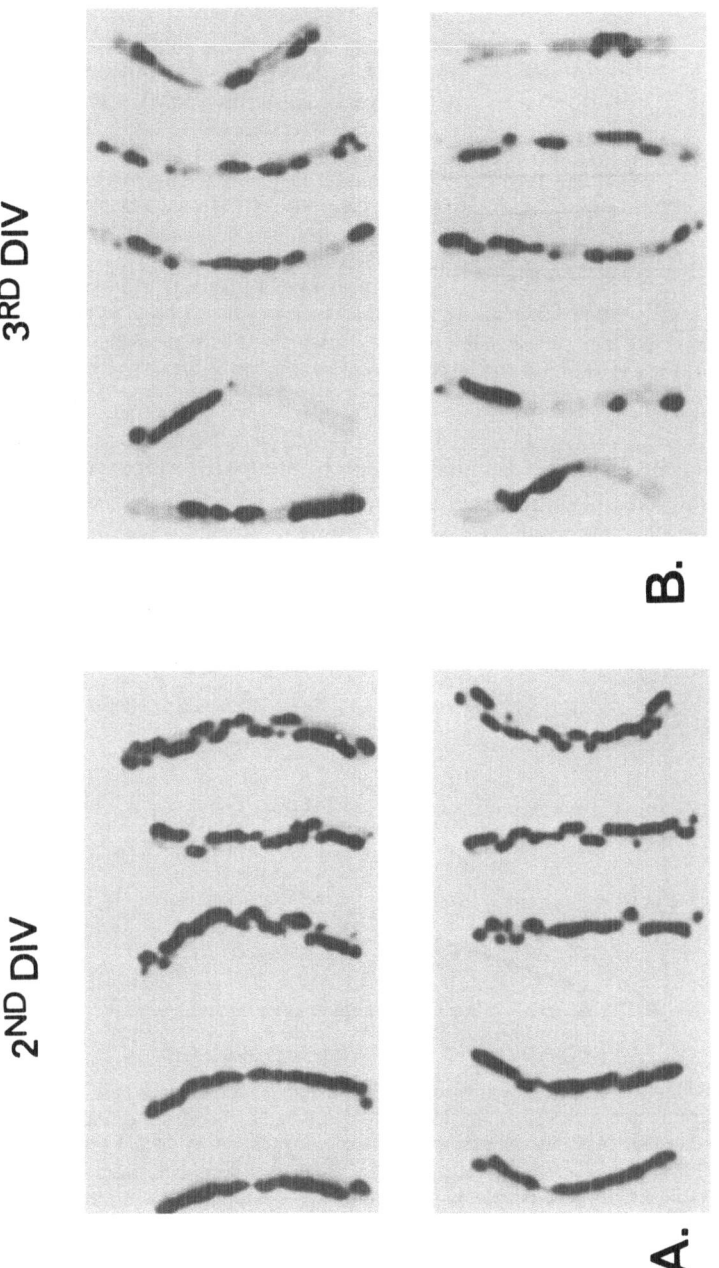

A.

B.

Fig. 13. Induction of SCE in second- and third-division CHO cell metaphases. CHO cells synchronized at the G1-S boundary were treated with 8-methoxypsoralen ($6 \times 10^{-6}$ M) plus light ($1.1 \times 10^{4}$ ergs/mm$^2$, mainly 365 nm) and were then allowed to replicate for (A) 32 or (B) 51 hours in BrdUrd ($2.5 \times 10^{-5}$ M). Each set of five chromosomes consists of two controls (at the left) and three chromosomes from cells treated before release in medium containing BrdUrd (at the right).[175]

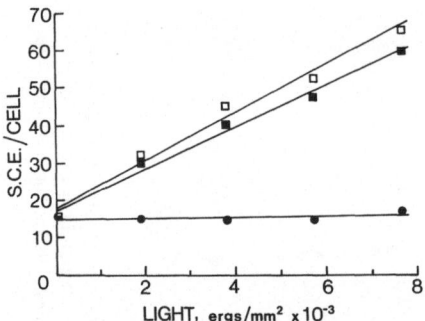

Fig. 14. SCE induction in CHO cells by 8-methoxypsoralen or tritiated 8-methoxypsoralen plus near UV light (320–370 nm). CHO monolayers were exposed to increasing doses of light 1 hr after additions [7.4 × 10⁻⁶ M 8-MeOP (□), 7.4 × 10⁻⁶ M [³H]-8-MeOP (■), or nothing (●)]. The cells were then placed in fresh medium containing 2.5 × 10⁻⁵ M BrdUrd, and the cells allowed to replicate twice (~28 hr) prior to harvest at metaphase. Slides were then subjected to a 33258 Hoechst plus Giemsa procedure and SCE per cell counted. The [³H]-8-MeOP was more than 85% as effective as the unlabeled 8-MeOP in inducing SCEs.

been reported by Ishii and Bender in cells treated with mitomycin C.[126] Thus, unremoved alkylation damage might underly the observation of Stetka *et al.*[284] that repeated exposure of rabbits to mitomycin C ultimately leads to persistently elevated SCE levels (in peripheral lymphocytes cultured *in vitro*). The persistence time for SCE induction appears to depend

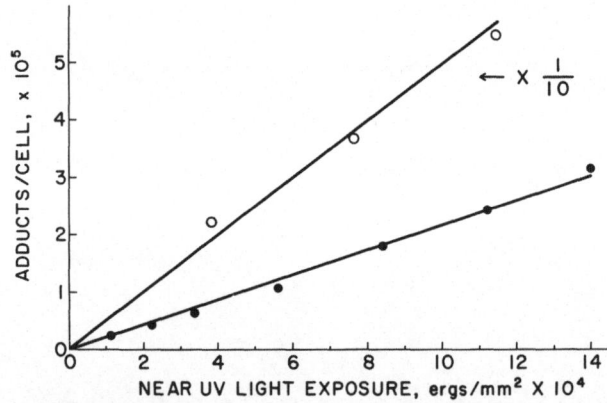

Fig. 15. DNA adducts in CHO cells exposed to [³H]-8-methoxypsoralen plus near UV light. Monolayers were treated with 7.4 × 10⁻⁶M [³H]-8-MeOP and higher doses of illumination of the type used in Fig. 14. Cells were then harvested, and nuclei isolated and subjected to pronase–RNse digestion. The number of [³H]-8-MeOP-DNA adducts was calculated from the amount of radioactivity precipitable on paper filters by trichloroacetic acid, the specific activity of the [³H]-8-MeOP (0.37 mCi/μM), and the tritium counting efficiency (45%). The slope of the line shown is 2.17 ± 0.05/ergs/mm². Since one damaged cell gives rise to two second-division metaphases, the yield of SCE per treated cell (using the data of Fig. 14) is 0.0110 ± 0.0007/ergs/mm² and the adduct/SCE ratio is 195 ± 18.

on the agent used. For example, Lambert[167] observed an elevation in the SCE rate in lymphocytes from patients treated even briefly with CCNU (1-(2-chloroethyl)-3-cyclohexyl-1-nitrosourea) several weeks after exposure, while SCE elevation following cyclophosphamide therapy was much more transient.

Shafer[269] has recently postulated that SCE formation involves the bypass of DNA cross-links during replication. While this model is compatible with the observation that 8-methoxypsoralen adducts are slowly removed by cells, it will now be important to determine whether, as predicted by Shafer, those adducts remaining after replication are still in the form of cross-links.

It is instructive to note that, since SCEs may reflect less than 1% of DNA adducts, and that chromosome breaks are less than 1% as frequent as SCE,[170,171] chromosome breaks may detect $10^{-4}$–$10^{-5}$ or less of the total DNA damage in a cell. The disparity between the numbers of DNA adducts, SCEs, and chromatid breaks might contribute to the multiplicity of results obtained by investigations comparing SCE-to-break ratios and the relative location of chromosome breaks and incomplete SCE following exposure of cells to different clastogens.

Consistent with an earlier suggestion by Heddle et al.,[107] nearly half of the breaks in chromosomes in lymphocytes from Fanconi's anemia patients treated at the start of S with mitomycin C occur at incomplete SCE sites (Fig. 16)[65,174,186] as do 25–50% of the breaks induced at the end of S by UV-irradiation of BrdUrd-substituted Chinese hamster cells.[137] Kihlman et al. have shown that, in Vicia, irradiation of chromosomes containing one BrdUrd-substituted chromatid (BT–TT) by near UV light produces breaks in the substituted (BT) chromatid but not in the unsubstituted (TT) chromatid, i.e., "trans"scission was rare, but occasional breaks very near SCE points were noted.[144,146] Chromosomes in which both chromatids contain BrdUrd (BT–BT) were much more sensitive to chromatid interchange, indicating that such exchanges require damage in both chromatids. Treatment of rat cells with dimethylbenzanthracene a few hours prior to harvest, i.e., at the end of S for the metaphases scored, gives a similar distribution of SCEs and breaks.[310] In other systems, breaks occur in the absence of SCE.[123,254] While an explanation of these divergent observations is not apparent, there is ample room within the confines of observed stoichiometry for a given combination of damage and cell response to cause SCE and chromosome breaks by completely or largely divergent paths.

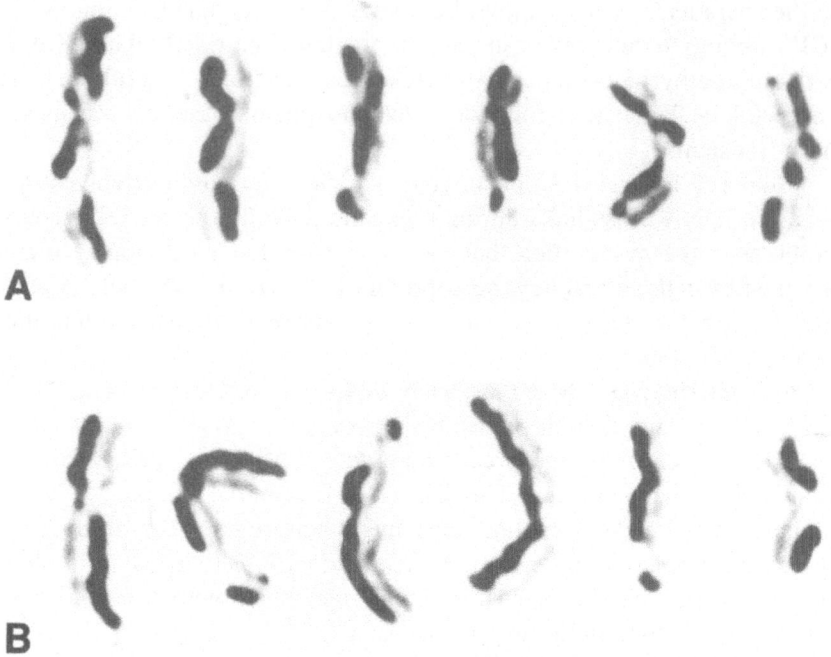

Fig. 16. Aberrations in chromosomes from Fanconi's anemia lymphocytes treated with mitomycin C. These chromosomes were selected from chromosomes from cells grown in medium containing $10^{-5}$ M BrdUrd, $10^{-4}$ M dC, $4 \times 10^{-7}$ FdUrd, and $6 \times 10^{-6}$ M Urd. Mitomycin C (0.03 µg/ml) was added for the third and final day of culture. Slides were first stained with 33258 Hoechst, subjected to intense illumination required for fluorescence photomicroscopy, washed, stained with Giemsa, and rephotographed. Chromosomes in the top row (A) exhibit chromatid breaks at sites of incomplete sister chromatid exchange, while those in the bottom row (B) exhibit breaks away from such sites. A comparable number of each type of chromatid breaks has been observed in such cells.[174]

Sister chromatid exchange formation appears to be tightly coupled to DNA synthesis. Wolff *et al.*[325] demonstrated that UV-damaged rodent cells needed to pass through S phase for SCE induction to be detected. Variation in SCE inducibility within the S phase was investigated by Kato,[135,138] who used near-UV light to induce SCEs in unsynchronized, BrdUrd-substituted Chinese hamster cells. The position of cells within S at the time of irradiation was estimated from the time between irradiation and metaphase collection, and by the extent of incorporation of a [³H]-dT pulse which was administered at the time of irradiation and then detected at metaphase. While SCEs induced at the end of S were observed to occur preferentially in late replicating regions, the efficiency of SCE induction appeared to be maximal near mid-S, coinciding with the maximum in the rate of DNA synthesis.

Analysis of SCE induction by 8-methoxypsoralen plus light in synchronized cells[175,180] led to a different conclusion, namely that SCE induction was maximal at the start of S and decreased progressively throughout the S phase (Fig. 17). The difference between this result and that of Kato[135] may be due to lack of cell synchrony in Kato's experiment or to a difference in the type of DNA damage effected. Preliminary evidence for the latter possibility has recently been presented by Shafer.[269] This possibility should be easy to test, e.g., by treating synchronized cells with BrdUrd plus light. Loss of coherence in cell phasing during S would tend to broaden the SCE versus S phase traverse curve, especially for data attributed to the start of S. For data obtained at the end of S, there was better agreement between the two studies; a need for DNA synthesis in a given chromosome region, subsequent to DNA damage, appeared

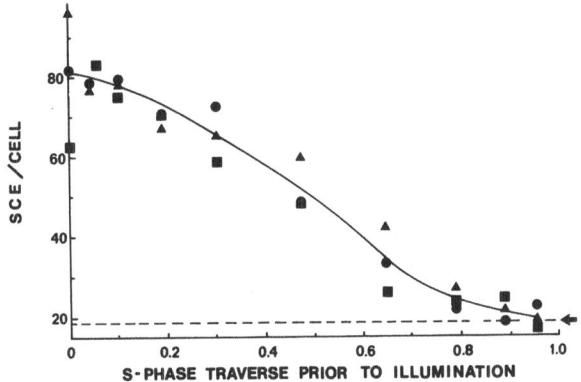

Fig. 17. Relative inducibility of SCEs in CHO cells during S phase. CHO cells were cultured in medium containing BrdUrd ($2.5 \times 10^{-5}$ M) during imposition of a hydroxyurea G1–S block, resulting in approximately one round of DNA labeling prior to the block. Cells were then released at G1–S by transfer to complete medium, containing BrdUrd ($2.5 \times 10^{-5}$ M), exposed to 8-methoxypsoralen ($6 \times 10^{-6}$ M) and near UV light ($1.1 \times 10^4$ ergs/mm²) at hourly intervals, and harvested at metaphase 12 hr after release. Data from three separate experiments (▲: ●: ■) are shown. 8-Methoxypsoralen alone has no effect on SCEs, although near UV light itself induces some SCEs in these BrdUrd substituted cells. The data are plotted to show SCE induction as a function of S-phase traverse. Amounts of [³H]-dT incorporation during 1-hr intervals were summed, and S-phase traverse was defined as the fraction of this total synthesis that had occurred *prior* to irradiation. Arrow, control SCE level.[175]

necessary for SCE induction. The molecular events accounting for the coupling between SCE induction and DNA synthesis, e.g., via a relationship to temporarily discontinuous segments of newly formed polynucleotide chains, remain to be determined, however.

## RELATIONSHIP OF SCE INDUCTION TO MUTAGENESIS

Implicit in many of the above studies is the assumption that SCE formation bears some relationship to DNA damage, repair, and mutagenesis. Certain evidence lends support to this idea. Carrano *et al.*[46] have observed an increase in mutations at the *HGPRT* (and *APRT*)[47] locus of the CHO cells in proportion to concentrations of ethylmethanesulfonate, ethylnitrosourea, mitomycin C, and proflavine, in concentration ranges also causing a linear response in SCE induction (Fig. 18). Compared with the other chemicals, relatively fewer mutations were observed with the bifunctional agent mitomycin C, or with its monofunctional, decarbamyl

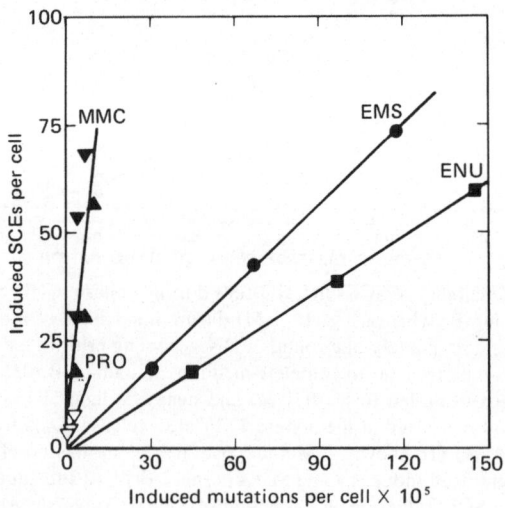

Fig. 18. The relationship between induced SCEs and induced mutations at the HGPRT locus in CHO cells (Carrano *et al.*[46]). Symbols: MMC (mitomycin C), EMS (ethylmethane sulfonate), ENU (ethylnitrosourea), and PRO (proflavine).

analogue.[47] Assuming the existence of 50,000 genes per cell, all with the same mutagenic susceptibility as *HGPRT*, Carrano *et al.* estimated that 0.01–1.0 mutation per SCE occurred during the first two S phases. It would seem desirable, though admittedly difficult, to develop a method of measuring SCE induction and mutagenesis in the same cells, to rule against the possibility that these two phenomena reflect disparate effects of alkylation in different members of a cell population. Other SCE inducers, e.g., *cis*-platinum (II) diamine dichloride[309] and cigarette-smoke condensate,[61] using various cell types and genetic loci, are being subjected to similar analysis. *trans*-Platinum (II) diamine dichloride, induces somewhat fewer SCEs than its *cis* derivative, and it appears to be relatively ineffective as a mutagen.[37] The net result of such studies will hopefully be a delineation not only of the parallels between SCEs and mutagenesis but also the point, if existent, at which, under special conditions, the processes leading to these two events diverge.

Alkylation by psoralen derivatives plus light, a powerful inducer of SCE formation[49,174,175,179,180,181,211,316] is known to stimulate DNA strand interchange in recombination-proficient but not in recombination-deficient (Rec A) bacteria.[53] This observation prompted the suggestion[171] that SCE formation in metaphase chromosomes was somehow analogous to recombinational repair[249,250] in bacteria. A feature complicating this analogy is the possible difference between DNA repair processes in bacterial and mammalian cells.[192] Putative associations between SCEs in animal or plant cells, recombinational repair in bacteria, and "error prone repair"[320] are thus far primarily speculative. Of potential interest, in this regard, is the claim[149] that the tumor promoter TPA (12-*O*-tetradecanoyl-phorbol-13-acetate) can induce SCEs. However, work from our laboratory,[198] using 0.3–3.0 μg/ml TPA, as well as that of Baker and associates (Baker, Thompson, and Carrano, unpublished), was unable to confirm this observation.

Another event, in addition to mutagenesis, paralleling SCE induction by clastogens is the release of SV40 virus from transformed cells. This has been demonstrated[131] in a number of different hamster kidney cell lines, using mitomycin C and EMS. A 10,000-fold greater concentration of EMS (relative to mitomycin C) was needed both for SCE induction and for virus induction. Again, parallelism between SCE induction and an associated process, i.e., virus induction, will no doubt be limited to a portion of each process, and points of pathway divergence will be as informative as the observation of similar initial steps.

# SISTER CHROMATID DIFFERENTIATION IN MEIOTIC CELLS

*In vivo* administration of BrdUrd has permitted sister chromatid differentiation (SCD) in meiotic cells. Previous studies of SCE in meiosis had utilized autoradiography,[226,300] which affords limited resolution. Initial success with BrdUrd incorporation was achieved in the X-Y bivalent of the mouse,[8] in which SCD was detected. However, meiotic interchange is not known to occur in the mouse X-Y pair, and only very limited sister chromatid differentiation was effected in autosomes, perhaps because of marked BrdUrd sensitivity of mouse meiotic tissue. Allen *et al.*[11] have investigated meiosis in the Armenian hamster, an animal in which meiotic interchange presumably occurs in the X-Y bivalent,[188] and have detected nonsister chromatid exchange, most likely due to meiotic recombination (Fig. 19). Very recently, Polani *et al.*[235] have described sister chromatid differentiation in female mouse meiotic tissue, using an *in vitro/in vivo* BrdUrd technique, and have detected meiotic exchange related to chiasmata formation as well as sister chromatid exchange.

BrdUrd–dye techniques have also been used to study meiotic interchange in locust chromosomes.[302,303] Assuming that all chiasmata reflected meiotic interchange, Tease and associates concluded that interchange between identically and nonidentically substituted chromatids were equally probable. Moreover, in the latter instance, in which interchange of differentially stained chromatids occurred, affording localization of the interchange position, no terminalization of synapsis beyond the exchange point was noted. If this observation of nonterminalization proves to be general, it will require reformulation of meiotic mechanisms. Tease has presented evidence that chiasma position is not BrdUrd-dependent, and Allen[6a] has observed sister chromatid differentiation and chromatid exchange at second meiotic metaphase in the Armenian hamster. Thus, terminalization arrest does not appear to be a BrdUrd-induced phenomenon. The relative incidence of SCEs in meiotic chromosomes, their induction by clastogens, as well as the precise location of SCEs and meiotic interchange relative to chromomeres are all questions, the answers to which are now within the range of technical capabilities. One distinction between SCEs and meiotic exchange may be the observation of Lin and Alfi[193] that SCEs in mouse chromosomes are very frequent in centric heterochromatin (though absent in heterochromatin in other systems), while

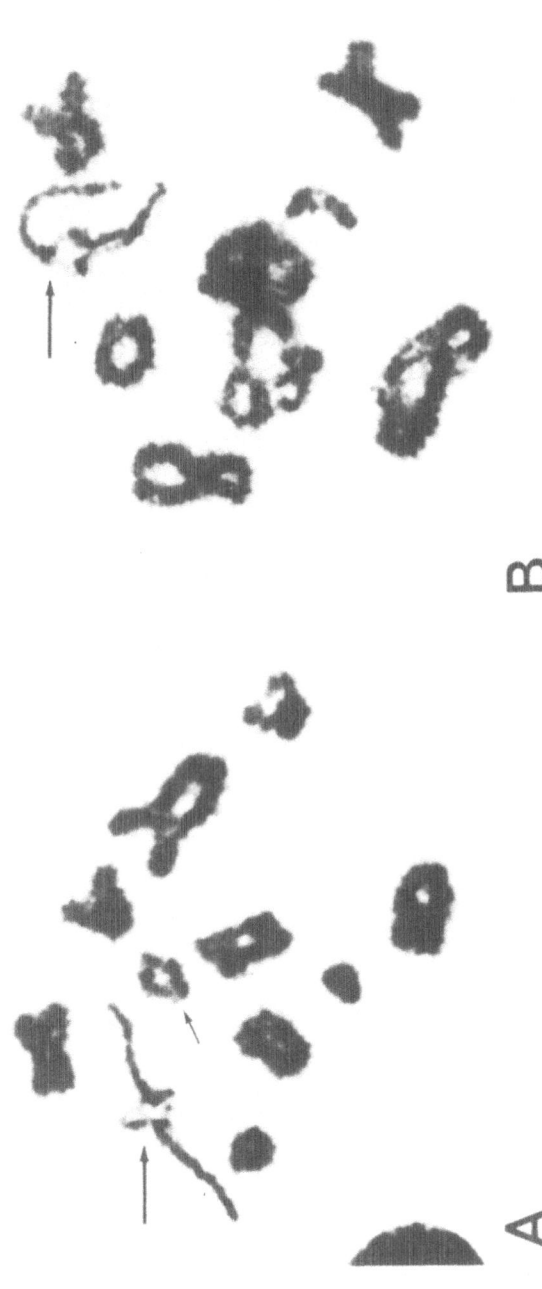

Fig. 19. Sister chromatid differentiation and chromatid interchange in Armenian hamster meiotic cells. The 40 to 45-g male Armenian hamsters, 1–1.05 years old, were implanted with 55-mg BrdUrd tablets; 16 days later, the cells were harvested and processed[1] as described previously. Sister chromatid differentiation is marked in the X–Y bivalent (large arrows) and is apparent in a few autosomes (small arrows). The X–Y bivalent in (B) shows uniformly light sister chromatids in synapsis with uniformly dark sister chromatids. This is most readily interpretable as reflecting a meiotic interchange.[11]

meiotic DNA synthesis, thought by Stern and Hotta to be related to meiotic interchange,[281] is virtually nonexistent in heterochromatin.[115]

## SISTER CHROMATID EXCHANGE FORMATION IN HERITABLE HUMAN DISEASES

Analysis of SCE formation has been used to differentiate between various inherited human diseases characterized by chromosome fragility and a predisposition for the development of neoplasia[91] (Table V). These diseases, which include Bloom's syndrome, Fanconi's anemia, and ataxia telangiectasia, presumably involve defects in DNA repair. The diseases potentially constitute test systems, with specific DNA repair defects, for dissecting the SCE process. Cells from another disease, xeroderma pigmentosum (see below), may permit extraordinarily sensitive clastogen detection. All four conditions listed above are rare, but they follow an autosomal recessive inheritance mode, and the respective heterozygotes amount to 1–2% of the total population.[294,295] For some conditions, het-

**TABLE V.** Sister Chromatid Exchange Levels in Selected Genetic Diseases

| Disorder | Baseline | Stressed[a] | Specific damaging agent | Reference |
|---|---|---|---|---|
| Fanconi's anemia | N[b] | ↓[c] | Mitomycin C | 186 |
| Bloom's syndrome | ↑ | ↑[d] | Ethylmethane sulfonate | 50, 92, 159 |
| Ataxia telangiectasia | N | N | X-ray, γ-ray | 82, 83, 105 |
| Xeroderma pigmentosum | | | | |
|   Groups A, B, C, and D | N | ↑[e] | UV; several alkylating agents | 52, 62, 326 |
|   Variant (post replication repair defect) | N | N | UV—caffeine-enhanced | 52, 62 |
| deSanctis–Cacchione | N | N | UV | 263 |

[a] SCE level seen in cells treated with specific damaging agent.
[b] N, Same level seen in normal individual with same treatment.
[c] ↓, Less than normal SCE increment in peripheral lymphocytes induced by mitomycin C; greater than normal increase in chromosomal aberrations caused by mitomycin C in both peripheral lymphocytes and dermal fibroblasts (and by diepoxybutane in fibroblasts[17]).
[d] ↑, Greater than normal SCE increment due to ethylmethane sulfonate.
[e] ↑, Greater than normal SCE increment caused by UV irradiation and by a variety of alkylating agents.

erozygotes also appear to be at an increased risk for certain forms of cancer,[293,294,295] and hence make up several percent of all individuals with those neoplastic conditions.

Cells from patients with Fanconi's anemia have been shown to be highly susceptible to killing[76,77] and to chromosome breakage[17,253,255] by bifunctional alkylating agents, and they appear to exhibit reduced ability to excise UV-[236] and gamma-irradiation products,[243] and DNA cross-links.[78] One recent report[110] has claimed that fibroblasts and lymphocytes from these patients are defective in DNA ligase (50% reduction) and data suggesting an intermediate reduction in lymphocytes from heterozygotes were presented. These data are of potential interest, though their interpretation must accommodate the report[227] that "normal" cells may differ among each other by as much as fourfold in DNA ligase activity.

Lymphocytes from Fanconi's anemia patients, while exhibiting essentially normal SCE frequencies in the presence of BrdUrd, respond to mitomycin C treatment with a subnormal increase in sister chromatid exchange formation (Table V).[186] This observation has now been independently confirmed.[82,273] The reduced stimulation of SCE formation by mitomycin C in Fanconi's anemia is associated with increased chromatid breakage. However, the relative contributions of mitomycin C monoadducts and cross-links to the SCE, chromosome breakage, and cell toxicity data have not yet been determined. Interestingly, approximately half of the breaks induced in FA lymphocytes by mitomycin C occurred at sites of incomplete sister chromatid exchange formation (Fig. 16),[176,186] a result substantiated by subsequent studies on Fanconi's anemia cells grown in the presence of BrdUrd but not treated with mitomycin C.[65] This observation is compatible with the hypothesis that the break increment and at least some of the exchange deficit in this particular disease are causally related.

Our initial studies[186] of lymphocytes from four patients with Fanconi'a anemia have been repeated, with similar though not identical results, on five other patients with this disease. However, while the general concept of a "stress test" involving exposure of Fanconi's anemia cells to a potential bifunctional alkylating agent may prove of some diagnostic value, the empirical nature of the present assay (SCE and chromosome breakage) suggests a need for some caution in the interpretation of the results. Moreover, fibroblasts from Fanconi's anemia patients show at most only a marginal deficit in SCE response, although chromosome breakage in the presence of mitomycin C is elevated, and the response in cells from different sources is heterogeneous (reference 186 and unpublished data). The basis of the different results with lymphocytes and fibroblasts is, at present, unknown. However, the data can probably be interpreted to suggest that Fanconi's anemia cells are defective in some form of DNA repair.

Abnormalities in short term SCE induction in heterozygotes from patients with Fanconi's anemia have not been detected. However, extended exposure of carriers to low levels of the potentially bifunctional alkylating agent diepoxybutane seems to elicit abnormally high chromosome breakage in both diseased and heterozygote cells.[17,18] This latter observation may reflect accumulation over several cell cycles of incompletely repaired DNA damage.

In Bloom's syndrome, the baseline SCE frequency is greatly elevated (Fig. 20).[50] This observation is consonant with German's previous[90] identification of Bloom's syndrome as a condition with increased somatic recombination, based on observation of quadriradial figures. Interestingly, quadriradials in Bloom's syndrome chromosomes, like SCEs in most systems, occur preferentially in a Q-negative band or at the junction of Q-negative and Q-positive bands.[160] It is not yet apparent how the SCE data relate to the retarded rate of DNA replication fork progression[93,103] or one report of increased sensitivity (based on DNA replication rates) to ultraviolet light[93] in these cells. One suggestion[103] is that the basic defect in Bloom's syndrome cells is manifest at the DNA synthesis growing point.

Bloom's syndrome cells do not show increased chromosome aberrations or abnormal unscheduled DNA synthesis following UV or $\gamma$-ray-induced damage.[69] Tice *et al.*[306] have observed an approximately 50% *elevation* in SCE frequencies in normal fibroblasts cocultivated with cells isolated from patients with Bloom's syndrome. One interpretation of these data is that a humoral factor is responsible for the SCE elevation in Bloom's syndrome. German *et al.*[92] reported that, in certain Bloom's syndrome patients, a subpopulation of lymphocytes does not exhibit elevated SCEs, perhaps suggesting that, if such a humoral factor exists, not all cells are equally susceptible. Van Buul *et al.*[312] found, in related experiments, that cocultivation of Bloom's syndrome fibroblasts with Chinese hamster cells led to a modest (~30%) *reduction* in SCEs in the Bloom's syndrome cells. Since this effect required the simultaneous presence of both cell types, the action of a humoral factor was considered to be un-

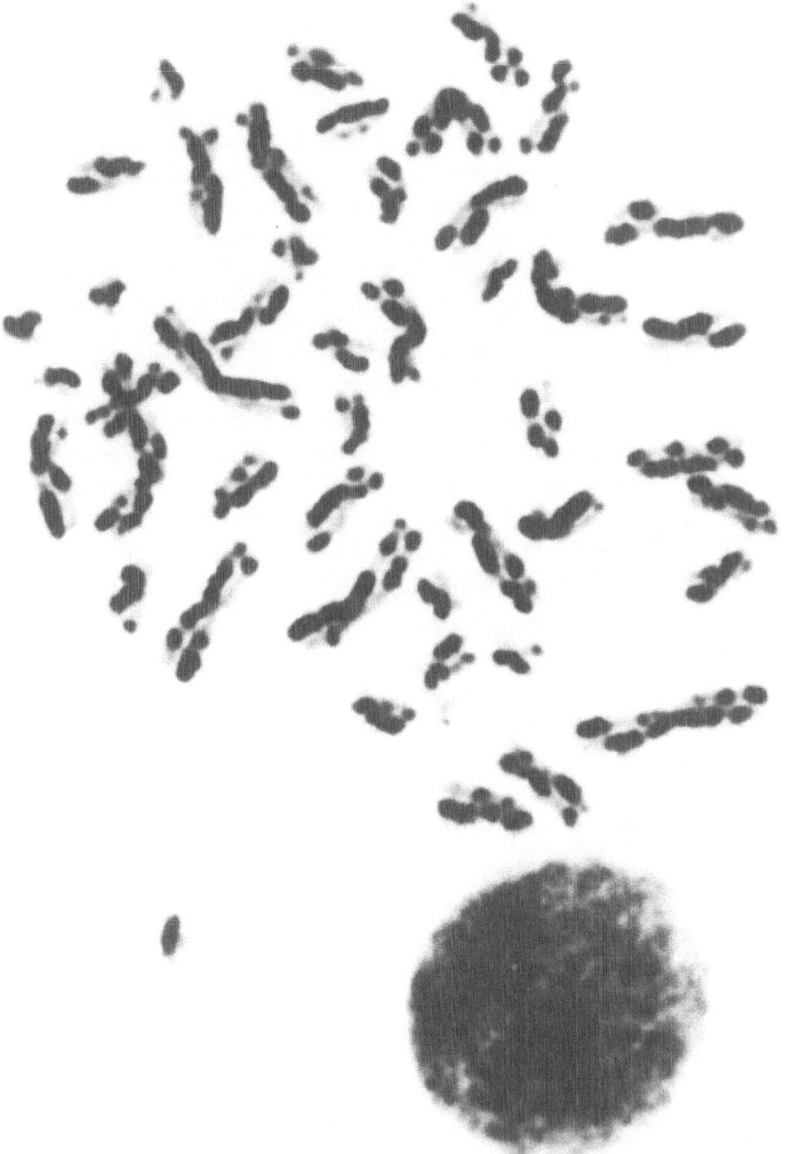

Fig. 20. Sister chromatid exchange formation in a peripheral lymphocyte from a patient with Bloom's syndrome. This cell replicated twice in medium containing BrdUrd. Slides were stained by a fluorescence plus Giemsa technique. An average of 95 SCEs per cell was observed in samples from this patient, compared to an average of approximately 15 SCEs per cell in controls.

likely. With regard to the cocultivation results, it will be important to determine the extent to which the large number of hamster cells present depleted the BrdUrd content of the medium. More recently, Bryant *et al.*[41a] reported that fusion products between Bloom's syndrome fibroblasts and normal fibroblasts exhibited an essentially normal SCE frequency. Bartram *et al.*[22] have recently shown that cocultivation of fibroblasts from patients with Bloom's syndrome with normal fibroblasts reduced the frequency of SCEs in the former cells, without affecting SCE formation in the latter. This effect was suggested to be due to a dialyzable factor. Identification of a chemical factor able to correct the SCE rate in Bloom's syndrome cells would provide an important tool for analysis of this condition.

Recently, Shiriashi and Sandberg[273] have shown that lymphocytes from a patient with Bloom's syndrome undergo a modest additional increase in SCEs upon exposure to mitomycin C. This increase may in part be limited by the high baseline level of SCEs ($\geq 100$/cell) and the existence of a saturation level of SCE formation (or detection) in a given cell. These workers also showed that SCE elevations could be detected in bone marrow, as well as blood cells, from patients with Bloom's syndrome,[272] and that there was little direct correlation between the distribution of SCEs and structural aberrations in chromosomes from patients with this disease. SCE frequencies in Bloom's syndrome fibroblasts are much lower ($\sim 50$/cell) than those in lymphocytes[280,306]; we have made similar observations on cells from two patients with this disease. Krepinsky *et al.*[159] have observed an unusually high sensitivity to SCE induction by monofunctional (EMS) alkylation in Bloom's syndrome lymphocytes, relative to alkylation by mitomycin C (potentially bifunctional), the response to which was described to be normal. However, since a large part of the mitomycin C damage may be due to monoadducts, the nature of the adduct, as well as (or perhaps, rather than) its functionality, may be responsible for accentuated SCE induction.

Patterson *et al.*[225] reported that cells from patients with ataxia telangiectasia exhibited a reduced ability to excise DNA bases damaged by high energy radiation. More recent studies[51] have indicated that the X-ray survival of cells from ataxia telangiectasia patients is well below normal, while survival of cells from heterozygotes was intermediate between that of cells from normal and diseased individuals. However, cells from ataxia telangiectasia patients show normal baseline SCE levels[83,105] as well as a normal SCE response after exposure to X-irradiation, MMC, EMS, and adriamycin.[82]

Cells from patients in complementation groups A, B, C, and D of xeroderma pigmentosum, another hereditary disease with a predisposition for neoplasia, hyperreact to UV irradiation,[21,52,62,263] or alkylating agents,[328] undergoing a much greater increase in SCEs than do identically treated normal cells. SCE induction by UV in lymphocytes from three patients with de Sanctis–Cacchione syndrome (xeroderma pigmentosum plus mental defects) has been found to be normal.[263] Xeroderma pigmentosum cells which exhibit SCE hyperinducibility also have a reduced ability to excise alkylation products (e.g., 6-$O$-methylguanine).[96] This is compatible with the idea that SCE results from DNA damage that has not been removed. However, the relative inducibility of SCE and chromosome breaks in xeroderma pigmentosum cells depends strongly on the type of DNA damage involved.[321,328]

It is interesting to note that, in xeroderma pigmentosum, a hyperinducibility in SCEs correlates with a hyperinducibility of mutations by similar agents.[201] Conversely, in Fanconi's anemia, the hypoinducibility in SCEs, more marked with mitomycin C than with ethylmethane sulfonate, is accompanied by a decrease in the ability of both of these alkylating agents to induce mutations.[75] Thus, even though SCE may reflect only a small fraction of the total damage caused to DNA, it is intriguing to speculate that, at least for certain types of DNA damage, the SCE-inducing component might ultimately prove to be extremely important biologically.

The availability of SCE, chromosome breakage and γ-ray survival analysis complements assays for deficient unscheduled DNA synthesis for the prenatal diagnosis of chromosomal fragility diseases. Published prenatal studies have thus far been limited to xeroderma pigmentosum,[242] and, more recently, Fanconi's anemia.[19] SCE and chromosome breakage studies on pregnancies at risk for Bloom's syndrome and Fanconi's anemia are probably being considered in several laboratories, and additional analogous work can be anticipated. At present, in the absence of an extensive data base on SCE behavior of amniotic fluid cells [which can be highly heterogeneous (see reference 112)], prenatal studies based on SCEs will typically rely on analogy with data on fibroblasts, and should probably be viewed conservatively. Also, in the case of Fanconi's anemia, SCE changes in fibroblasts are minimal, and other data, e.g., alkylating agent-induced structural aberrations,[17,18,19] are important. However, in spite of present limitations, prospects are reasonably good for future utility of cytogenetic studies in the prenatal diagnosis of chromosome fragility diseases.

SCE frequencies have been examined in a number of other human diseases, as well as in a variety of chromosomal abnormalities, generally with weakly positive or negative results. In a subpopulation of bone marrow (and to a lesser extent peripheral blood cells) from patients with megaloblastic anemia, the SCE frequency is elevated.[151] However, SCE formation in one patient with Cockayne's syndrome, a condition in which cells are hypersensitive to both UV light and mitomycin C,[111] appears to be normal,[52] and SCEs in Down's syndrome have been reported to be normal in one study,[330] elevated in a second,[191] and normal in the presence of only BrdUrd but hyperinducible by X-rays and mitomycin C[29] in a third. Also, SCE induction by vaccinia virus appears to be defective in cells from some patients with Down's syndrome.[154] Similarly, SCE frequencies in most individuals with either supernumerary or structurally abnormal chromosomes appear to be normal,[6,290] although isolated examples of abnormal karyotypes with slightly elevated SCEs have been observed.[6] Some of these discrepancies may reflect very slight age dependence of SCE frequencies,[142] different culture conditions, e.g., serum types,[140] the preferential killing of diseased cells by BrdUrd (leading to a higher effective dose of BrdUrd), or perhaps more likely, variations between SCEs in different normal individuals or different samplings from the same individual.[6,57,73,174]

The relationship between aging and sister chromatid exchange frequencies has been examined by Schneider *et al.* Baseline SCE frequencies are not altered by aging either *in vitro* (in late passage cultured cells) or *in vivo*[158,258,259,260] using cells from old individuals, or on examining SCEs formed *in vivo* in old animals. However, with one exception, fewer clastogen induced SCEs were observed in older cells. Assuming that all cells sustained equal levels of drug induced damage, this would suggest that whatever mechanism is responsible for SCE formation is diminished with age. The results obtained with aging cells bear at least a superficial resemblance to some of the data obtained on material from patients with Fanconi's anemia.[186] In both cases, the impact of ascertainment bias in cell scoring due to differential cell survival following clastogen exposure remains to be determined.

# STUDIES OF THE MECHANISM OF SCE FORMATION

Various approaches have been used to investigate the mechanism of SCE formation. For example, factors influencing the extent of SCE induction by different agents have been studied, and considerable effort has been focused on chemical identification of DNA interchange corresponding to sister chromatid exchange formation. However, current knowledge about the actual mechanism of SCE formation remains sketchy.

Kato[137] has examined SCE inducibility in unsynchronized Chinese hamster cells that were allowed to incorporate BrdUrd for one cycle and grow a second cycle in the presence or absence of BrdUrd. SCE induction at a time approximating the last few hours of the second S phase was effected by irradiation with near UV light. Only a small additional increase in SCE was observed in those cells which had incorporated BrdUrd for the second S phase, prompting the suggestion that SCE induction might have multiple pathways, at least one of which was independent of the degree of BrdUrd substitution. However, if SCE induction in a particular chromosome region requires DNA synthesis following damage,[175] then only the regions that had not replicated a second time at the time of irradiation would be susceptible to SCE induction. These would be unifilarily substituted with BrdUrd, independent of the growth protocol used, and no difference in SCE induction would be expected in the two types of cells, whatever the specific mechanisms involved.

Kato[137] also examined the effect of caffeine on SCE induction, and found it to inhibit induction in cells which had undergone one round of BrdUrd incorporation but to stimulate SCE induction, when present during the second S phase, in cells which incorporated BrdUrd for two cycles. Interpretation of this result will depend on the chromosomal location of these additional SCEs. Kato has previously reported[132] that caffeine inhibited SCE induction by UV in Chinese hamster cells, prompting analogy with postreplication repair, while other workers have observed either a potentiation[316] of an inhibition[314] of SCE frequencies with caffeine. Vogel and Bauknecht[314] stressed the importance of the toxicity of caffeine and its effect on selection of metaphases for scoring. Recently Ishii and Bender[127] have determined that SCE potentiation by caffeine requires that the caffeine be added with or soon after the SCE inducer. Also, Basler et al.[23] observed that caffeine increased SCE frequencies *in vivo* in

Chinese hamster bone marrow cells. Caffeine may well exert multiple effects which might be very difficult to dissect.

SCE induction, like mutagenesis[247] may also be influenced by agents, e.g., cysteine,[5] capable of trapping free radicals. However, these results, like those in which the enzymes superoxide dismutase and catalase protect cells from chromosome breakage,[216,217,218] probably deal more with the chemistry of the inducing agent than with alterations in cellular response to the damage induced. A complicating factor is the ability of reducing agents such as ascorbate[85] to induce SCEs. Perhaps, intermediate products formed during reactions deactivating radicals can cause DNA damage. The mechanism by which selenium under some conditions can induce SCEs,[240] and in some cases suppress SCE induction,[128] is not clear at present.

Two types of experimental approaches have been used to search for DNA interchange corresponding to sister chromatid exchange. Both utilize cells which have incorporated BrdUrd for less than one cycle, and thus contain DNA substituted in only one strand. Following sister strand exchange, junctions of substituted and unsubstituted polynucleotide should result and appear as material of intermediate density in alkaline CsCl gradients.[246] The Holliday model[114] for DNA recombination (Fig. 21) also predicts segments of double-substituted heavy–heavy (HH) and light–light (LL) DNA at interchange sites in neutral CsCl gradients.

Rommelaere and Miller-Faures[246] reported the detection of Chinese hamster DNA with intermediate density in alkaline CsCl gradients. However, most of this material exhibited rapid renaturation following neutralization, a result expected for cross-linked DNA. If DNA from the Chinese hamster cells was centrifuged in neutral CsCl, approximately 0.1% of the material exhibited density greater than that of hybrid, heavy–light (HL) DNA and interpretable as containing segments of bifilarly substituted, heavy–heavy (HH) DNA. The amount of this DNA was increased 4-fold by UV irradiation (100 ergs/mm$^2$) prior to BrdUrd incorporation, but the amount of DNA detected was more than 10 times that expected from the number of SCE in these cells.

Moore and Holliday[209] similarly detected 0.1–0.2% "heavy–heavy" DNA from rapidly growing CHO cells cultured not quite one cycle in medium containing BrdUrd. Mitomycin C, when administered in highly toxic amounts (1 μg/ml) five hours prior to harvest, appeared to increase both "heavy–heavy" DNA and SCE. Again, the amount of "heavy–heavy" DNA was much more than expected for the number of SCE observed.

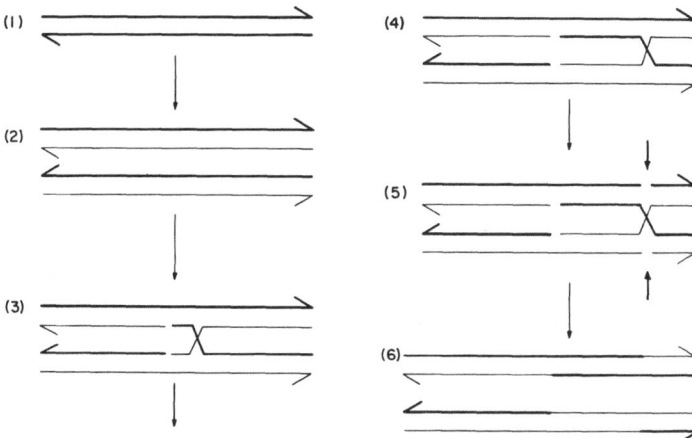

Fig. 21. Formation of heavy–heavy DNA after one cycle of BrdUrd incorporation, according to the Holliday model[114,209] for DNA interchange. Complementary DNA strands are synthesized from a duplex template (1) using BrdUrd (thin line) in place of thymidine (dark line) yielding hybrid density DNA (HL) (2). Following the introduction of single-strand breaks in each duplex, recombination is initiated by the crossing-over of a single strand from one molecule to pair with the complementary strand of the sister DNA duplex, generating a heteroduplex overlap (3). Branch migration can extend the heteroduplex region (4). Recombinant DNA molecules are produced if single strand breaks are introduced into the two outer DNA strands, enabling the two DNA molecules to separate (5). The final product (after the nicks are sealed by ligase) consists of two recombinant DNA molecules with a heteroduplex region in each at the site of exchange (6). At one site there is a small region of HH DNA (DNA containing BrdUrd in both strands); at the other side there is a region of LL DNA (DNA containing TdR in both strands).

An increased amount (6- to 10-fold over a baseline of 0.04%) of "heavy–heavy" DNA in Bloom's syndrome fibroblasts, relative to normal human fibroblasts, has recently been described by Waters et al.[319] and hypothesized to be associated with the elevated SCE frequency in these cells.

In further experiments in which synchronized CHO cells were employed, unusually dense DNA was observed, but it had some properties not expected for HH DNA.[197,198a] Cells which had incorporated BrdUrd for one cycle exhibited a small amount (0.4 ± 0.2%) of DNA banding with a density expected for HH DNA, but this was not increased by addition of sufficient mitomycin C (0.03 μg/ml, at the start of S) to more than triple the SCE frequency (Fig. 22). Significantly, the dense DNA persisted after a subsequent round of replication in the absence of BrdUrd (calling its bifilar substitution into question), and material with a similar

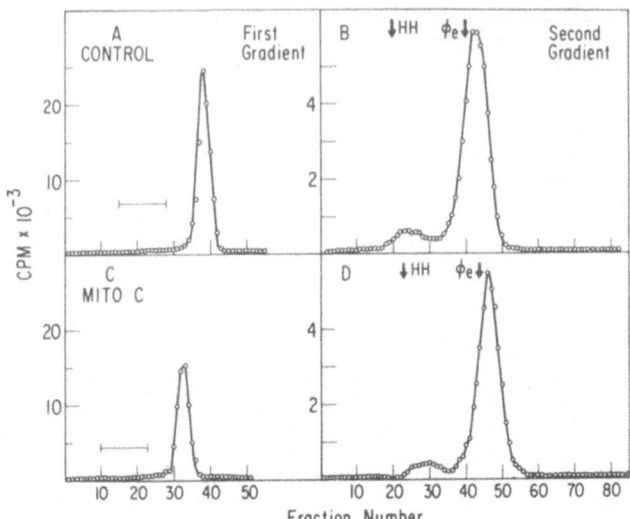

Fig. 22. Density gradient analysis of CHO DNA after one cycle of BrdUrd incorporation. Synchronized CHO cells were released into medium containing [³H]-BrdUrd (5 mCi/ml, 2 × 10⁻⁵ M), and colcemid (0.45 μg/ml) was added after 8 hr. DNA was isolated from metaphase cells 4 hr later, sheared and centrifuged to equilibrium in CsCl. Three-drop fractions were collected and aliquots (10%) were counted: (A) control; (C) 0.03 μg/ml mitomycin C added at the time of release from Gl–S. The indicated fractions were centrifuged with ¹⁴C-labeled DNA and 2-drop fractions were collected onto filters. The second gradients are shown in (B) no mitomycin C; (D) + mitomycin C. The arrows mark the expected position of HH DNA (HH) and the actual position of φₑ DNA. Total radioactivity (CPM): (A) 1.1 × 10⁶, with 6.6 × 10³ in dense DNA (0.65%); (C) 6.7 × 10⁵, with 4.9 × 10³ in dense DNA (0.73%).[197]

density shift from the main band DNA was seen in cells which incorporated [³H]-dT (but not BrdUrd). Moreover, Loveday's recent results[198a] have shown that the "heavy" DNA interacts differently with certain base-specific dyes than does main band DNA, and the former may in fact be a cryptic satellite DNA species. Removal of this (?satellite) DNA might conceivably enable detection of true HH DNA due to SCE formation. While Loveday's data do not rule out the existence of the "heavy–heavy" DNA predicted by the Holliday model, and they do not account for the observations of Waters *et al.*,[319] they suggest that the biochemical evidence thus far claimed for this DNA in CHO cells may be weak, and that additional experiments are necessary to clarify the chemical events associated with DNA interchange during SCE formation.

In spite of the extensive data on SCE formation, the mechanism of the SCE process is unknown. Rather than construct a detailed model from current, incomplete information, an attempt will be made to outline those constraints which, at present, might be placed on future models. Relevant data include the restriction of strands involved in exchanges by the need to conserve DNA polarity, the coupling of SCEs with DNA replication, and the location of SCEs at junctions between cytologically distinct chromatin types, e.g., Q-positive/Q-negative bands or euchromatin/heterochromatin. Numerous reports of unusually high or low SCE frequencies within heterochromatin suggest that SCE formation is somehow sensitive to DNA sequence repetition, a result potentially compatible with suggestions[278] that SCE formation may, via unequal crossing over, mediate[161] alterations in the amount of repeated DNA in individual chromatids. Perhaps the orientation of any such DNA-exchange-related sequence repetition, i.e., tandem vs. inverted, might determine whether or not a DNA interchange led to a visible SCE or to an alteration in chromatid DNA content.

A more definitive evaluation of the Holliday model as it relates to SCEs is essential. In addition to other factors, it might be noted that this model, which envisions recombinational events to involve staggered DNA interchange, may be more appropriate for meiotic recombination, which occurs *after* semiconservative DNA synthesis is complete, than SCEs, which presumably occur *during* DNA synthesis, perhaps at the growing point of semiconservative DNA replication. Interchange of only one polynucleotide chain at a DNA synthesis growing point might create a double helical discontinuity capable of producing a chromatid break. The cross-link bypass model for SCE formation might circumvent this problem, but does not account for the ability of monofunctional alkylating agents or single strand breaks caused by light plus BrdUrd to induce SCEs. Analysis of the fate of cross-links during DNA replication and SCE formation might permit a more definitive evaluation of this model.

The relatively low proportion of DNA damage sites (by 8-methoxypsoralen) converted into SCEs suggests that SCE is just one of many sequelae, perhaps involving special DNA repair machinery, to several different types of DNA damage. A requirement for special types of DNA sequence repeats at the site of DNA damage in order for the damage response to cause an SCE might in part account for this low relative frequency. Such a constraint would be consistent with SCE localization data. Elucidation of the type of sequence repeat, if any, involved in SCE formation might also ultimately relate to the junctional structure and extent of double helical DNA interchange occurring as part of the exchange process.

ACKNOWLEDGMENTS. Research in the authors' laboratory reviewed in this article was supported by grants (GM 21121 and HD 04807, CD-36D, and 1-353, from the National Institutes of Health, the American Cancer Society, and the National Foundation March of Dimes, respectively). S. L. and K. L. are recipients of a Research Career Development Award (GM 00122, from the National Institute of General Medical Sciences) and a postdoctoral fellowship (PF-1223, from the American Cancer Society), respectively. We thank Dr. Stephen Bloom for making available to us some of his unpublished data on SCE induction in chick embryos and Dr. A. V. Carrano and associates for permission to include their data comparing SCE induction and mutagenesis.

# REFERENCES

1. Aaronson, M. W., Nichols, W. W., Miller, R. C., and Meadows, A. T., Sister chromatid exchange in childhood cancer, Lake Yamanaka SCE Conference, July, 1978.
2. Abe, S., and Sasaki, M., Chromosome aberrations and sister chromatid exchanges in Chinese hamster cells exposed to various chemicals, *J. Nat. Cancer Inst.* **58**:1635–1641 (1977).
3. Abe, S., and Sasaki, M., Studies in chromosomal aberrations and sister chromatid exchanges induced by chemicals, *Proc. Jpn. Acad.* **53**:46–49 (1977).
4. Adolph, K., Cheng, S. M., Paulson, J. R., and Laemmli, J. K., Isolation of a protein scaffold from mitotic Hela cell chromosomes, *Proc. Nat. Acad. Sci. USA* **74**:4937–4941 (1977).
5. Abramovsky, I., Vorsanger, G., and Hirschhorn, K., Sister chromatid exchange induced by X-ray of human lymphocytes and the effect of L-cysteine, *Mutat. Res.* **50**:93–100 (1978).
6. Alhadeff, B., and Cohen, M. M., Frequency and distribution of sister chromatid exchanges in human peripheral lymphocytes, *Israel J. Med. Sci.* **12**:1440–1447 (1976).
6a. Allen, J. W., BrdU-dye characterization of late replication and meiotic recombination in Armenian hamster germ cells, *Chromosoma* **74**: 189–207 (1979).
7. Allen, J. W., and Latt, S. A., Analysis of sister chromatid exchange formation *in vivo* in mouse spermatogonia as a new test system for environmental mutagens, *Nature (London)* **260**:449–451 (1976).
8. Allen, J. W., and Latt, S. A., *In vivo* BrdU–33258 Hoechst analysis of DNA replication kinetics and sister chromatid exchange formations in mouse somatic and meiotic cells, *Chromosoma* **58**:325–340 (1976).
9. Allen, J. W., Shuler, C. F., Mendes, R. W., and Latt, S. A., A simplified technique

for *in vivo* analysis of sister chromatid exchanges using 5-bromodeoxyuridine tablets. *Cytogenet. Cell Genet.* **18**:231–237 (1977).

10. Allen, J. W., Shuler, C. F., and Latt, S. A., Extension of BrdU-dye analysis of DNA replication and sister chromatid exchange formation to *in vivo* systems. *Stadler Symp.* **9**:9–36 (1977).

11. Allen, J. W., Shuler, C. F., and Latt, S. A., BrdU tablet methodology for *in vivo* studies of DNA synthesis, *Somat. Cell Genet.* **4**:393–405 (1978).

12. Alves, P., and Jonasson, J., New staining method for the detection of sister chromatid exchanges in BrdU labelled chromosomes, *J. Cell Sci.* **32**:185–195 (1978).

13. Ames, B. N., McCann, J., and Yamasaki, E., Methods for detecting carcinogens and mutagens with the salmonella/mammalian-microsome mutagenicity test, *Mutat. Res.* **31**:347–364 (1975).

14. Angell, R. R., and Jacobs, P. A., Lateral asymmetry in human constitutive heterochromatin, *Chromosoma* **51**:301–310 (1975).

15. Angell, R. R., and Jacobs, P. A., Lateral asymmetry in human constitutive heterochromatin: Frequency and inheritance, *Am. J. Hum. Genet.* **30**:144–152 (1978).

16. Arndt-Jovin, D., and Jovin, T. M., Analysis and sorting of live cells according to DNA content, *J. Histochem. Cytochem.* **25**:585–589 (1977).

17. Auerbach, A. D., and Wolman, S. R., Susceptibility of Fanconi's anemia fibroblasts to chromosome damage by carcinogens, *Nature (London)* **261**:494–496 (1976).

18. Auerbach, A. D., and Wolman, S. R., Carcinogen-induced chromosome breakage in Fanconi's anemia heterozygous cells, *Nature (London)* **271**:69–71 (1978).

19. Auerbach, A. D., Warburton, D., Bloom, A. D., and Chaganti, R. S. K., Prenatal diagnosis of the Fanconi anemia gene by cytogenetic methods, *Am. J. Hum. Genet.* **31**:77–81 (1979).

20. Balaban-Malenbaum, G. and Gilbert, F., Origin of double minute chromosomes in human neuroblastoma cells, *Am. J. Hum. Genet.* **29**:21A (1978).

21. Bartram, C. R., Koske-Westphal, T., and Passarge, E., Chromatid exchange in ataxia telangiectasia, Bloom's syndrome, Werner's syndrome, and xeroderma pigmentosum. *Ann. Hum. Genet.* **40**:79–86 (1976).

22. Bartram, C. R., Rudiger, H. W., and Passarge, E., Frequency of sister chromatid exchanges in Bloom's syndrome fibroblasts reduced by cocultivation with normal cells. *Hum. Genet.* **46**:331–334 (1979).

23. Basler, A., Bachmann, U., Roszinsky-Kocher, G., and Rohrborn, G., Effects of caffeine on sister-chromatid exchanges (SCE) *in vivo*, *Mut. Res.* **59**:209–214 (1979).

24. Bauknecht, T., Vogel, W., Bayer, U., and Wild, D., Comparative *in vivo* mutagenicity testing by SCE and micronucleus induction in mouse bone marrow, *Hum. Genet.* **35**:299–307 (1977).

25. Bayer, U., The *in vivo* induction of sister chromatid exchanges in the bone marrow of the Chinese hamster II. N-nitrosodiethylamine (DEN) and N-isopropyl-α-(2-methyl-hydrazino)-p-toluamide (Natulan), two carcinogenic compounds with specific mutagenicity problems, *Mutat. Res.* **56**:305–309 (1978).

26. Bayer, U., and Bauknecht, Th., The dose dependence of sister chromatid exchanges in the *in vivo* bone marrow test with Chinese hamsters induced by 3-hydrocarbons, *Experientia* **33**:25 (1977).

27. Beek, B., and Obe, G., The human leukocyte test system. VI. The use of sister chromatid exchanges as possible indicators for mutagenic activities, *Humangenetik* **29**:127–134 (1975).

28. Benedict, W. F., Banerjee, A., and Venkatesan, N., Cyclophosphamide induced on-

cogenic transformation, chromosomal breakage, and sister chromatid exchange following microsomal activation, *Cancer Res.* **38**:2922–2924 (1978).

29. Biederman, B., and Bowen, P., Sister chromatid exchanges in Down syndrome, *Mamm. Chrom. Newsletter* **18**:12 (1977).

30. Bigger, C. A. H., Tomaszewski, J. W., and Dipple, A., Differences between products of binding of 7,12-dimethylbenz(α)anthracene to DNA in mouse skin and in a rat liver microsomal system, *Biochem. Biophys. Res. Commun.* **80**:229–235 (1978).

31. Bloom, S., Chick embryos for detecting environmental mutagens, in: Chemical *Mutagens*, Vol. 5 (A. Hollaender and F. DeSerres, eds.), pp. 203–232, Plenum Press, New York (1978).

32. Bloom, S. E., Detection of sister chromatid exchanges *in vivo* using avian embryos, in: *Cytogenetic Testing of Environmental Mutagens* (T. C. Hsu, ed.) (1979) (in press).

33. Bloom, S. E., and Hsu, T. C., Differential fluorescence of sister chromatids in chicken embryos exposed to 5-bromo-deoxyuridine, *Chromosoma* **51**:261–267 (1975).

34. Bloomfield, C. D., Kurvink, K., Levitt, S., and Cervenka, J., Sister chromatid exchange (SCE) in lymphocytes from patients with malignant lymphomas, *Cancer Res.* **19**, Abstr. No. 503 (1978).

35. Boobis, A. R., Reinhold, C., and Thorgiersson, S. S., Induction of aryl hydrocarbon (benzo(α)pyrene) hydroxylase and 2-acetylaminofluorene *N*-hydroxylase by polycyclic hydrocarbons in regenerating liver from inbred strains of mice, *Biochem. Pharm.* **26**:1501–1505 (1977).

36. Bostock, C. J., and Christie, S., Analysis of the frequency of sister chromatid exchange in different regions of chromosomes of the kangaroo rat, *Chromosoma* **56**:275–287 (1976).

37. Bradley, M. O., Hsu, T. C., and Harris, C. C., Varying relationships between sister chromatid exchanges, mutagenicity, and DNA damage (Abstract Ed-14), *10th Annual Meeting, Environmental Mutagenesis Society*, March, 1979.

38. Brewen, J. G., and Peacock, W. J., Restricted rejoining of chromosomal subunits in aberration formation. A test for subunit dissimilarity, *Proc. Nat. Acad. Sci. USA* **62**:389–394 (1968).

39. Brewen, J. G., and Peacock, W. J., The effect of tritiated thymidine on sister chromatid exchange in a ring chromosome, *Mutat. Res.* **7**:433–440 (1969).

40. Brown, R. L., and Crossen, P. E., Increased incidence of sister chromatid exchanges in Rauscher leukemia virus infected mouse embryo fibroblasts, *Exp. Cell Res.* **103**:418–420 (1976).

41. Brown, R. F., and Wu, Y., Induction of sister chromatid exchanges in Chinese hamster cells by chlorpropamide, *Mutat. Res.* **56**:215–217 (1977).

41a. Bryant, E. M., Hoehn, H., and Martin, G. M., Normalization of sister chromatid exchange frequencies in Bloom's syndrome by euploid cell hybridization, *Nature (London)* **279**:795–796 (1979).

42. Burgdorf, W., Kurvink, K., and Cerevenka, J., Elevated sister chromatid exchange rate in lymphocytes of subjects treated with arsenic, *Hum. Genet.* **36**:69–72 (1977).

43. Burkholder, G. D., Reciprocal Giemsa staining of late DNA replicating regions produced by low and high pH sodium phosphate, *Exp. Cell Res.* **111**:489–492 (1978).

44. Burkholder, G. D., and Wang, H. C., Electron microscopy of differentially BrdU-substituted sister chromatids treated with sodium phosphate, *Chromosoma* **70**:101–107 (1978).

45. Carrano, A. V., and Johnston, G. R., The distribution of mitomycin C-induced sister chromatid exchanges in the euchromatin and heterochromatin of the Indian muntjac, *Chromosoma* **64**:97–107 (1977).

46. Carrano, A. V., Thompson, L. H., Lindl, P. A., and Minkler, J. L., Sister chromatid exchange as an indicator of mutagenesis, *Nature (London)* **271**:551–553 (1978).
47. Carrano, A. V., Thompson, L. H., Stetka, D. G., Minkler, J. L., Mazrimas, J. A., and Fong, S., DNA crosslinking, sister chromatid exchange, and specific locus mutations, *Mutat. Res.* **63**:175–188 (1979).
48. Carrano, A. V., and Wolff, S., Distribution of sister chromatid exchanges in the euchromatin and heterochromatin of the Indian muntjac, *Chromosoma* **53**:361–369 (1975).
49. Carter, D. M., Wolff, K., and Schnedl, W. J., 8-methoxypsoralen and UVA promote sister chromatid exchanges, *J. Invest. Dermatol.* **67**:548–551 (1976).
50. Chaganti, R. S. K., Schonberg, S., and German, J., A manyfold increase in sister chromatid exchanges in Bloom's syndrome lymphocytes, *Proc. Nat. Acad. Sci. USA* **71**:4508–4512 (1974).
51. Chen, P. C., Lavin, M. F., Kidson, C., and Moss, D., Identification of ataxia telangiectasia heterozygotes, a cancer prone population, *Nature (London)* **274**:484–486 (1978).
52. Cheng, W. S., Tarone, R. F., Andrews, A. D., Whang-Peng, J. S., and Robbins, J. H., Ultraviolet light-induced sister chromatid exchanges in xeroderma pigmentosum and in Cockayne's syndrome lymphocyte cell lines, *Cancer Res.* **38**:1601–1609 (1978).
53. Cole, R. S., Repair of DNA containing intrastrand cross-links in *Escherichia coli*: Sequential excision and recombination, *Proc. Nat. Acad. Sci. USA* **70**:1064–1068 (1973).
54. Comings, D. E., Isolabelling not compatible with single stranded model, *Nature New Biol.* **229**:24–25 (1971).
55. Comings, D. E., The distribution of sister chromatids at mitosis in Chinese hamster cells, *Chromosoma* **29**:428–433 (1970).
56. Craig-Holmes, A. P., and Shaw, M. W., Effects of six carcinogens on SCE frequency and cell kinetics in cultured human lymphocytes, *Mutat. Res.* **46**:375–384 (1977).
57. Crossen, P. E., Drets, M. E., Arrighi, F. E., and Johnston, D. A., Analysis of the frequency and distribution of sister chromatid exchanges in cultured human lymphocytes, *Hum. Genet.* **35**:345–352 (1977).
58. Darzynkiewicz, A., Andreeff, M., Traganos, F., Sharpless, T., and Melamed, M. R., Discrimination of cycling and noncycling lymphocytes by BUdR-suppressed acridine orange fluorescence in a flow cytometric system, *Exp. Cell Res.* **115**:31–36 (1978).
59. DeRaat, W. K., The induction of sister chromatid exchanges by cyclophosphamide in the presence of differently induced microsomal fractions of rat liver, *Chem. Biol. Int.* **19**:125–131 (1977).
60. DeRaat, W. K., Induction of sister chromatid exchanges by styrene and its presumed metabolite styrene oxide in the presence of rat liver homogenate, *Chem. Biol. Interact.* **20**:163–170 (1978).
61. DeRaat, W. K., Comparison of the induction by cigarette smoke condensates of sister chromatid exchanges in Chinese hamster cells and of mutations in *Salmonella typhimurium*, *Mut. Res.* **66**:253–259 (1979).
62. DeWeerd-Kastelein, E. A., Keijzer, W., Rainaldi, G., and Boostma, D., Induction of sister chromatid exchanges in xeroderma pigmentosum cell after exposure to ultraviolet light, *Mutat. Res.* **45**:253–261 (1977).
63. Djordjevic, B., and Szybalski, W., Genetics of human cell lines. III. Incorporation of 5-bromo- and 5-iododeoxyuridine into the deoxyribonucleic acid of human cells and its effect on radiation sensitivity, *J. Exp. Med.* **112**:509–531 (1960).
64. Dolfini, S. F., Sister chromatid exchanges in *Drosophila melanogaster* cell lines *in vitro*, *Chromosoma* **69**:339–347 (1978).

65. Dutrillaux, B., Couturier, J., Viegas-Pequignot, E., and Schaison, G., Localization of chromatid breaks in Fanconi's anemia, using three consecutive stains. *Hum. Genet.* **37**:65–71 (1977).

66. Dutrillaux, B., Fosse, A. M., Prieur, M., and LeJeune, J., Analyses des échanges de chromatides dans les cellules somatiques humaines. *Chromosoma* **48**:327–340 (1974).

67. Dutrillaux, B., Laurent, C., Couturier, J., and LeJeune, J., Coloration des chromosomes humains par l'acridine orange après traitement par 5-bromodéoxyuridine. *C. R. Acad. Sci. Ser. D* **276**:3179–3181 (1973).

68. Emanuel, B. S., Compound lateral asymmetry in human chromosome 6: BrdU-dye studies of 6q12 → 6q14, *Am. J. Hum. Genet.* **30**:153–159 (1978).

69. Evans, H. J., Adams, A. C., Clarkson, J. M., and German, J., Chromosome aberrations and unscheduled DNA synthesis in X- and UV-irradiated lymphocytes from a boy with Bloom's syndrome and a man with xeroderma pigmentosum, *Cytogenet. Cell Genet.* **20**:124–140 (1978).

70. Evans, L. A., Kevin, M. J., and Jenkins, E. C., Human sister chromatid exchange caused by methylazoxymethanol acetate, *Mutat. Res.* **56**:51–58 (1977).

71. Fabricant, J. D., Hofnung, M. J., and Kelly, F., Sister chromatid exchange induction by mitomycin C is deficient in embryonal carcinoma cells (Abstract EC-14), 10th Annual Meeting, Environmental Mutagenesis Society, March, 1979.

72. Faed, M. J. W., and Mourelatos, D., Enhancement by caffeine of sister chromatid exchange frequency in lymphocytes from normal subjects after treatment by mutagens, *Mutat. Res.* **49**:437–440 (1978).

73. Falek, A., Madden, J. J., and Shafer, D. A., Interindividual differences in mutagenic sensitivity in human lymphocytes, *Am. J. Hum. Genet.* **30**:118A (1978).

74. Farrel, S. A., and Worton, R. C., Chromosome loss is responsible for segregation at the HPRT locus in Chinese hamster cell hybrids, *Somat. Cell Genet.* **3**:539–551 (1977).

75. Finkelberg, R., Buchwald, M., and Sminovich, L., Decreased mutagenesis in cells from patients with Fanconi's anemia, *Am. J. Hum. Genet.* **29**:42a (1977).

76. Finkelberg, R., Thompson, M. W., and Siminovich, L., Survival after treatment with EMS, X-rays, and mitomycin C of skin fibroblasts from patients with Fanconi's anemia, *Am. J. Hum. Genet.* **26**:30a (1974).

77. Fujiwara, Y. and Tatsumi, M., Repair of mitomycin C damage to DNA in mammalian cells and its impairment in Fanconi's anemia cells, *Biochem. Biophys. Res. Commun.* **66**:592–598 (1975).

78. Fujiwara, Y., Tatsumi, M., and Sasaki, M. S., Cross-link repair in human cells and its possible defect in Fanconi's anemia cells, *J. Mol. Biol.* **113**:634–649 (1977).

79. Funes-Cravioto, F., Kolmodin-Hedman, B., Lindsten, J., Nordenskjolo, M., Apata Gayon, G., Lambert, B., Norberg, G., Olin, R., and Swensson, A., Chromosome aberrations and sister chromatid exchanges in workers in chemical laboratories and a rotoprinting factory and in children of women laboratory workers, *Lancet* **ii**:322–325 (1977).

80. Furukawa, M., Sirianni, S. R., Tan, J. C., Huang, C. C., Sister chromatid exchanges and growth inhibition by the flame retardant Tris (2,3 dibromopropyl phosphate) in Chinese hamster cells, *J. Nat. Canc. Inst.* **60**:1179–1181 (1978).

81. Galley, W. C. and Purkey, R. M., Spin-orbital probes of biomolecular structure. A model DNA-acridine system, *Proc. Nat. Acad. Sci. USA* **69**:2198–2202 (1972).

82. Galloway, S. M., Ataxia telangiectasia: The effects of chemical mutagens and X-rays on S.C.E. in blood lymphocytes, *Mutat. Res.* **45**:343–349 (1977).

83. Galloway, S. M., and Evans, H. J., Sister chromatid exchange in human chromosomes from normal individuals and patients with ataxia telangiectasia, *Cytogenet. Cell Genet.* **15**:17–29 (1975).

84. Galloway, S. M. and Evans, H. J., Asymmetrical C-bands and satellite DNA in man, *Exp. Cell Res.* **94**:454–459 (1975).

85. Galloway, S. M. and Painter, R. B., Vitamin C is positive in DNA synthesis inhibition and sister chromatid exchange tests, *Mutat. Res.* **60**:321–327 (1979).

86. Galloway, S., and Wolff, S., The relationship between chemically induced sister chromatid exchanges and chromatid breakage, *Mutat. Res.* **61**:297–307 (1979).

87. Gatti, M., Pimpinelli, S., Santini, G., and Olivieri, G., Lack of spontaneous sister chromatid exchange (S.C.E.) in somatic cells of *Drosophila melanogaster*, *Genetics* **91**:255–274 (1979).

88. Gaynor, A. L., and Carter, D. M., Greater promotion in sister chromatid exchanges by trimethylpsoralen than by 8-methoxypsoralen in the presence of UV-light, *J. Invest. Dermat.* **71**:257–259 (1978).

89. Gebhart, E., and Kappauf, H., Bleomycin and sister chromatid exchanges in human lymphocyte chromosomes, *Mutat. Res.* **58**:121–124 (1978).

90. German, J., Cytological evidence for crossing-over *in vitro* in human lymphoid cells, *Science* **144**:298–301 (1964).

91. German, J., Genes which increase chromosomal instability in somatic cells and predispose to cancer, *Prog. Med. Genet.* **8**:61–101 (1972).

92. German, J., Schonberg, S., Loue, E., and Chaganti, R. S. K., Bloom's syndrome. IV. Sister chromatid exchanges in lymphocytes, *Am. J. Hum. Genet.* **29**:248–255 (1977).

93. Gianelli, F., Benson, P. F., Pawsey, S. A., and Polani, P. E., Ultraviolet light sensitivity and delayed DNA-chain maturation in Bloom's syndrome fibroblasts, *Nature (London)* **265**:466–469 (1977).

94. Gibas, Z., and Limon, J., Isolabeling of the long arm of the human Y chromosome demonstrated by the FPG technique, *Chromosoma* **69**:113–120 (1978).

95. Gibson, D. A., and Prescott, D. M., Induction of sister chromatid exchanges in chromosomes of rat kangaroo cells by tritium incorporated into DNA, *Exp. Cell Res.* **74**:397–402 (1972).

96. Goth-Goldstein, R., Repair of DNA damage by alkylating carcinogens is defective in xeroderma pigmentosum-derived fibroblasts, *Nature (London)* **267**:81–92 (1977).

97. Goto, K., Akematsu, T., Shimazu, H., and Sugiyama, T., Simple differential Giemsa staining of sister chromatids after treatment with photosensitive dyes and exposure to light and the mechanism of staining, *Chromosoma* **53**:223–230 (1975).

98. Goto, K., Maeda, S., Kano, Y., Sugiyama, T., Factors involved in differential Giemsa staining of sister chromatids, *Chromosoma* **66**:351–359 (1978).

99. Gratzner, H. G., Pollack, A., Ingram, D. J., and Lief, R. C., Deoxyribonucleic acid replication in single cells and chromosomes by immunologic techniques, *J. Histochem. Cytochem.* **24**:34–39 (1976).

100. Grisham, J. W., in: *Drugs and Cell Cycle* (A. M. Zimmerman, G. M. Padilla, and I. Z. Cameron, eds.), pp. 95–136, Academic Press, New York (1973).

101. Gurtoo, H. L., Bejba, N., and Minowada, J., Properties, inducibility, and an improved method of analysis of aryl hydrocarbon hydroxylase in cultured human lymphocytes, *Cancer Res.* **35**:1235–1243 (1975).

102. Gurtoo, H. L., Minowada, J., Paigen, B., Parker, N. B., and Hayner, N. T., Factors influencing the measurement and the reproducibility of aryl hydrocarbon hydroxylase activity in cultured human lymphocytes, *J. Nat. Cancer Inst.* **59**:787–798 (1977).

103. Hand, R., and German, J., Bloom's syndrome: DNA replication in cultured fibroblasts and lymphocytes, *Hum. Genet.* **38**:297–306 (1977).

104. Hansteen, I. L., Hillestad, L., Thiis-Evensen, E., and Heldas, S. S., Effects of vinyl chloride in man; a cytogenetic follow-up study, *Mutat. Res.* **51**:271–278 (1978).

105. Hatcher, N. H., Brinson, P. S., Hook, E. B.: Sister chromatid exchanges in ataxia telangiectasia, *Mutat. Res.* **35**:333–336 (1976).
106. Hayashi, K., and Schmid, W., The rate of sister chromatid exchanges parallel to spontaneous chromosome breakage in Fanconi's anemia and to trenimon-induced aberrations in human lymphocytes and fibroblasts, *Humangenetik* **29**:201–206 (1975).
107. Heddle, J. A., Whissel, D., and Bodycote, J. D., Changes in chromosome structure induced by radiation: a test of the two chief hypotheses, *Nature (London)* **221**:159–160 (1969).
108. Henderson, P. T., and Kersten, K. J., Metabolism of drugs during rat liver regeneration, *Biochem. Pharmacol.* **19**:2343–2351 (1970).
109. Herreros, B. and Giannelli, F., Spatial distribution of old and new chromatid subunits and frequency of chromatid exchanges in induced human lymphocyte endoreduplications, *Nature (London)* **182**:286–288 (1967).
110. Hirsch-Kauffmann, M., Schweiger, M., Wagner, E. F., and Sperling, K., Deficiency of DNA ligase activity in Fanconi's anemia, *Hum. Genet.* **45**:25–32 (1978).
111. Hoar, D. I. and Waghorne, C. W., DNA repair in Cockayne syndrome, *Am. J. Hum. Genet.* **30**:590–601 (1978).
112. Hoehn, H., Bryant, E. M., Karp, L. E., and Martin, G. M., Cultured cells from diagnostic amniocentesis in second trimester pregnancies. I. Clonal morphology and growth potential, *Ped. Res.* **8**:746–754 (1974).
113. Hollander, D. H., Tockman, M. S., Liang, Y. W., Borgaonkar, D. S., and Frost, J. K., Sister chromatid exchanges in the peripheral blood of cigarette smokers and in lung cancer patients; and the effect of chemotherapy, *Hum. Genet.* **44**:167–171 (1978).
114. Holliday, R., A mechanism for gene conversion in fungi, *Genet. Res.* **5**:282–304 (1964).
115. Hotta, Y., and Stern, H., Absence of satellite DNA synthesis during meiotic prophase in mouse and human spermatocytes, *Chromosoma* **69**:323–330 (1978).
116. Hsu, T. C., and Pathak, S., Differential rates of sister chromatid exchanges between euchromatin and heterochromatin, *Chromosoma* **58**:269–273 (1976).
117. Huang, C. C., Induction of a high incidence of damage to the X chromosomes of *Rattus (Mastomys) natalensis* by base analogues, viruses and carcinogens, *Chromosoma* **23**:162–179 (1967).
118. Huang, C. C., and Furukawa, M., Sister chromatid exchanges in human lymphoid lines cultured in diffusion chambers in mice, *Exp. Cell Res.* **111**:458–461 (1978).
119. Hunke, M. H. and Carpenter, N. J., Effects of diphenylhydantoin on the frequency of sister chromatid exchanges in human lymphocytes, *Am. J. Hum. Genet.* **30**:83A (1978).
120. Hutchinson, F., The lesions produced by ultraviolet light in DNA containing 5-bromouracil, *Q. Rev. Biophys.* **6**:201–246 (1973).
121. Huttner, K. M. and Ruddle, F. H., Study of mitomycin C-induced chromosomal exchange, *Chromosoma* **56**:1–13 (1975).
122. Igali, S., Bridges, B. A., Ashwood-Smith, M. J., and Scott, B. R., Mutagenesis in *E. coli*. IV. Photosensitization to near UV by 8-methoxypsoralen, *Mutat. Res.* **9**:20–30 (1970).
123. Ikushima, T., Role of sister chromatid exchanges in chromatid aberration formation, *Nature (London)* **268**:235–236 (1977).
124. Ikushima, T., and Wolff, S., Sister chromatid exchanges induced by light-flashes to 5-bromodeoxyuridine and 5-iododeoxyuridine-substituted Chinese hamster chromosomes, *Exp. Cell Res.* **87**:15–19 (1974).
125. Ishidate, M. and Odashima, S., Chromosome tests with 134 compounds on Chinese hamster cells *in vitro*—a screening for chemical carcinogens, *Mutat. Res.* **48**:337–354 (1977).

126. Ishii, Y., and Bender, M., Factors influencing the frequency of mitomycin C-induced sister chromatid exchanges in 5-bromodeoxyuridine substituted human lymphocytes in culture, *Mutat. Res.* **51**:411–418 (1978).

127. Ishii, Y., and Bender, M., Caffeine inhibition of prereplication repair of mitomycin C-induced DNA damage in human peripheral lymphocytes, *Mutat. Res.* **51**:419–425 (1978).

128. Jacobs, M. M., Inhibitory effects of selenium on 1,2-dimethylhydrazine and methylazoxymethanol colon carcinogenesis, *Cancer* **40**:2557–2564 (1977).

129. Kakati, S., Abe, S., and Sandberg, A. A., Sister chromatid exchange in Philadelphia chromosome (Ph)-positive leukemia, *Cancer Res.* **38**:2918–2921 (1978).

130. Kanda, N., and Kato, H., A simple technique for *in vivo* observation of SCE in mouse ascites tumor and spermatogonial cells, *Exp. Cell Res.* **118**:431–435 (1979).

131. Kaplan, J. C., Zamansky, G. B., Black, P. H., and Latt, S. A., Parallel induction of sister chromatid exchanges and infectious virus from SV-40 transformed cells by alkylating agents, *Nature (London)* **271**:662–663 (1978).

132. Kato, H., Induction of sister chromatid exchanges by UV light and its inhibition by caffeine, *Exp. Cell Res.* **82**:382–390 (1973).

133. Kato, H., Spontaneous sister chromatid exchanges detected by BudR-labelling method, *Nature (London)* **251**:70–72 (1974).

134. Kato, H., Induction of sister chromatid exchanges by chemical mutagens and its possible relevance to DNA repair, *Exp. Cell Res.* **85**:239–247 (1974).

135. Kato, H., Possible role of DNA synthesis in function of sister chromatid exchanges, *Nature (London)* **252**:739–741 (1974).

136. Kato, H., Is isolabelling a false image?, *Exp. Cell Res.* **89**:416–420 (1974).

137. Kato, H., Mechanisms for sister chromatid exchanges and their relation to the production of chromosome aberrations, *Chromosoma* **59**:179–191 (1977).

138. Kato, H., Spontaneous and induced sister chromatid exchanges as revealed by the BudR-labelling method, *Int. Rev. Cytol.* **37**:55–95 (1977).

139. Kato, H., and Sandberg, A. A., Effects of herpes simplex virus on sister chromatid exchange and chromosome abnormalities in human diploid fibroblasts, *Exp. Cell Res.* **109**:423–427 (1977).

140. Kato, H., and Sandberg, A. A., The effect of sera on sister chromatid exchanges *in vitro*, *Exp. Cell Res.* **109**:445–448 (1977).

141. Kato, H., and Shimada, H., Sister chromatid exchanges induced by mitomycin C: A new method of detecting DNA damage at the chromosomal level, *Mutat. Res.* **28**:459–464 (1975).

142. Kato, H., and Stich, N. F., Sister chromatid exchanges in aging and repair-deficient human fibroblasts, *Nature (London)* **260**:447–448 (1976).

143. Kihlman, B. A., Sister chromatid exchanges in *Vicia faba*. II. Effects of thiotepa, caffeine, and 8-ethoxy caffeine in the frequency of S.C.E.s, *Chromosoma* **51**:11–18 (1975).

144. Kihlman, B. A., Andersson, H. C., and Natarajan, A. T., Molecular mechanisms in the production of chromosomal aberrations: Studies with the 5-bromodeoxyuridine-labelling method, in: *Chromosomes Today*, Vol. 6 (A. de Chapelle and M. Sorsa, eds.), pp. 287–296, Elsevier/North Holland, Amsterdam (1977).

145. Kihlman, B. A., and Kronberg, D., Sister chromatid exchanges in *Vicia Faba* I. Demonstration by a modified fluorescence plus Giemsa (FPG) technique, *Chromosoma* **51**:1–10 (1975).

146. Kihlman, B. A., Natarajan, A. T., and Andersson, H. C., Use of the 5-bromodeoxyuridine-labelling technique for exploring mechanisms involved in the formation of chromosomal aberrations, *Mut. Res.* **52**:181–198 (1978).

147. Kihlman, B. A., and Sturelid, S., Effects of caffeine on the frequencies of chromosomal aberrations and sister chromatid exchanges induced by chemical mutagens in root tips of *Vicia faba*, *Hereditas* **88**:35–41 (1978).

148. Kim, M. A., Chromatid Austausch und Heterochromatin Veränderungen menschlicher Chromosomen nach BrdU-Markierung, *Humangenetik* **25**:179–188 (1974).

149. Kinsella, A. R., and Radman, M., Tumor promoter induces sister chromatid exchanges: Relevance to mechanisms of carcinogens, *Proc. Natl. Acad. Sci. USA* **75**:6149–6153 (1978).

150. Kligerman, A. D., and Bloom, S. E., Sister chromatid differentiation and exchanges in adult mudminnows (*Umbra limi*) after *in vivo* exposure to 5-bromodeoxyuridine, *Chromosoma* **56**:101–109 (1976).

151. Knuutila, S., Helmined, E., Vuopio, P., and de La Chapelle, A., Increased sister chromatid exchange in megaloblastic anemia. Studies on bone marrow cells and lymphocytes, *Hereditas* **89**:175–181 (1978).

152. Knuutila, S., Helmined, E., Vuopio, P., and de la Chapelle, A., Sister chromatid exchanges in human bone marrow cells. I. Control subjects and patients with leukemia, *Hereditas* **88**:189–196 (1978).

153. Knuutila, S., Maki-Paakkanen, J., Kahkonen, M., and Hookanen, G., An increased frequency of chromosomal changes and S.C.E.s in cultured blood lymphocytes of 12 subjects vaccinated against smallpox, *Hum. Genet.* **41**:89–96 (1978).

154. Knuutila, S., Harkki, A., Ellimaki, K., and Salunen, R., Decreases sister chromatid exchange in Down's syndrome after measles vaccination, *Hereditas* **90**:149–150 (1979).

155. Korenberg, J. R., and Freedlender, E., Giemsa technique for the detection of sister chromatid exchanges, *Chromosoma* **48**:355–360 (1974).

156. Kram, D., Bynum, G. D., Senula, G. C., and Schneider, E. L., *In utero* detection of sister chromatid exchanges: A new assay for transplacental mutagens, *Nature (London)* **279**:531 (1979).

157. Kram, D., and Schneider, E. L., Reduced frequencies of mitomycin C-induced sister chromatid exchanges in AKR mice, *Hum. Genet.* **41**:45–51 (1978).

158. Kram, D., Schneider, E. L., Tice, R. R., and Gianas, P., Aging and sister chromatid exchange I. The effect of aging on mitomycin-C induced sister chromatid exchange frequencies in mouse and rat bone marrow cells *in vivo*, *Exp. Cell Res.* **114**:471–475 (1978).

159. Krepinsky, A. B., Heddle, J. A., Rainbow, A. J., and Kwok, E., Sensitivity of Bloom's syndrome cells to specific mutagens (Abstract Ed-14), 10th Annual Meeting, Environmental Mutagenesis Society, March, 1979.

160. Kuhn, E. M., Mitotic chiasmata and other quadriradials in mitomycin C-treated Bloom's syndrome lymphocytes, *Chromosoma* **66**:287–297 (1978).

161. Kurnit, D. M., Satellite DNA and heterochromatin variants. The case for unequal mitotic crossing over, *Hum. Genet.* **47**:169–186 (1979).

162. Kurvink, K., Bloomfield, C. D., and Cervenka, J., Sister chromatid exchange in patients with viral disease, *Exp. Cell Res.* **113**:450–453 (1978).

163. Kurvink, K., Bloomfield, C. D., Keenen, K. M., Levitt, S., and Cervenka, J., Sister chromatid exchange in lymphocytes from patients with malignant lymphoma, *Hum. Genet.* **44**:137–144 (1978).

164. Lambert, B., Hansson, K., Lindsten, J., Sten, M., and Werelius, B., Bromodeoxyuridine-induced sister chromatid exchanges in human lymphocytes, *Hereditas* **83**:163–174 (1976).

165. Lambert, B., Linblad, A., Nordenskjold, M., and Werelius, B., Increased frequency of sister chromatid exchanges in cigarette smokers, *Hereditas* **88**:147–149 (1978).

166. Lambert, B., Morad, M., Bredberg, A., Swanbeck, G., and Thyresson-Hok, M., Sister chromatid exchanges in patients treated with psoralen and UV light, *Mutat. Res.* **46**:228–229 (1977).

167. Lambert, B., Ringborg, U., and Lindblad, A., Prolonged increase of sister-chromatid exchanges in lymphocytes of melanoma patients after CCNA treatment, *Mut. Res.* **59**:295–300 (1979).

168. Langenbach, R., Freed, H. J., Raveh, D., and Huberman, E., Cell specificity in metabolic activation of aflatoxin B and benzo($\alpha$)pyrene to mutagens for mammalian cells, *Nature (London)* **276**:277–280 (1978).

169. Latt, S. A., Microfluorometric detection of deoxyribonucleic acid replication in human metaphase chromosomes, *Proc. Nat. Acad. Sci. USA* **70**:3395–3399 (1973).

170. Latt, S. A., Localization of sister chromatid exchanges in human chromosomes, *Science* **185**:74–76 (1974).

171. Latt, S. A., Sister chromatid exchanges, indices of human chromosome damage and repair: detection by fluorescence and induction by mitomycin C, *Proc. Nat. Acad. Sci. USA* **71**:3162–3166 (1974).

172. Latt, S. A., Longitudinal and lateral differentiation of metaphase chromosomes based on the detection of DNA synthesis by fluorescence microscopy, in: *Chromosomes Today*, Vol. 5 (P. L. Pearson and K. R. Lewis, eds.), pp. 367–394, Wiley, New York (1976).

173. Latt, S. A., Fluorescent probes of chromosome structure and replication, *Can. J. Genet. Cytol.* **19**:603–623 (1977).

174. Latt, S. A., and Juergens, L., Determinants of sister exchange frequencies in human chromosomes, in: *Population Cytogenetics* (E. B. Hood and I. Porter, eds.), pp. 217–236, Academic Press, New York (1976).

175. Latt, S. A., and Loveday, K. S., Characterization of sister chromatid exchange induction by 8-methoxypsoralen plus near UV light, *Cytogenet. Cell Genet.* **21**:184–200 (1978).

176. Latt, S. A., and Stetten, G., Spectral studies on 33258 Hoechst and related bisbenzimidazole dye, useful for fluorescent detection of deoxyribonucleic acid synthesis, *J. Histochem. Cytochem.* **24**:24–33 (1976).

177. Latt, S. A., and Wohlleb, J. C., Optical studies of the interaction of 33258 Hoechst with DNA, chromatin, and metaphase chromosomes, *Chromosoma* **52**:297–316 (1975).

178. Latt, S. A., George, Y. S., and Gray, J. W., Flow cytometric analysis of BrdU-substituted cells stained with 33258 Hoechst, *J. Histochem. Cytochem.* **25**:927–934 (1977).

179. Latt, S. A., Allen, J. W., Rogers, W. E., and Juergens, L. A., *In vitro* and *in vivo* analysis of sister chromatid exchange formation, in: *Handbook of Mutagenicity Test Procedures* (B. Kilbey, C. Ramel, and W. Nichols, eds.), pp. 275–291, Elsevier/North Holland, Amsterdam (1977).

180. Latt, S. A., Allen, J. W., Shuler, C., Loveday, K. S., and Monroe, S. H., The detection and induction of sister chromatid exchanges, in: *Molecular Human Cytogenetics, VII ICN-UCLA Symposium on Molecular and Cellular Biology* (R. S. Sparkes, D. E. Comings, and C. F. Fox, eds.), pp. 315–334, Plenum Press, New York (1977).

181. Latt, S. A., Allen, J. W., and Stetten, G., *In vitro* and *in vivo* analysis of chromosome structure replications, and repair using BrdU–33258 Hoechst techniques, in: *International Cell Biology, 1976–1977*, Rockefeller University Press, New York (1977).

182. Latt, S. A., Davidson, R. L., Lin, M. S., and Gerald, P. S., Lateral asymmetry in the fluorescence of human Y chromosomes stained with 33258 Hoechst, *Exp. Cell Res.* **87**:425–429 (1974).

183. Latt, S. A., Munroe, S. H., Disteche, C., Rogers, W. E., and Cassell, D. M., Uses

of fluorescent dyes to study chromosome structure and replication, in: *Chromosomes Today*, Vol. 6 (A. de La Chapelle and M. Sorsa, eds.), pp. 27–36, Elsevier, Amsterdam (1977).

184. Latt, S. A., Schreck, R. R., Loveday, K. S., and Shuler, C. F., *In vitro* and *in vivo* analysis of sister chromatid exchange, *Pharmacol. Rev.* (1979) (in press).

185. Latt, S. A., Schreck, R. R., Loveday, K. S., and Shuler, C. F., Sister chromatid exchange analysis: Methodology, applications and interpretation, in: *Cytogenetic Testing of Environmental Mutagens* (T. C. Hsu, ed.), (1979) (in press).

186. Latt, S. A., Stetten, G., Juergens, L. A., Buchanan, G. R., and Gerald, P. S., Induction by alkylating agents of sister chromatid exchanges and chromatid breaks in Fanconi's anemia, *Proc. Nat. Acad. Sci. USA* **72**:4066 (1975).

187. Latt, S. A., Stetten, G., Juergens, L. A., Willard, H. F., and Scher, C. D., Recent developments in the detection of deoxyribonucleic acid synthesis by 33258 Hoechst fluorescence, *J. Histochem. Cytochem.* **23**:493–505 (1975).

188. Lavappa, K. S., and Yerganian, G., Spermatogonial and meiotic chromosomes of the Armenian hamster *Cricetulus migratius*, *Exp. Cell Res.* **61**:159–172 (1970).

189. Lau, Y. F., Hittleman, W. N., and Arrighi, F. E., Sister chromatid differential staining pattern in prematurely condensed chromosomes, *Experientia* **32**:917–918 (1976).

190. Legator, M. S., and Malling, H. V., The host-mediated assay, a practical procedure for evaluating potential mutagenic agents in mammals, in: *Chemical Mutagens*, Vol. 2 (A. Hollaender, ed.), pp. 569–589, Plenum Press, New York (1971).

191. Lezana, E. A., Bianchi, N. O., Bianchi, M. S., and Zabala-Suarez, J. E., Sister chromatid exchanges in Down syndrome and normal human beings, *Mutat. Res.* **45**:85–90 (1977).

192. Lehmann, A. R., and Bridges, B. A., DNA repair, *Essays Biochem.* **13**:71–119 (1977).

193. Lin, M. S. and Alfi, O. S., Detection of sister chromatid exchanges by 4'-6-diamidino-2-phenylindole fluorescence, *Chromosoma* **57**:219–225 (1976).

194. Lin, M. S., Comings, D. E., and Alfi, O. S., Optical studies of the interaction of 4'-6-diamidino-2-phenylindole with DNA and metaphase chromosomes, *Chromosoma* **60**:15–25 (1977).

195. Lin, M. S., Latt, S. A., and Davidson, R. L., Microfluorometric detection of asymmetry in the centromeric region of mouse chromosomes, *Exp. Cell Res.* **86**:392–394 (1974).

196. Loewe, H., and Urbanietz, J., Basisch substituierte 2,6-Bisbenzimidazolderivate, eine neue chemotherapeutisch active Körperklasse, *Arzneim. Forsch.* **24**:1927–1933 (1974).

197. Loveday, K. S., and Latt, S.A., Search for DNA interchange corresponding to sister chromatid exchanges in Chinese hamster ovary cells, *Nuc. Acid Res.* **5**:4087–4104 (1978).

198. Loveday, K. S., and Latt, S. A., The effect of a tumor promoter, 12-*O*-tetradecanoyl-phorbol-13-acetate (TPA) on sister chromatid exchange formation in cultured Chinese hamster cells, *Mut. Res.* **67**:343–348 (1979).

198a Loveday, K. S., and Latt, S. A., Is there biochemical evidence for sister chromatid exchange formation?, *Am. J. Hum. Genet.* **31**:103A (1979).

199. McCann, J., Choi, E., Yamaski, E., and Ames, B. N., Detection of carcinogens as mutagens in the salmonella/microsome test; assay of 300 chemicals, *Proc. Nat. Acad. Sci. USA* **72**:5135–5139 (1975).

200. McKenzie, W. H., and Hall, S. H., Conventional aberration and sister chromatid exchange analysis of human lymphocytes exposed to ozone *in vivo*, *Am. J. Hum. Genet.* **30**:73A (1978).

201. Maher, V. M., Ouelette, L. M., Curren, R. D., and McCormick, J. J., Frequency of

ultraviolet light-induced mutations is higher in xeroderma pigmentosum variant cells than in normal cells, *Nature (London)* **261:**593–595 (1976).

202. Marin, G., and Prescott, D. M., The frequency of sister chromatid exchanges following exposure to varying doses of ³H-thymidine or X-rays, *J. Cell Biol.* **21:**159–167 (1964).
203. Marquardt, H., and Bayer, U., The induction *in vivo* of sister chromatid exchanges in the bone marrow of the Chinese hamster, *Mutat. Res.* **56:**169–176 (1977).
204. Martin, C. N., McDermid, A. D., and Garner, R. C., Testing of known carcinogens and noncarcinogens for their ability to induce unscheduled DNA synthesis in HeLa cells, *Cancer Res.* **38:**2621–2627 (1978).
205. Mutsushima, T., Sanamura, M., Umezawa, K., and Sigimura, T., Induction of SCE by quercetin and suppression of SCE by elastatinal, a microbial protease, Meeting on SCEs, Lake Yamanaka, Japan, July, 1978.
206. Mazrimas, J. A., and Stetka, D. G., Direct evidence for the role of incorporated BudR in the induction of sister chromatid exchanges, *Exp. Cell Res.* **117:**23–30 (1978).
207. Meyn, M. S., Rossman, T., and Troll, W., A protease inhibitor blocks SOS functions in *Escherichia coli*: Antipain prevents repressor inactivation, ultraviolet mutagenesis, and filamentous growth, *Proc. Nat. Acad. Sci. USA* **74:**1152–1156 (1977).
208. Miller, R. C., Aaronson, M. M., and Nichols, W. W., Effects of treatment on differential staining of BrdU labeled metaphase chromosomes: three way differentiation of M₃ chromosomes, *Chromosoma* **55:**1–11 (1976).
208a Monticone, R. E., and Schneider, E. L., Induction of sister chromatid exchanges in human cells by fluorescent light, *Mutat. Res.* **59:**215–221 (1979).
209. Moore, P. D., and Holliday, R., Evidence for the formation of hybrid DNA during mitotic recombination in Chinese hamster cells, *Cell* **8:**573–579 (1976).
210. Morgan, W. F., and Crossen, P. E., The frequency and distribution of sister chromatid exchanges in human chromosomes, *Hum. Genet.* **38:**271–278 (1977).
211. Mourelatos, D., Faed, J. J. W., and Johnson, B. E., Sister chromatid exchanges in human lymphocytes exposed to 8-methoxypsoralen and long wave UV radiation prior to incorporation of bromodeoxyuridine, *Experientia* **33:**1091–1093 (1977).
212. Natarajan, A. T., Tates, A. D., Van Buul, P. P. W., Meijers, M., and DeVogel, N., Cytogenetic effects of mutagens/carcinogens, after activation in a microsomal system *in vitro*. I. Induction of chromosome aberrations and sister chromatid exchanged by diethylnitrosamine (DEN) and dimethylnitrosamine (DMN) in CHO cells in the presence of rat liver microsomes, *Mutat. Res.* **37:**83–90 (1976).
213. Nevstad, N. P., Sister chromatid exchanges and chromosome aberrations induced in human lymphocytes by the cytostatic drug adriamycin, *in vivo* and *in vitro*, *Mutat. Res.* **57:**253–258 (1978).
214. Nichols, W. W., Bradt, C. I., Toji, L. H., Godley, M., and Segawa, M., Induction of sister chromatid exchanges by transformation with simian virus 40, *Cancer Res.* **38:**906–964 (1978).
215. Nilsson, K., and Ponten, J., Classification and biological nature of established human hematopoietic cell lines, *Int. J. Cancer* **15:**321–341 (1975).
216. Nordenson, I., Beckman, G., and Beckman, L., The effect of superoxide dismutase and catalase on radiation-induced chromosome breaks, *Hereditas* **80:**125–126 (1976).
217. Nordenson, I., Effect of superoxide dismutase and catalase on spontaneously occurring chromosome breaks in patients with Fanconi's anemia, *Hereditas* **86:**147–150 (1977).
218. Nordenson, I., Chromosome breaks in Werner's syndrome and their prevention *in vitro* by radical-scavenging enzyme, *Hereditas* **87:**151–154 (1977).
219. Obe, G., and Ristow, H., Acetaldehyde, but not ethanol induces sister-chromatid exchanges in Chinese hamster cells in vitro, *Mutat. Res.* **56:**211–213 (1977).

220. Otter, M., Palmer, C. G., and Baehner, R. L., Elevated sister chromatid exchange rate in childhood acute lymphoblastic leukemia, *Cancer Res.* **19,** Abstract No. 808 (1978).
221. Pal, K., Tierney, B., Gover, P. L., and Sims, P., Induction of sister chromatid exchanges in Chinese hamster ovary cells treated *in vitro* with non-K-region dihydrodiols of 7-methylbenz(α)anthracene and benzo(α)pyrene, *Mutat. Res.* **30:**367–375 (1978).
222. Palitti, F., and Becchetti, A., Effect of caffeine on sister chromatid exchanges and chromosomal aberrations induced by mutagens in Chinese hamster cells, *Mutat. Res.* **45:**157–159 (1977).
223. Palmer, C. G., 5-Bromodeoxyuridine-induced constrictions in human chromosomes, *Can. J. Genet. Cytol.* **12:**816–830 (1970).
224. Pathak, S., Ward, O. G., and Hsu, T. C., Rate of sister chromatid exchanges in mammalian cells differing in diploid numbers, *Experientia* **33:**875–876 (1977).
225. Patterson, M. C., Smith, B. P., Lohman, P. H., Anderson, A. K., and Fishman, L., Defective excision repair of X-ray damaged DNA in human (ataxia telangiectasia) fibroblasts, *Nature (London)* **260:**444–446 (1976).
226. Peacock, W. J., Replication, recombination, and chiasmata in *Gonices australasiae, Genetics* **65:**593–617 (1970).
227. Pedrini, A. M., Dalpra, L., Ciarrocchi, G., Pedrali Noy, G. C. F., Spadari, S., Nuzzo, F., and Falaschi, A., Levels of some enzymes acting on DNA in xeroderma pigmentosum, *Nuc. Acids Res.* **1**(2):193–202 (1974).
228. Peleg, L., Raz, E., and Ben-Ishai, R., Changing capacity for DNA excision repair in mouse embryonic cells *in vitro, Exp. Cell Res.* **104:**301–307 (1976).
229. Pera, R., and Mattias, P., Labelling of DNA and differential sister chromatid staining after BrdU treatment *in vivo, Chromosoma* **57:**13–18 (1976).
230. Perry, P., Use of sister chromatid exchange techniques for cytological detection of mutagen carcinogen exposure. *Mutat. Res.* **46**(Abstr.):205 (1977).
231. Perry, P., Chemical mutagens and sister chromatid exchange, in: *Chemical Mutagens,* Vol. 6 (A. Hollaender and F. deSerres, eds.), Plenum Press, New York (1979).
232. Perry, P., and Evans, H. J., Cytological detection of mutagen-carcinogen exposure by sister chromatid exchange, *Nature (London)* **258:**121–124 (1975).
233. Perry, P. E., and Searle, C. E.; Induction of sister chromatid exchanges in Chinese hamster cells by the hair dye constituents 2-nitro-*p*-phenylene diamine and 4-nitro-1-phenylenediamine, *Mutat. Res.* **56:**207–210 (1977).
234. Perry, P., and Wolff, S., New Giemsa method for differential staining of sister chromatids, *Nature (London)* **261:**156–158 (1974).
235. Polani, P. E., Crolla, J. A., Seller, M. J., and Moir, F., Meiotic crossing over exchange in the female mouse visualized by BUdR substitution. *Nature (London)* **278:**348–349 (1979).
236. Poon, P. K., O'Brien, R. L., and Parker, J. W., Defective DNA repair in Fanconi's anemia, *Nature (London)* **250:**223–225 (1974).
237. Popescu, N. C., Turnbull, D., and DiPaolo, J. A., Sister chromatid exchanges/chromosome aberration analysis with the use of several carcinogens and noncarcinogens, *J. Nat. Canc. Inst.* **59:**289–293 (1977).
238. Potten, C. S., Hume, W. J., Reid, P., and Cairns, J., The segregation of DNA in epithelial stem cells, *Cell* **15:**899–906 (1978).
239. Raposa, T., Sister chromatid exchange studies for monitoring DNA damage and repair capacity after cytostatics *in vitro* and in lymphocytes of leukaemic patients under cytostatic therapy, *Mutat. Res.* **57:**241–251 (1978).
240. Ray, J. H., and Altenburg, L. C., Cytogenetic effects of activated selenium, *Am. J. Hum. Genet.* **30:**92A (1978).

241. Razin, S. V., Mantieva, V. L., and Georgiev, G. P., DNA adjacent to attachment points of deoxyribonucleoprotein fibril to chromosomal axial structure is enriched in reiterated base sequences, *Nuc. Acids Res.* **5**:4737–4751 (1978).

242. Regan, J. D., Stetlow, R. B., Kaback, M. M., Klein, E., Xeroderma pigmentosum: A rapid sensitive method for prenatal diagnosis, *Science* **174**:147–150 (1971).

243. Remsen, J. F., and Cerutti, P. A., Deficiency of gamma ray excision repairs in skin fibroblasts from patients with Fanconi's anemia, *Proc. Nat. Acad. Sci. USA* **73**:2419–2423 (1976).

244. Renault, G., Pot-Deprun, J., and Chouroulinkov, I., Induction d'échanges entre chromatides soeurs *in vivo* sur les cellules de moelle osseuse de souris AKR. *C. R. Acad. Sci. Ser. D* **286**:887–890 (1978).

245. Ristow, H., and Obe, G., Acetaldehyde induces cross-links in DNA and causes sister chromatid exchanges in human cells, *Mutat. Res.* **58**:115–119 (1978).

246. Rommelaere, J., and Miller-Faures, A., Detection by density equilibrium centrifugation of recombinant-like DNA molecules in somatic mammalian cells, *J. Mol. Biol.* **98**:195–218 (1975).

247. Rosin, M. P., and Stich, H. F., The inhibitory effect of cysteine on the mutagenic activities of several carcinogens, *Mutat. Res.* **54**:73–81 (1978).

248. Rudiger, H. W., Kohl, F., Mangeles, W., Von Wichert, P., Bartram, C. R., Wohler, W., and Passarge, E., Benzpyrene induces sister chromatid exchanges in cultured human lymphocytes, *Nature (London)* **262**:290–292 (1976).

248a Rudiger, H. W., Haenisch, F., Metzler, M., Oesch, F., and Glatt, H. R., Metabolites of diethylstilbesterol induce sister chromatid exchange in human cultured fibroblasts, *Nature (London)* **281**:392–394 (1979).

249. Rupp, W. D., and Howard-Flanders, P., Discontinuities in the DNA synthesis in an excision defective strain of *Escherichia coli* following ultraviolet irradiation, *J. Mol. Biol.* **31**:291–304 (1968).

250. Rupp, W. D., Wilde, C. E., III, Reno, D. L., and Howard-Flanders, P. J., Exchanges between DNA strains in ultraviolet irradiated *Escherichia coli*, *J. Mol. Biol.* **61**:25–44 (1971).

251. Russev, G., and Tsanev, R., Application of precursors adsorbed onto activated charcoal for labeling of mammalian DNA *in vivo*, in: *Methods in Cell Biology*, Vol. IX (Prescott, D. M., ed.), pp. 115–122, Academic Press, New York (1975).

252. Sakanishi, S., and Takayama, S., Reverse differential staining of sister chromatid after substitution with BUdR and incubation in sodium phosphate solution, *Exp. Cell Res.* **115**:448–450 (1978).

253. Sasaki, M., Is Fanconi's anemia defective in a process essential to the repair of DNA crosslinks?, *Nature (London)* **257**:501–503 (1975).

254. Sasaki, M. S., Sister chromatid exchange and chromatid interchange as possible manifestation of different DNA repair processes, *Nature (London)* **269**:623–625 (1977).

255. Sasaki, M. S., and Tonomura, A., A high susceptibility of Fanconi's anemia to chromosome breakage by DNA crosslink agents, *Cancer Res.* **33**:1829–1835 (1973).

256. Scheres, J. M. J. C., Hustinx, T. W. J., Ruttem, F. J., and Merkx, G. F. M., "Reverse" differential staining of sister chromatids, *Exp. Cell Res.* **109**:466–468 (1977).

257. Schneider, E. L., Chaillet, J., and Tice, R., *In vivo* BrdU labelling of mammalian chromosomes, *Exp. Cell Res.* **100**:396–399 (1976).

258. Schneider, E. L. and Gilman, B., Sister chromatid exchanges and aging III. The effect of donor age on mutagen-induced sister chromatid exchange in human diploid fibroblasts, *Hum. Genet.* **46**:57–63 (1979).

259. Schneider, E. L., Kram, D., Nakanishi, Y., Monticone, R. E., Tice, R. R., Gilman,

G. A., and Nieder, M. L., The effect of aging on sister chromatid exchange, *Mech. Ageing Dev.* **9**:303–311 (1979).

260. Schneider, R. L., and Monticone, R. E., Cellular aging and sister chromatid exchange II. Effect of *in vitro* passage of human fetal lung fibroblasts on baseline and mutagen induced sister chromatid exchange frequency level, *Exp. Cell Res.* **115**:269–276 (1978).

261. Schneider, E. L., Sternberg, H., and Tice, R. R., *In vivo* analysis of cellular replication, *Proc. Nat. Acad. Sci. USA* **74**:2041–2044 (1977).

262. Schonwald, A. D., Bartram, C. R., and Rudiger, H. W., Benzpyrene-induced sister chromatid exchanges in lymphocytes of patients with lung cancer, *Hum. Genet.* **36**:261–264 (1977).

263. Schonwald, A. D. and Passarge, E., UV-light induced sister chromatid exchanges in xeroderma pigmentosum lymphocytes, *Hum. Genet.* **36**:213–218 (1977).

264. Schreck, R. R., Paika, I. J., and Latt, S. A., *In vivo* induction of sister chromatid exchanges (S.C.E.) in liver and marrow cells by drugs requiring metabolic activation, *Mutat. Res.* **64**:315–328 (1979).

265. Schubert, I., Sturelid, S., Dobel, P., and Rieger, R., Intra-chromosomal distribution patterns of mutagen-induced SCEs and chromatid aberrations in reconstructed karyotypes of *Vicia faba*, *Mut. Res.* **59**:27–38 (1979).

266. Schvartzman, J., and Cortes, F., Sister chromatid exchanges in *Allium cepa*, *Chromosoma* **62**:119–131 (1977).

267. Schwartz, A. L., Cole, F. S., Fiedorek, R., Matthews, D., Paika, I., Frantz, I. D., and Latt, S. A., Effect of phototherapy on sister chromatid exchange in premature infants, *Lancet* **ii**:157–158 (1978).

268. Schwarzacher, H. G., and Schnedl, W., Endoreduplication in human fibroblast cultures, *Cytogenetics* **4**:1–18 (1965).

269. Shafer, D. A., Replicative bypass model of sister chromatid exchanges, implications for Bloom's syndrome and Fanconi's anemia, *Hum. Genet.* **39**:177–190 (1977).

270. Shiriashi, Y., Chromosome aberrations induced by monomeric acrylamide in bone marrow and germ cells of mice, *Mutat. Res.* **57**:313–324 (1978).

271. Shiriashi, Y., The sister chromatid exchange and the DNA repair replication in human chromosomes, *Proc. Jpn. Acad.* **54**(Ser. B):179–182 (1978).

272. Shiriashi, Y., Freeman, A. I., and Sandberg, A. A., Increased sister chromatid exchange in bone marrow and blood cells from Bloom's syndrome, *Cytogenet. Cell Genet.* **17**:162–173 (1976).

273. Shiriashi, Y., and Sandberg, A. A., Effects of mitomycin C on normal and Bloom's syndrome cells, *Mutat. Res.* **49**:239–248 (1978).

274. Shiriashi, Y., and Sandberg, A. A., The relationship between sister chromatid exchanges and chromosome aberrations in Bloom's syndrome, *Cytogenet. Cell Genet.* **18**:13–23 (1977).

275. Shuler, C. F., and Latt, S. A., Sister chromatid exchange test in Chinese hamster cheek pouch mucosa, *J. Dental Res.* **578**:211 (1978).

276. Shuler, C. F. and Latt, S. A., Sister chromatid exchange induction resulting from systemic, topical and systemictopical presentations of carcinogens, *Cancer Res.* **39**:2510–2514 (1979).

277. Sirianni, S. R., and Huang, C. C., Sister chromatid exchange induced by promutagens/carcinogens in Chinese hamster cells cultured in diffusion chambers in mice, *Proc. Soc. Exp. Biol. Med.* **158**:269–274 (1978).

278. Smith, G. P., Evolution of repeated DNA sequences by unequal crossover, *Science* **191**:528–535 (1976).

279. Solomon, E., and Bobrow, M., Sister chromatid exchanges: A sensitive assay of agents damaging human chromosomes, *Mutat. Res.* **30**:273–278 (1975).

280. Sperling, K., Goll, U., Kunze, J., Ludtke, E. K., Tolksdorf, M. and Obe, G., Cytogenetic investigations in a new case of Bloom's syndrome, *Hum. Genet.* **31**:47–52 (1976).

281. Stern, H., and Hotta, Y., Biochemical controls of meiosis, *Ann. Rev. Genet.* **7**:37–66 (1973).

282. Stern, R. S., Thibodeau, L. A., Kleinerman, R. A., Parrish, J. A., and Fitzpatrick, T. B., Risk of cutaneous carcinoma in patients treated with oral methoxsalen photochemotherapy for psoriasis, *New Eng. J. Med.* **300**:809–318 (1979).

283. Stetka, D., and Carrano, A. V., The interaction of Hoechst 33258 and BrdU substituted DNA in the formation of sister chromatid exchanges, *Chromosoma* **63**:21–31 (1977).

284. Stetka, D. G., Minkler, J., and Carrano, A. V., Induction of long-lived chromosome damage as manifested by sister chromatid exchange in lymphocytes of animal exposed to mitomycin-C, *Mutat. Res.* **51**:383–396 (1978).

285. Stetka, D. G., and Wolff, S., Sister chromatid exchanges as an assay in genetic damage induced by mutageniccarcinogens I. *In vivo* test for compounds requiring metabolic activation, *Mutat. Res.* **41**:333–342 (1976).

286. Stetka, D. G., and Wolff, S.: Sister chromatid exchanges as an assay for genetic damage induced by mutageniccarcinogens. II. *In vitro* test for compounds requiring metabolic activation, *Mutat. Res.* **41**:343–350 (1976).

287. Stetten, G., Latt, S. A., and Davidson, R. L., 33258 Hoechst enhancement of the photosensitivity of bromodeoxyuridine-substituted cells, *Somat. Cell Genet.* **2**:285–290 (1976).

288. Stetten, G., Davidson, R. L., and Latt, S. A., 33258 Hoechst enhances the selectivity of the bromodeoxyuridine-light method of isolating contitional lethal mutants, *Exp. Cell Res.* **108**:447–452 (1977).

289. Stoll, C., Borgaonkar, D., and Levy, J. M., Effect of vincristine on sister chromatid exchanges of normal human lymphocytes, *Cancer Res.* **36**:2710–2713 (1976).

290. Stoll, C., Borgaonkar, D. S., and Bigel, P., Sister chromatid exchanges in balanced translocational carriers and in patients with unbalanced karyotypes, *Hum. Genet.* **37**:27–32 (1977).

291. Swartzendruber, D. G., Microfluorometric analysis of cellular DNA following incorporation of bromodeoxyuridine, *J. Cell Physiol.* **90**:445–454 (1977).

292. Swartzendruber, D. G., A bromodoexyuridine (BudR)–mithramycin technique for detecting cycling and noncycling cells by flow microfluorometry, *Exp. Cell Res.* **109**:439–443 (1977).

293. Swift, M., Fanconi's anemia in the genetics of neoplasia, *Nature (London)* **230**:370–373 (1971).

294. Swift, M., Malignant neoplasms in heterozygous carriers of genes for certain autosomal recessive syndrome, in: *Genetics of Human Cancer* (J. J. Mulvihill, R. W. Miller, and J. E. Fraumeni, Jr., eds.), pp. 209–215, Raven Press, New York (1977).

295. Swift, M., Sholman, L., Perry, M., and Chase, C., Malignant neoplasms in the families of patients with ataxia telangiectasis, *Cancer Res.* **36**:209–216 (1976).

296. Takayama, S., and Sakanishi, S., Differential Giemsa staining of sister chromatids after extraction with acids, *Chromosoma* **64**:109–115 (1977).

297. Takehisa, S., and Wolff, S., Induction of sister chromatid exchanges in Chinese hamster cells by carcinogenic mutagens requiring metabolic activation, *Mutat. Res.* **45**:263–270 (1977).

298. Takehisa, S., and Wolff, S., The induction of sister chromatid exchanges in Chinese hamster ovary cells by prolonged exposure to 2-acetylaminofluorene and S-9 mix, *Mutat. Res.* **58**:103–106 (1978).

299. Taylor, J. H., Sister chromatid exchanges in tritiumlabelled chromosomes, *Genetics* **43**:515–529 (1958).

300. Taylor, J. H., Distribution of tritium-labelled DNA among chromosomes during meiosis I. Spermatogenesis in the grasshopper, *J. Cell Biol.* **25**:57–67 (1965).

301. Taylor, J. H., Woods, P. S., and Hughes, W. L., The organization and duplication of chromosomes as revealed by autoradiographic studies using tritium-labelled thymidine, *Proc. Nat. Acad. Sci. USA* **43**:122–128 (1957).

302. Tease, C., Cytological detection of crossing-over in BudR substituted meiotic chromosomes using the fluorescent plus Giemsa technique, *Nature (London)* **272**:823–824 (1978).

303. Tease, C., and Jones, G. H., Analysis of exchanges in differentially stained meiotic chromosomes of *Locusta migratoria* after BrdU-substitution and FPG staining. I. Crossover exchanges in monochiasmate bivalents, *Chromosoma* **69**:163–178 (1978).

304. Thust, R., Warzok, R., Grund, E., and Mendel, J., Use of human-liver microsomes from kidney-transplant donors for the induction of chromatid aberrations and sister-chromatid exchanges by means of pre-carcinogens in Chinese hamster cells *in vitro*, *Mutat. Res.* **51**:397–402 (1978).

305. Tice, R., Chaillet, J., and Schneider, E. L., Evidence derived from sister chromatid exchanges of restricted rejoining of chromatid sub-units, *Nature (London)* **256**:642–644 (1975).

306. Tice, R., Windler, G., and Rary, J. M., Effect of cocultivation on sister chromatid exchange frequencies in Bloom's syndrome and normal fibroblast cells, *Nature (London)* **273**:538–540 (1978).

307. Treiff, N. M., Cantell-Fort, G., Smart, V. B., Kempen, R. R., and Kilian, D. J., Appraisal of fluorometric assay hydrocarbon (benzo($\alpha$)pyrene) hydroxylase in cultured human lymphocytes, *Brit. J. Canc.* **38**:335–338 (1978).

308. Trosko, J. E., Chu, E. H. Y., and Carrier, W. C., The induction of thymidine dimers in ultraviolet-irradiated mammalian cells, *Radiat. Res.* **24**:667–672 (1965).

309. Turnbull, D., Popescu, N. C., DiPaolo, J. A., and Myhr, B. C., *cis*-Platinum (II) diamine dichloride causes mutation, transformation, and sister chromatid exchanges in cultured mammalian cells, *Mut. Res.* **66**:267–275 (1979).

310. Ueda, N., Uenaka, H., Akematsu, T., and Sugiyama, T., Parallel distribution of sister chromatid exchanges and chromosome aberrations, *Nature (London)* **262**:581–583 (1976).

311. Utakoji, T., and Hosoda, K., High-concentration thymidine and sister chromatid exchanges in Chinese hamster cells *in vitro*, Lake Yamanaka SCE Conference, July, 1978.

312. van Buul, P. P. W., Natarajan, A. T., and Verdegaal-Immerzeel, A. M., Suppression of the frequencies of sister chromatid exchanges in Bloom's syndrome fibroblasts by co-cultivation with Chinese hamster cells, *Hum. Genet.* **44**:187–189 (1978).

313. Vogel, W., and Bauknecht, T., Differential chromatid staining by in vivo treatment as a mutagenicity test system, *Nature (London)* **260**:448–449 (1976).

314. Vogel, W., and Bauknecht, Th., Effects of caffeine on sister chromatid exchange (S.C.E.) after exposure to UV light or triaziquone studies with a fluorescence plus Giemsa (FPG) technique, *Hum. Genet.* **40**:193–198 (1978).

315. Vosa, C. G., Sister chromatid exchange bias in *Vicia Faba* chromosomes, in: *Current Chromosome Research* (K. Jones and P. E. Brandham, eds.), pp. 105–114 Elsevier/North-Holland, Amsterdam (1977).

316. Waksvik, H., Brogger, A., and Stene, J., Psoralen/UVA treatment and chromosomes. I. Aberrations and sister chromatid exchange in human lymphocytes *in vitro* and synergism with caffeine, *Hum. Genet.* **38:**195–207 (1977).

317. Walen, K. H., Spatial relationships in the replication of chromosomal DNA, *Genetics* **51:**915–929 (1965).

318. Walker, A. P., and Dumars, K. W., Commonly used pediatric drugs, sister chromatid exchanges, and the cell cycle, *Am. J. Hum. Genet.* 110A (1978).

319. Waters, R., Regan, J. D., and German, J., Increased amounts of hybrid (heavy/heavy) DNA in Bloom's syndrome fibroblasts, *Biochem. Biophys. Res. Comm.* **83**(2):536–541 (1978).

320. Witkin, E. M., Ultraviolet mutagenesis and inducible DNA repair in *Escherichia coli*, *Bacteriol. Rev.* **40:**869–907 (1976).

321. Wolff, S., Sister chromatid exchanges, *Ann. Rev. Genet.* **11:**183–201 (1977).

322. Wolff, S., and Perry, P., Differential Giemsa staining of sister chromatids and the study of sister chromatid exchanges without autoradiography, *Chromosoma* **48:**341–353 (1974).

323. Wolff, S., and Perry, P., Insights of chromatid structure from sister chromatid exchange ratios and the lack of both isolabelling and heterolabelling as determined by the FPG technique, *Exp. Cell Res.* **93:**23–30 (1975).

324. Wolff, S., and Rodin, B., Saccharin-induced sister chromatid exchanges in Chinese hamster and human cells, *Science* **200:**543–545 (1978).

325. Wolff, S., Bodycote, J., and Painter, R. B., Sister chromatid exchanges induced in Chinese hamster cells by UV irradiation at different stages of the cell cycle: The necessity of cells to pass through S, *Mutat. Res.* **25:**73–81 (1974).

326. Wolff, S., Bodycote, J., Thomas, G. H., and Cleaver, J. E., Sister chromatid exchanges in xeroderma pigmentosum cells that are defective in DNA excision repair or post-replication repair, *Genetics* **81:**349–355 (1975).

327. Wolff, S., Lindsley, D. L., and Peacock, W. J., Cytological evidence for switches in polarity of chromosomal DNA, *Proc. Nat. Acad. Sci. USA* **73:**877–881 (1976).

328. Wolff, S., Rodin, B., and Cleaver, J. E., Sister chromatid exchanges induced by mutagenic carcinogens in normal and xeroderma pigmentosum cells, *Nature (London)* **265:**345–347 (1977).

329. Yamamoto, M., and Miklos, G. L. G., Genetic studies on heterochromatin in *Drosophila melanogaster* and their implications for the functions of satellite DNA, *Chromosoma* **66:**71–98 (1978).

330. Yu, C. W., and Borgaonkar, D. S., Normal rate of sister chromatid exchange in Down syndrome, *Clin. Genet.* **11:**397–401 (1977).

331. Yunis, J. J., and Sanchez, O., High resolution of human chromosomes, *Science* **191:**1268–1270 (1976).

332. Yunis, J. J., Sawyer, J. R., and Ball, D. W., The characterization of high-resolution G-banded chromosomes of man, *Chromosoma* **67:**293–307 (1978).

333. Zack, G. W., Rogers, W. E., and Latt, S. A., Automatic measurement of sister chromatid exchange frequency, *J. Histochem. Cytochem.* **25:**741–753 (1977).

334. Zakharov, A. F., and Egolina, N. A., Asynchrony of DNA replication and mitotic spiralization along heterochromatic portions of Chinese hamster chromosomes, *Chromosoma* **23:**365–385 (1968).

335. Zakharov, A. F., and Egolina, N. A., Differential spiralization along mammalian mitotic chromosomes I. BUdR-revealed differentiates in Chinese hamster chromosomes, *Chromosoma* **38:**341–355 (1972).

336. Zimmerman, A. M., Stich, H., and San, R., Nonmutagenic action of cannabinoids *in vitro*, *Pharmacology* **16:**333–343 (1978).

*Chapter 5*

# Genetic Disorders of Male Sexual Differentiation

Kaye R. Fichman, Barbara R. Migeon, and
Claude J. Migeon

*Department of Pediatrics, Divisions of
Pediatric Endocrinology and Pediatric Genetics
The Johns Hopkins University
School of Medicine and Hospital
Baltimore, Maryland 21205*

## NORMAL MALE DIFFERENTIATION IN THE FETUS

There are many complex interactions that contribute to the events that characterize normal sexual differentiation in the male. Although many of the pertinent steps have not yet been defined, recent studies have provided some insights. A review of our current knowledge of these events will serve as a basis for further discussion of the abnormalities in sexual differentiation and their genetic basis.

### The Neutral Stage

In the three-week embryo of either sex, the primitive germ cells can be found in the yolk sac near its union with the allantois.[159] Anlagen of the gonads appear in the four-week human embryo as the genital ridges, a pair of longitudinal swellings in the posterior wall of the coelomic cavity medial to the anlagen for the urinary system.[47] By the sixth week, having migrated along the allantois through the dorsal mesentery, the germ cells reach the genital ridge where they interact with the mesenchyme.[159] Simultaneously, the coelomic epithelium of the genital ridge proliferates and invaginates into the underlying mesenchyme to form the primitive sex cords.[52,56,64]

At the beginning of the sixth week, both males and females have two systems of potential genital ducts, the wolffian and müllerian ducts.[155] The former is originally part of the excretory tubular system of the kidney, the portion nearest the gonad being the potential genital duct. Only in the male will it connect to the gonad.[152]

The müllerian duct develops as an invagination of the coelomic epithelium near the genital ridge. At the cranial end of each duct is a funnel-shaped orifice which opens into the coelomic cavity.[65] These ducts are lateral to the wolffian ducts and have no connection to the gonads. Distally, the ducts fuse in the midline forming the uterovaginal canal that terminates in the posterior medial aspect of the pouch known as the urogenital sinus.[65]

## Differentiation of the Fetal Testes

The first step in normal male differentiation is the transformation of the bipotential primitive gonad into a testis. This transformation occurs even in individuals with more than one X chromosome as long as a Y chromosome is present, indicating that the Y chromosome is the important determinant of male gonadal differentiation. Although the nature of the gene product specified by the Y chromosome is not known, there have been suggestions that the initiation of testicular differentiation is attributable to a cell surface component identified serologically as the HY antigen. The HY antigen has been found in tissues of the male of many species.[149] The antigen is a weak one, and the assay is difficult. There are some dosage effects related to the number of Y chromosomes in the karyotype, suggesting a relationship with that chromosome,[150] but the antigen has been found in individuals with functional ovaries.[149] The reader is referred to recent reviews for more detailed discussion.[19,107,148]

Under the influence of the product of the Y chromosome, the primitive sex cords of the gonad in the male surround the germ cells as they reach the genital ridge.[66] The cords then proliferate into a network and penetrate deeply into the medullary portion of the gonad.[52] By the seventh week, the cords lose their connection to the coelomic surface epithelium and a thick layer of connective tissue, the *tunica albuginea*, forms over the gonads.[155] The epithelial portion of the cord develops into both the lining cells of the seminiferous tubules and the adjacent sertoli cells.[52,91] The testicular mesenchyme of the gonad gives rise to the leydig cells which are responsible for steroid production.[152]

## Functions of the Fetal Testes

There are at least two important functions for the fetal testes: the production of testosterone by the leydig cells and the elaboration of the müllerian inhibiting factor (MIF).

### Elaboration of Müllerian Inhibiting Factor (MIF)

The cells of the fetal testes secrete a product which acts locally to cause the regression of the müllerian duct structures on the same side as the gonad.[65] The regression which begins at 62 to 65 days involves obliterating the opening of the duct into the coelomic cavity (which would have been the abdominal ostium of the fallopian tube in the female), narrowing the lumen of the duct, and replacing it with fibrous tissue. These changes provide the basis of the bioassay for the müllerian inhibiting factor.[65] Cocultivation of müllerian duct explants from fetal rats with human fetal testicular tissue results in duct regression.[65] The cocultivation assay has been used to show that the sertoli cells are the source of MIF.[16,65] A protein with MIF activity and with a molecular weight of 200–320 × 10³ has been isolated from the incubation medium.[65] Although the precise time has not been determined, there seems to be a critical period during which the müllerian ducts are sensitive to MIF. Studies of human testicular explants from abortuses of various ages have shown that antimüllerian duct activity is lost during the perinatal period.

### Production of Testosterone

The differentiation of the fetal gonad in the male is not androgen-dependent. However, it is clear that further masculinization is mediated by androgenic hormones. Testosterone and its metabolite dihydrotestosterone (DHT) are the hormones necessary to effect masculinization of the wolffian ducts and external genitalia.[64,132,139,158] Testosterone is produced in the leydig cells in the interstitium of the testes.[56] Based on studies of testicular tissue incubated with labeled precursors, the onset of testosterone production correlates well with the first appearance of these cells in the fetus at 65 days.[16] In fact, the concentration of testosterone in fetal serum parallels the proliferation of leydig cells. It rises to nearly adult male levels at 14–18 weeks of gestation, when the leydig cells are most prominent and account for more than half the volume of the testes.[158] The testosterone production decreases at 20–24 weeks as the leydig cells diminish. These cells are virtually undetectable histologically soon after birth[157] even though significant plasma testosterone levels are found in males at two to four postnatal months.

As in the adult, testosterone is synthesized in the fetal testes from acetate and cholesterol (Fig. 1). A series of three enzymes—20-hydroxylase, 22-hydroxylase, and 20,22-desmolase—transform cholesterol into pregnenolone, the precursor of all steroid hormones in man. Three additional enzyme systems—3β-hydroxysteroid dehydrogenase, 17-hydroxylase, and 17,20-desmolase—are needed for the conversion of pregnenolone to androstenedione. This steroid has 19 carbons, and is therefore considered an androgen. However, to acquire biological activity, androstenedione must be metabolized to testosterone by 17-ketosteroid reductase. In both males and females, estrogens are synthesized from androstenedione and/or testosterone as precursors.

## Gonadotropin Regulation

The fetal leydig cells, like those of the adult, must be stimulated by gonadotropins to produce testosterone. Androgen production is initally induced by human chorionic gonadotropin (HCG) derived from the placenta. The peak concentration of HCG in fetal blood occurs at 8–10 weeks of gestation and levels reach a nadir at 17–19 weeks.[159] Concomitant with the decline in HCG is an increase in luteinizing hormone (LH) of fetal pituitary origin. The LH is first detected in the fetal pituitary at 10 weeks and is more abundant at 20–24 weeks.[67] The secretion of LH is under the control of a peptide hormone of hypothalamic origin, LH-releasing hormone (LHRH).[67] The female fetus has more LH activity than the male, whose lower level has been attributed to negative feedback regulation by testosterone.[67] Receptors for androgens are present in the hypothalamus at this time, whereas receptors for estrogens do not appear until later in development.[67,80]

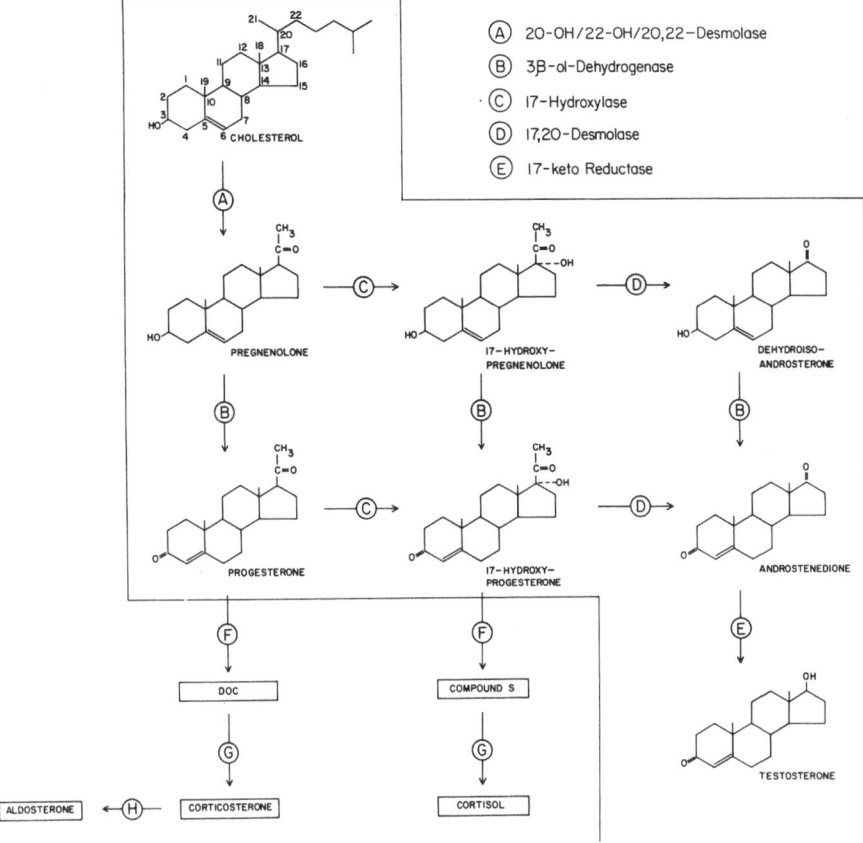

Fig. 1. Diagram showing steps in the synthesis of testosterone from cholesterol. The line encloses those steps occurring in the testis. (A) through (E) represent the enzymatic reactions necessary for this conversion. The adrenal is capable of carrying out all of those reactions except the formation of testosterone from androstenedione which occurs only in the testes. The adrenal also has the enzymes (F,G,H) necessary for the synthesis of glucocorticoids (mainly cortisol) and mineralocorticoids (mainly aldosterone).

The LH and HCG molecules are each composed of an α and a β subunit. The α subunits of both hormones are nearly identical in their amino acid composition. Many of the amino acid sequences of the β subunits of LH and HCG are homologous, but it is this subunit that confers biologic and immunologic specificity.[53] Another gonadotropin, follicle-stimulating hormone (FSH), regulates the activity of sertoli cells and may be important in MIF production. Its concentration in the fetus parallels that of LH and it is also under the regulation of LHRH.[67]

## Function of Androgen Target Cells

Cells that are stimulated by androgens to carry out functions which do not occur otherwise have been called target cells. Many extratesticular cells responsive to androgens have been identified and these include those which carry out functions normally associated with male differentiation (i.e., genitalia, internal ducts, prostate) and those which do not (bone marrow, liver, kidney). Target cells in females have the potential for response if androgens are present.

How target cells function in response to androgens is not well understood but certain insights have been obtained. Androgenic effects are mediated by means of a cytosol receptor which is specific for androgens. Subsequently, the receptor hormone complex is translocated to the nucleus where it is believed to interact with a specific acceptor, presumably a nonhistone protein. This interaction makes gene(s) responsible for androgenic effects available for transcription.[108,109,154]

The first step in most target cells is to metabolize testosterone to a more potent androgen. Although testosterone itself induces the growth of certain androgen target tissues, such as the genital ducts,[64,129,158] it must be converted to dihydrotestosterone (DHT) to initiate certain androgenic effects such as differentiation of the external genitalia in the male.[155]

### 5α-Reductase Activity

Dihydrotestosterone is formed from testosterone in a single step reaction mediated by the enzyme 5α-reductase.[130] When skin slices or cultured skin fibroblasts from normal individuals are incubated with labeled testosterone, several 5α-reduced metabolites including DHT are rapidly formed (see Fig. 2). The enzyme is present in numerous tissues but its activity is greatest in prostate, genital ducts, tissues of the external genitalia, liver, and hypothalamus.[23,80,129,132]

Recently it has been suggested that there are two different 5α-reductase enzyme activities. The major enzyme activity with a pH optimum of 5.5 is found only in genital skin fibroblasts while the other at pH 7–9

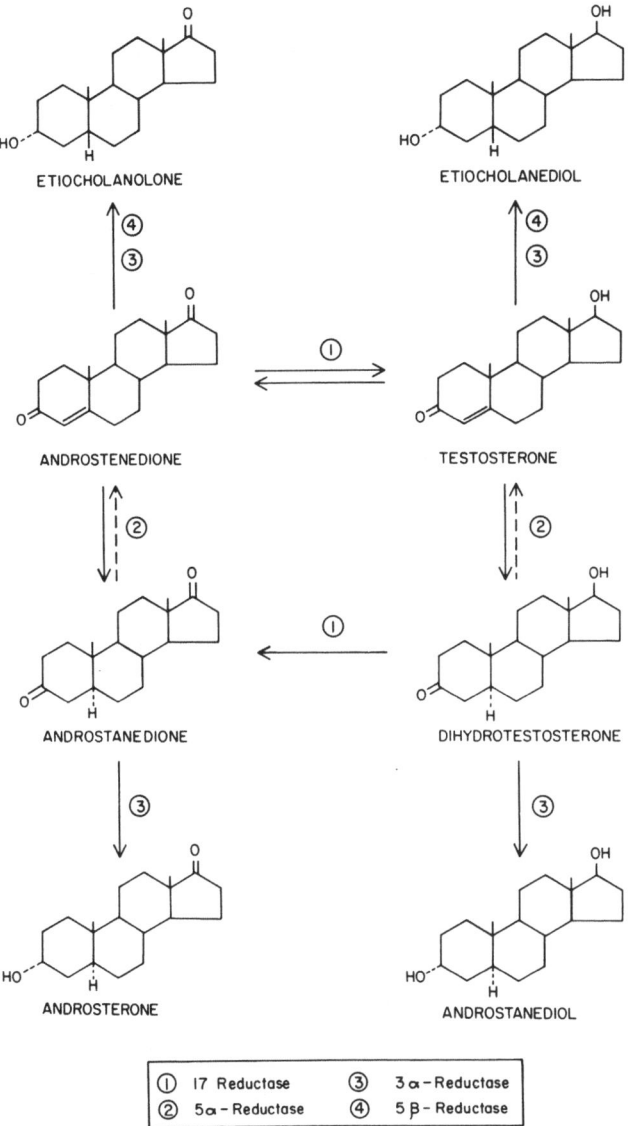

ETIOCHOLANOLONE

ETIOCHOLANEDIOL

ANDROSTENEDIONE

TESTOSTERONE

ANDROSTANEDIONE

DIHYDROTESTOSTERONE

ANDROSTERONE

ANDROSTANEDIOL

| ① | 17 Reductase | ③ | 3 α – Reductase |
| ② | 5α – Reductase | ④ | 5 β – Reductase |

Fig. 2. Diagram showing the metabolism of testosterone to etiocholanolone and androsterone in the liver, which normally yields equal amounts of each metabolite. A deficiency of 5α-reductase results in a relative excess of etiocholanolone in the urine.

is present in all skin fibroblasts.[103] Patients with 5α-reductase deficiency lack the enzyme activity with pH optimum 5.5 suggesting that this is the important one in normal masculinization.[102,118]

Target cells from the liver have, in addition to 5α-reductase activity, an active 5β-reductase; both enzymes are involved in the normal catabolism of testosterone in that tissue[62,117] (Fig. 2).

## Androgen Receptor Activity

Receptors for androgens have been demonstrated in several androgen-sensitive organs from various species[13,35,87,88,89] Cultured human skin fibroblasts also contain specific androgen receptor activity[72,157] which is heat-labile and trypsin sensitive indicating its protein nature.[72] The receptor activity is distributed equally between cytosolic and nuclear components of the cells.[35,72,89] Androgen receptors have a high affinity for DHT and 5α-androstane-3α,17β-diol (see Fig. 3). Testosterone can also be bound by the receptor, but with less affinity.[86]

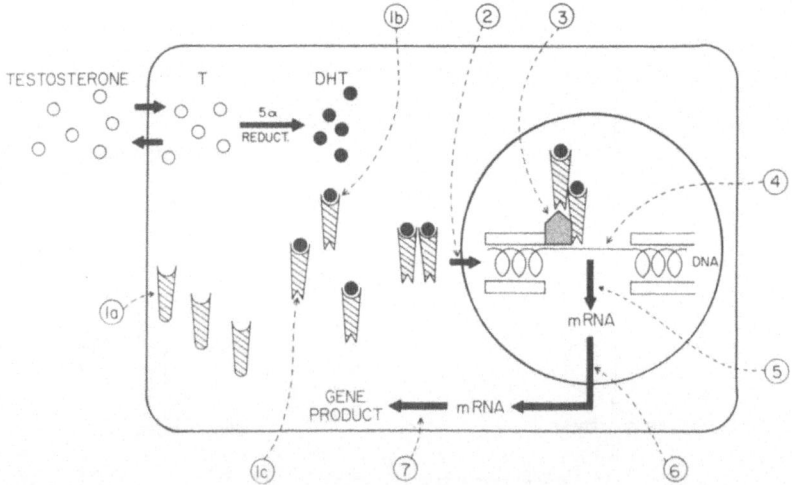

Fig. 3. Diagram of a target cell depicting steroid hormone action based on available experimental evidence. Numbers refer to sites where mutations might result in androgen insensitivity. (1) Mutations affecting cytosol receptor protein include (a) absent protein, (b) abnormal protein with respect to DHT binding site, (c) abnormal protein with respect to acceptor binding site. (2) Defect in translocation of hormone receptor complex to nucleus, (3) Abnormalities of nuclear acceptor site (4) Abnormal regulatory molecules. (5) Abnormal transcription of nuclear mRNA. (6) Abnormal mRNA processing. (7) Abnormal translation of androgen-dependent protein.

The binding affinity of a receptor for a steroid reflects the tightness with which the steroid is bound to the receptor and is expressed as a dissociation constant or $K_d$, (the concentration of unlabeled steroid that will displace 50% of the bound labeled steroid). The mean binding affinity of the androgen receptor for DHT in genital skin fibroblasts is the same for normal males and females at every age.[72,101]

The binding capacity ($B_{max}$) estimates the number of receptor sites present in the tissue. The capacity varies with the origin of skin fibro-blasts, the mean $B_{max}$ for genital skin (labia, prepuce) being $883 \pm 622 \times 10^{-18}$ mol/μg DNA which is greater than that of nongenital skin ($478 \pm 318 \times 10^{-18}$ mol/μg DNA).[98] However, there is no sex- or age-related difference. In fact, the $B_{max}$ for DHT binding in genital skin fibroblasts from fetuses of either sex is comparable to that of adult sexual skin.[142a]

## Androgen-Mediated Effects in the Fetus

### Maturation of the Wolffian Ducts

As the müllerian system degenerates, differentiation of the wolffian system is taking place under the local influence of testosterone produced in the adjacent testis.[129] The portion of the wolffian duct nearest to the testis (along with the ductuli efferentes) convolutes to form the epididymis. Distally the duct continues as the ductus deferens. Where the ductus joins the urogenital sinus, a dilatation develops to form the seminal vesicle.[66] These effects seem to occur under the influence of testosterone rather than its 5α-reduced product, DHT, as the cells of the developing wolffian ducts have not yet acquired 5α-reductase activity.[132,155] These cells bind testosterone so that the development of the wolffian ducts is probably mediated by the androgen receptor.

### Masculinization of the External Genitalia

Although the development of the wolffian ducts is effected by diffusion of the androgen from the adjacent gonad, the masculinization of the external genitalia is effected by blood born androgens; hence it is a true hormonal effect.[155,156] At six weeks of gestation, the external genitalia in both males and females consists of swellings of the perineum. Anteriorly there is a prominence, the genital tubercle, and on either side of it the urethral folds, which meet posteriorly to form the rim of the anal orifice.[64,139] The first manifestation of masculinization, visible at 65–70 days, is an increase in the distance from the genital tubercle to the anal portion of the folds.[139] Subsequently, the folds fuse in the midline to form the scrotum. Simultaneously, the genital tubercle lengthens to become the phallus and the urethral folds, having fused, invaginate along the phallus to form the penile urethra.[139]

While testosterone is responsible for the development of the internal ducts, DHT is the androgen involved in masculinization of the external genitalia. In fact, the tissues of the external genitalia contain 5α-reductase activity at the earliest stages of differentiation, and this activity is comparable to that found in adult target tissues.[155]

## ABNORMAL MALE SEX DIFFERENTIATION

Normal male sexual differentiation depends upon appropriate function at each step in the process. The first requirement is the presence of a Y chromosome or related gene product(s). Subsequently, the fetal testes must be able to produce müllerian inhibiting factor and to respond to gonadotropin stimulation with the production of those gene products necessary for masculinization.

We begin with disorders related to abnormalities of the sex chromosomes. These are usually not considered in a discussion of male pseudohermaphroditism and are included because of their relevance to a discussion of male differentiation. This is followed by disorders of sex differentiation associated with a normal male karyotype, which are properly classified as male pseudohermaphroditism (Table I). This group can be subdivided according to the specific step in which the error occurs. The first are abnormalities of the fetal gonads which interfere in various degrees with one or both of the functions of the fetal testes, i.e., the production of MIF and the secretion of testosterone. The essential role of gonadotropins in testosterone production is evident from the abnormalities resulting from a deficiency of gonadotropin activity. A number of inborn errors result from deficiencies of enzymes necessary for the production of testosterone by the fetal leydig cells. Some of these enzymes are needed for the biosynthesis of both cortisol in the adrenals and tes-

TABLE I. Classification of Male Pseudohermaphroditism

Dysgenesis of fetal gonads associated with normal karyotype
   XY Gonadal dysgenesis
   Congenital anorchia
   Leydig cell agenesis
   Deficiency of MIF
Abnormalities of gonadotropins
   Hypopituitarism
   Kallman's syndrome
   Abnormal endogenous LH
   Deficiency of gonadotropin receptor
   Probable delayed development of the HCG/LH Receptor
Deficiencies of enzymes needed for the biosynthesis of testosterone
   Defects involving both the adrenal glands and the testes
      Deficiency of 20-hydroxylase, 22-hydroxylase or 20,22-desmolase
      Deficiency of 3-hydroxysteroid dehydrogenase
      Deficiency of 17-hydroxylase
   Deficiencies of enzymes of testicular origin
      Deficiency of 17,20-desmolase
      Deficiency of 17-ketosteroid reductase
Abnormalities of androgen target cells
   Deficiency of $5\alpha$-reductase
   Syndromes of androgen insensitivity

tosterone in the testes, whereas others are primarily involved in testosterone biosynthesis. The remaining disorders of male differentiation result from mutations affecting the target cells for androgens rather than hormone production. These include the deficiency of an enzyme necessary to convert testosterone to a more potent androgen and abnormalities in the androgen receptor.

## Genetic Considerations

Every step in the process of male sex differentiation is under genetic control and the number of relevant genes is large. Little is known about those which regulate differentiation and migration of germ cells, determine the onset of meiosis, or specify structural components of the male genitourinary tract. However, we do know that initiation of male gonadal differentiation requires the Y chromosome, hence implicating at least one Y-linked product. Studies of individuals with androgen insensitivity have revealed the presence of at least one important male-determining gene on the X chromosome. Other important gene products are those specifying gonadotropins and their receptors, those elaborating the product responsible for inhibition of müllerian ducts, and those involved in the synthesis of androgens.

The contribution to our knowledge of normal events in differentiation is readily apparent from studies of individuals with defective masculinization. The availability of mutations affecting steps in the process have elucidated the normal pathway for the biosynthesis of androgens and their relative virilizing efficiency, as well as the role of androgen receptors in mediating hormone action. Observations of male pseudohermaphrodites have revealed important differences between differentiation in the fetus and at puberty.

Inborn errors are easily recognizable when defects in a metabolic pathway can be demonstrated. Single point mutations are responsible for those metabolic errors of testosterone biosynthesis or disorders where a defective protein product has been demonstrated. However, it is likely that many of the other developmental disorders of male differentiation are also single-gene-determined, and these represent a reservoir from which new inborn errors will be drawn.

For many of the disorders associated with male pseudohermaphroditism it is difficult to determine the nature of the mutation and its mode of transmission or if it is genetic at all. First of all, it is difficult to make a specific diagnosis. Whether the underlying basis for the disorder is an enzyme deficiency or androgen insensitivity, the clinical phenotype is the same—some degree of inadequate masculinization. The mutations affect differentiated functions and, therefore, pertinent tissues are not easily available for study. In most cases the diagnosis is based on secondary effects of the mutation rather than the direct demonstration of an abnormal primary gene product. Furthermore, there is significant variability in the expression of these mutations, even within members of the same family.

The distinction between partial or complete forms of a disorder is generally based upon similarities among members of the same family in clinical expression (the degree of masculinization *in utero* and at puberty), as well as quantities of secondary gene products. Only with respect to androgen-binding protein has it been possible to demonstrate quantitative differences between partial and complete forms of the disorder. Although many of these disorders may be attributable to abnormal rather than absent protein products, observations of this kind have been reported only for LH and 5α-reductase.

Even when a specific diagnosis has been made, it is difficult to discover the mode of transmission. The frequency of affected individuals is often low; therefore, the number of informative families is small and the problem is compounded by small family size. Furthermore, in many cases only males are ascertained. Females with the mutant gene are infrequently identified, even if homozygous, because the mutant phenotype is inadequate masculinization. In addition, affected males do not reproduce. Unless there are affected individuals in more than one generation, the occurrence of the disorder in two sibs (although indicating a probable genetic influence) does not discriminate between alternative modes of transmission—or between genetic and maternal causes in a common intrauterine environment.*

Although we assume that most of the inborn errors of testosterone biosynthesis are recessive, other disorders may be transmitted as dominants. Autosomal dominant transmission with expression limited to males is demonstrable if the relevant locus is assigned to a specific chromosome or if the gene product responsible for the abnormal phenotype in the male is as deficient in all cells of the female. The demonstration of close linkage to an X-chromosomal locus would provide compelling evidence for X-linkage.

While none of the disorders has been recognized as multifactorial, there is at least one good candidate. Genetic susceptibility to testicular injury is suggested by the familial aggregation and variable phenotype within families in some cases of congenital anorchia. One would expect that genetically determined drug sensitivities might lead to developmental anomalies of the genitalia and ducts. There has been some suggestion that exposure to progestins, which compete with DHT for receptor sites, may be responsible for some cases of hypospadias.[1] On the other hand, the male fetus is exposed normally to high levels of a potent antiandrogen, estrogen, in the maternal circulation. However, estrogens compete only weakly for androgen binding sites, if at all. It may be that drugs which interfere with masculinization of the fetus must compete strongly with androgens for specific binding sites.

---

* It is interesting to note that McKusick solves the dilemma in the case of congenital anorchia by assigning (on the basis of the same set of observations) two numbers to this disorder, one as an autosomal recessive, the other as an X-linked trait.[95]

The effect of inbreeding is readily seen in families from the Dominican Republic with 5α-reductase deficiency. The apparent lack of ethnic concentration of individuals with other disorders may reflect the relatively small numbers of individuals affected with any single disorder.

## Chromosomal Abnormalities

There are many chromosomal abnormalities that do not permit the normal development of a testis. Although the XO karyotype is not identified with male pseudohermaphroditism, the associated phenotype has provided evidence for the importance of the Y chromosome for masculinization. In its absence, development of the bipotential gonad proceeds in the female direction. The ovaries of fetuses with XO karyotypes at 12 weeks of gestation are similar to those of normal females of the same age, even with respect to the number of germ cells.[26,136] Therefore, a single X chromosome is sufficient for the initiation of normal female development and it is the Y chromosome which induces differentiation away from the female direction.[107]

### Abnormalities of the Y Chromosome

Deletions of the short arm of the Y chromosome are associated with a female phenotype and streak gonads. This is also true for isochromosomes of the long arm of the Y. In contrast, deletions of the distal part of the long arm of the Y chromosome are found among normal men and are not associated with infertility. These observations have supported the hypothesis that the testis-determining locus on the Y chromosome is situated on or near the short arm.[76]

In individuals with a dicentric Y chromosome in which duplication of the long arm occurs, the phenotype is variable and may be normal. However, infants with ambiguous genitalia have been reported with this karyotype. Many of these had a coexisting XO cell line and were therefore mosaic for the dicentric Y.[76]

### XYY Karyotype

Males with an XYY karyotype are generally taller than the average male population. Their sexual development is usually normal. However, patients with ambiguous genitalia have been reported.[41] There is a high incidence of infertility secondary to oligospermia and testicular biopsies have shown variable tubular diameter with hyalinization of the tubular membranes and reduced numbers of spermatids and mature sperm.[10] Meiotic studies of these individuals have been generally unsuccessful because of the maturation arrest.[59,137,144] There is one report of transmission of the XYY karyotype from father to son.[143]

## Mixed Gonadal Dysgenesis with Chromosomal Mosaicism

This term is applied to males with abnormal gonads ranging from bilateral streaks to bilateral dysgenetic testes. There may be a streak on one side, and a dysgenetic gonad on the other. The karyotype is usually XO/XY, but XX/XY has also been reported.[53] Conceivably, these karyotypes may be associated with a perfectly normal testicular development, but these individuals are not likely to be ascertained. The masculinization of the external genitalia is variable, reflecting the severity of the testicular dysfunction in the fetus. Most of the cases are sporadic, but a few familial cases have been reported.[37,58]

## Klinefelter's Syndrome and Related Variants

The influence of additional X chromosomes on the expression of the Y chromosome is seen in individuals with 47 chromosomes including XXY. Although cryptorchidism and hypospadias may occur, the external genitalia of these males is usually normal, at least in infancy. Delayed puberty is a frequent occurrence and small testicular size becomes apparent in adulthood. Eunuchoid body habitus and gynecomastia are common.[77] Testosterone levels are minimally decreased while FSH and LH are markedly elevated. Although at birth the testicular histology is normal, there is progressive loss of germ cells and hyalinization of the seminiferous tubules, so that infertility is the most common presenting complaint among affected adults. The Y chromosome, despite the presence of *two* X chromosomes, is able to effect normal testicular development *in utero*; however, an X-linked gene in double dose leads to progressive loss of germ cells and the eventual destruction of the seminiferous tubules. Mosaicism for XXY has been noted to ameliorate the testicular abnormalities and such individuals may be fertile.[77]

Nondisjunction during meiosis in the germ cells of either parent has been implicated in the etiology of Klinefelter's syndrome.[53,133] In some pedigrees, studies of other X-linked markers have indicated that in at least 70% of the cases both of the X chromosomes are of maternal origin.[53] In these cases there is evidence for maternal age effect.[53] In the remaining cases, one of the X chromosomes as well as the Y was contributed by the father and there is no evidence for an age effect.[53,133]

## Other X Polysomies

Individuals with more than two X chromosomes along with the Y have testicular abnormalities similar to those observed in Klinefelter's syndrome, but somatic abnormalities are noted as well. Patients with four Xs and a Y (XXXXY) have mental deficiency, radioulnar dysostosis and more severe genital abnormalities than in classical Klinefelter's syndrome.[77] Hypospadias, bifid scrotum, cryptorchidism, and micropenis are frequently present, and the deficiency of androgens is notable.[77] Because only one X chromosome is active in each somatic cell of these patients, it is not clear why there are somatic abnormalities. Conceivably, the presence of somatic abnormalities may be related to the timing of X inactivation in these cells and may indicate that two or more X chromosomes were expressed prior to inactivation. Alternatively, some part of the X chromosome may escape inactivation.[131]

## Triploidy

Triploidy is among the most frequent chromosomal abnormalities occurring in approximately 1% of all conceptions.[105] Although it is usually lethal and results in spontaneous abortion, a few fetuses survive up to the third trimester. In contrast to the situation in Klinefelter's syndrome, triploid individuals with an XXY karyotype usually have ambiguous genitalia, specifically a small phallus, hypospadias, bifid scrotum, and cryptorchidism.[105] In the majority of triploids surviving early gestation, two of the X chromosomes are active in each somatic cell and may explain the ambiguity of the genitalia. However, the sex chromosome complement of germ cells in triploids is the same as that in Klinefelter's syndrome. Among the other abnormalities in triploids are adrenal hypoplasia and agenesis of the corpus callosum.[105] Whether the lack of pituitary and/or adrenal hormones or the extra autosomes in target cells is responsible for the incomplete masculinization of triploids remains to be determined.[135]

## Male Differentiation Associated with Inappropriate Karyotype (XX Males) (26985)*

More than 40 individuals have been reported who have a male phenotype associated with an XX karyotype.[31,32,68,119] The phenotype is very much like that of patients with Klinefelter's syndrome including the testicular histology. These individuals demonstrate the detrimental influence of two X chromosomes on testicular function. The nature of the Y-like product responsible for inducing fetal testicular development is unknown. Conceivably there may be a mutation at an autosomal locus which results in a product able to induce male differentiation of the primitive gonad. A pedigree consistent with a paternally transmitted autosomal gene influencing testicular development has been reported.[68] Alternatively, the pertinent segment of the Y chromosome may have been translocated to an X or an autosome, or there may be mosaicism for an XY cell line which has not been demonstrated (see Addendum at the back of the book).

## True Hermaphroditism (23560)

True hermaphroditism is characterized by the presence of well-differentiated elements of both male and female gonads in the same subject. There may be a testis on one side and an ovary on the other, an ovotestis one side and a male or female gonad on the other, or bilateral ovotestes. Most of these myxoploid individuals have an XX sex chromosome complement although some are XY or XX/XY mosaics. The phenotype depends to some extent on which gonadal tissue predominates but most subjects have ambiguous genitalia.[82,99,124]

Rosenberg has reported a family with three true hermaphrodite sibs whose karyotypes, including that of cultured gonadal tissue, were 46 XX.[124] It may be that familial XX true hermaphroditism is transmitted as an autosomal recessive mutation coding for a gene product that induces differentiation along male lines. These individuals resemble the XX phenotypic male except that their gonads have not been completely mascu-

---

* Refers to McKusick assigned number.[95]

linized, perhaps attributable to a difference in virilizing effect of the autosomal product. Alternatively, the pedigree is compatible with an interchange between X and Y during spermatogenesis.[38] In this case, the paternal X carries a pertinent small piece of Y chromosome. X inactivation in the somatic cells of the gonad of affected individuals could account for the myxoploid gonad.

With regard to the less common XY true hermaphroditism, a pedigree has been reported with individuals whose fathers were brothers. Another family has two affected sibs. Despite the absence of consanguinity, an autosomal recessive mutation inhibiting normal testicular differentiation seems likely.[82] There are also now at least five reports of XX/XY hermaphrodites in whom blood group studies have confirmed the presence of chimerism.[112] One would expect histologic differences in the gonads of mosaic and nonmosaic hermaphrodites, but none have been described.[135]

## Male Pseudohermaphroditism

Male pseudohermaphroditism is defined as the condition of incomplete masculinization of the external genitalia in a karyotypically normal XY male. We have classified male pseudohermaphroditism as shown in Table I.

### Dysgenesis of Fetal Gonads Associated with Normal Karyotype (Table II)

Gonadal dysgenesis is a general term denoting defective development of the embryonic gonad. The term dysgenetic gonad refers to a range of disorders including fibrotic or streak gonads. rudimentary gonads with some histopathologic elements recognizable as abortive testes, and the absence of any detectable gonad or ducts. In some cases the testis may appear normal but is functionally ineffective in terms of testosterone or MIF production. Usually the genital ducts and external genitalia are also abnormal. The extent of these abnormalities is related to the nature and timing of the gonadal defect.

**XY Pure Gonadal Dysgenesis (30610).** Since 1974 there have been more than 90 reports of male pseudohermaphrodites with a normal XY karyotype and marked gonadal dysgenesis.[27,29,37,39,42,45,92,121,134,141] The typical features are female external genitalia and ducts (attributable to lack of müllerian inhibitory factor), and bilateral streak gonads. Plasma androgens are in the female range. The incidence of gonadal tumors is high, approaching 60% by the age of 30 years.[39,42,92]

Various hypotheses have been invoked to explain XY pure gonadal dysgenesis, including agenesis of the gonadal anlagen, failure of germ cell migration or early attrition of germ cells, absence of the Y-linked testicular organizing gene, or an inhibitor of the Y gene product.[45,134]

In some families there is an aggregation of affected males.[27,29,39,45,141] Studies of these families have supported transmission of the condition through unaffected females as an X-linked mutation or an autosomal trait whose expression is limited to males. In either case, the mutant product is one which modified Y chromosome function.[45] If X-linked, it indicates that there are X-linked loci in addition to that of the androgen receptor which contribute to testicular function. Linkage studies might be helpful in this respect.

**XY Partial Gonadal Dysgenesis.** This is probably a variant of the previous syndrome. These individuals have some clitoral enlargement and their plasma testosterone levels are greater than those of normal females. As in pure gonadal dysgenesis, there is a familial incidence with conventional evidence for X-linkage in some families.[141] However, there is significant phenotypic variability within members of the same family, some having bilateral fallopian tubes, while others have unilateral well-developed wolffian ducts.[29,141] Furthermore, in some pedigrees there are both individuals with a completely female phenotype as well as those with ambiguous genitalia, indicating that the complete and partial forms can occur in the same sibship,[12,27] and suggesting the presence of modifying genes.

**Cogenital Anorchia (20695) (30165).** More than 50 cases of male pseudohermaphroditism have been attributed to "congenital anorchia," which is also referred to as the "syndrome of vanishing testes."[2] These individuals usually have a small but well-defined penis and an empty scrotum or unilateral cryptorchidism. The absence of müllerian structures and the presence of male internal ducts, as well as some virilization of the external genitalia support the existence of a functional testis in early fetal life. Two patients were reported with low levels of testosterone, implying the presence of ectopic leydig cells.[75] Others who lacked gonadal tissue had ambiguous external genitalia and müllerian remnants, as well as wolffian structures. Presumably testicular degeneration in these individuals occurred somewhat earlier in fetal development.

**TABLE II. Characteristics of Disorders Resulting in Male Pseudohermaphroditism[a]**

| Disorder | External genitalia in infancy[b] | Internal ducts[b] | Gonadal tissue | Phenotype at puberty | Testicular androgens at puberty[b] | Mode of transmission | Salient feature[b] |
|---|---|---|---|---|---|---|---|
| Pure XY gonadal dysgenesis | F | F | Streak | Infantile | − | X-linked/autosomal recessive/Autosomal dominant limited to males | Streak gonad, F-genitalia |
| Partial XY gonadal dysgenesis | A | M or F | Dysgenetic testes | Partial masculinization | − | X-linked/autosomal recessive/Autosomal dominant limited to males | Dysgenetic gonad |
| Congenital anorchia | M or A | M | None | Infantile | − | c | |
| Leydig cell agenesis | F or A | M | Testes | Partial masculinization or infantile | − | c | Absence of leydig cells in otherwise normal testes |
| MIF deficiency | M | M and F | Testes | Normal masculinization | N | X-linked/autosomal recessive | Müllerian derivatives in otherwise normal male |
| LH deficiency, Kallman's syndrome (CRM−) | M or A | M | Testes | Partial masculinization, gynecomastia | − | X-linked/autosomal recessive | − LH (+ response to exogenous HCG) |

| | | | | | | |
|---|---|---|---|---|---|---|
| LH deficiency (CRM+) | F or A | M | Testes | Infantile | − | c | +LH (+ response to exogenous HCG) |
| Deficient LH receptors | F | M | Testes | Infantile | − | Autosomal recessive | −HCG binding to receptor in testicular tissue |
| Delayed LH receptors | A | M | Testes | Normal masculinization | N | c | |
| 5α-Reductase deficiency | F or A | M | Testes | Nearly normal masculinization | +T (−DHT) | Autosomal recessive | −Enzyme activity in genital skin fibroblasts |
| Complete androgen insensitivity, DHT receptor − | F | M | Testes | Infantile/gynecomastia | ++ | X-linked | −DHT binding activity in genital fibroblasts |
| Complete androgen insensitivity, DHT receptor + | F | M | Testes | Infantile/gynecomastia | ++ | c | ++T +DHT binding activity in genital skin fibroblasts |
| Inborn errors of testosterone biosynthesis | | | | See Table III | | | |

[a] Information based on patients reported in the literature.
[b] Abbreviations: F, female; M, male; A, ambiguous; N, normal quantity; −, decreased to absent; +, increased.
[c] Insufficient information.

Most cases are sporadic; however, there are reports of families with unilateral cryptorchidism but otherwise normal external genitalia in two affected sibs. Puberty progressed normally with compensatory hypertrophy of the right gonad. In one family affected sibs had blind-ending testicular blood vessels and rudimentery vasa deferentia on the affected side.[2] Affected identical twins have also been reported, one with bilateral anorchia and the other with unilateral cryptorchidism.[55] The familial occurrence suggests the presence of a gene(s) conveying susceptibility to intrauterine testicular torsion or other vascular injury.[55]

Two affected sibs from another family had bilateral anorchia and also lacked genital ducts.[114] The phenotype therefore was completely female except for amenorrhea, and the lack of breast development and pubic hair. This condition may represent complete failure of gonadal and duct anlagen development in which case it could be considered gonadal agenesis.[114,122]

**Leydig Cell Agenesis.**    Leydig cell agenesis has been implicated as a cause of male pseudohermaphroditism.[14,22] An affected male with female genitalia was ascertained because of primary amenorrhea and lack of breast development. The labia majora were fused posteriorly and inguinal gonads were evident. The only internal organs found at laparotomy were testes, each with an epididymis and vas deferens. Microscopic examination of the testes revealed normal-appearing sertoli cells and hyalinized seminiferous tubules with occasional immature germ cell but a complete absence of leydig cells, confirmed by electron microscopy. The testosterone level was consistent with the absence of leydig cells, being low even for a female and not altered by HCG stimulation or castration. Although FSH levels were in the normal range, serum LH was significantly elevated.[14] These findings are compatible with an absence of leydig cells in the fetal testis. If leydig cells had been present and functional at that time, then greater masculinization of the external genitalia would have occurred. The development of the vas deferens and epididymis has been attributed to androgens of adrenal origin.[14,22] Because the two reported cases were sporadic the role of genetic factors cannot be determined.

**Deficiency of Müllerian Inhibiting Factor (Persistent Müllerian Duct Syndrome) (26155).**    The independent functioning of the two endocrine activities of the testes is readily apparent in individuals whose testosterone production is normal but who have defective müllerian inhibition. These phenotypic males are ascertained because of chance occurence of inguinal hernias and/or cryptorchid testes. The hernia sac usually contains a fallopian tube and uterus along with a normal testis ("hernia uteri inguinale").[147] The müllerian structures are always bilateral.[8] The testicular histology is normal and appropriate for age.[8,138,147,153] At puberty masculinization occurs normally. The condition may be due to a failure of MIF production or an insensitivity of the end organs to MIF. At this time there is no means to discriminate between alternatives.

More than 70 cases with persistent müllerian duct syndrome have been reported, largely as sporadic occurrences and frequently at autopsy as an incidental finding.[138,147] However, there are at least seven families with two affected males.[8,21] The parents in two cases were related, suggesting autosomal recessive transmission.[8,147] In another family, the two affected half sibs had different fathers, compatible with X-linked or autosomal dominant inheritance.[137]

Although müllerian ducts in an XY male may be due to a specific lack of MIF activity, it may also result from defective development of the fetal testes in which case these are associated abnormalities of the external genitalia.

## Abnormalities of Gonadotropins

High levels of chorionic gonadotropins and precursors of testosterone synthesis derived from the placenta are required for adequate leydig cell function during the first trimester of gestation. In the second and third trimesters, however, this function is supplemented by the gonadotropins produced in the fetal pituitary.

**Deficiency of Fetal Gonadotropin Secretion.** Anencephalic male infants with poor pituitary development show disturbances in penile and scrotal development and descent of the testes.[81] Although infrequent, a micropenis anomaly has been associated with *idiopathic hypopituitarism*.[81] The hypogonadism related to gonadotropin deficiency may not be detected until puberty, when lack of secondary sex characteristics becomes apparent.

The association of underdeveloped genitalia with anosmia occurs in *Kallman's syndrome* (24420). Anosmia is secondary to maldevelopment or absence of the olfactory lobes, which have neuronal connections with the hypothalamus.[28] It is not clear whether this syndrome is due to defective gonadotropin secretion, or to abnormal regulation of this secretion by the hypothalamus. It is likely that both kinds of deficiencies occur as some individuals are able to secrete gonadotropins after clomiphene stimulation.[106] Although some cases of Kallman's syndrome appear to be sporadic, others are familial. There is evidence for genetic heterogeneity.[106] In some families the observations are consistent with X-linkage. Transmitting females show partial or complete anosmia and some of them have low gonadotropin production. However, a large kindred with affected males and females has been reported in which there was a high rate of consanguinity.[106] The phenotype of affected individuals varied—not all having the complete syndrome. In this case, the mutation was probably transmitted as an autosomal recessive.

**Abnormal Endogenous LH.** Defective masculinization has been attributed to a mutation affecting the structure of luteinizing hormone.[9,111] The two unrelated affected males had poorly masculinized external genitalia.[9,111] Biopsy of testicular tissue in one male revealed sparse leydig cells and a maturation arrest in spermatogenesis. Serum testosterone was low but increased 15-fold after HCG stimulation. Although FSH was normal, LH was significantly elevated. The administration of either HCG or exogenous LH was effective in inducing androgen production and secondary male sex characteristics.[9] The association of low testosterone levels with high levels of immunoreactive LH and the prompt response of the leydig cells to exogenous HCG suggests an abnormality in the endogenous LH molecule which precludes its biological activity.

One of the affected males belonged to a kindred with consanguinity in two generations.[9] Affected females were not apparent but three maternal uncles had a history of infertility. Two had low testosterone levels but their response to HCG was not evaluated. This pedigree supports an autosomal recessive mode of inheritance or an X-linked disorder with fortuitous consanguinity.[9]

**Deficiency of Gonadotropin Receptor (30618).** A deficiency of the gonadotropin receptor in leydig cells has been proposed as the cause of male pseudohermaphroditism in three sibs.[116] Their endogenous levels of LH were elevated but plasma testosterone remained low even after stimulation with HCG. LH increased in response to luteinizing releasing factor and could be suppressed by exogenous testosterone. The leydig cells were poorly differentiated and did not bind labeled LH.[116] On the basis of these limited observations, the inheritance pattern cannot be determined.

**Probable Delayed Development of the HCG/LH Receptor.** Two families, each with two sibs affected with male pseudohermaphroditism, have been reported. [96] In each case, the probands were considered normal females at birth despite borderline clitoromegaly and slight fusion of the labial folds posteriorly. At puberty, there was marked enlargement on the clitoris, along with development of a muscular habitus, deep voice, acne, and facial hair. Plasma levels of testosterone, DHT, and other androgens were in the normal range for males of their age so that it is unlikely that an inborn error of testosterone metabolism was involved. In fact, incubation of testicular tissue with labeled precursors indicated normal testosterone production. The 5α-reductase and DHT binding protein activities were normal, as was serum LH, but FSH was elevated. [96]

The appearance of the external genitalia prior to puberty suggests defective masculinization in the first trimester of fetal life, at a time when activity of the leydig cell is primarily regulated by placental HCG. The normal response to endogenous gonadotropins at puberty indicates that masculinization was inadequate only *in utero*. It has been postulated that the insufficient testosterone production *in utero* was due to a deficiency of HCG. [96] If this were the case, then the deficiency must be limited to the hormone's role in stimulating fetal leydig cells as there must have been appropriate HCG to maintain the pregnancy.

Alternatively, the failure of testosterone production in the fetus resulted from a delay in the development of HCG/LH receptors on the membrane of the leydig cells. This kind of timing defect in the maturation of HCG/LH receptors has been proposed. [96]

## Deficiencies of Enzymes Needed for the Biosynthesis of Testosterone (Table III)

Normal male sexual development is dependent upon the availability of testosterone. Figure 1 shows the steps involved in the synthesis of testosterone from cholesterol. Inborn errors have been described at each of these steps. In some cases, the enzyme deficiency has been demonstrated directly in the tissue in which the pathway is active. For others, the diagnosis has been based on the pattern of urinary metabolites. Characteristically, this pattern involves the accumulation of substrate for the enzyme and a reduction in the amount of product of the reaction catalyzed by the enzyme.

The phenotype in all cases is defective masculinization because none of the testosterone precursors is able to initiate sufficient androgenic ac-

TABLE III. Characteristics of Defects in Testosterone Biosynthesis Resulting in Male Pseudohermaphroditism[a,b]

| Deficient enzyme | Phenotype of affected males | | Biochemical phenotype | | | | | | Phenotype at puberty | Mode of transmission | Salient features |
|---|---|---|---|---|---|---|---|---|---|---|---|
| | External genitalia | Ducts | Progesterone | 17-OH Progesterone | Cortisol | Aldosterone | Adrenal androgens | Testicular androgens | | | |
| 20-Hydroxylase or 22-hydroxylase or 20,22-desmolase | F or A | M | - | - | - | - | - | - | Usually lethal in infancy | Autosomal recessive | Addisonian crisis |
| 3β-Hydroxysteroid dehydrogenase | F, M, or A | M | - | - | - | - | + (as DHEA) | - | Usually lethal in infancy (one treated 12-yr male) | Autosomal recessive | Addisonian crisis |
| 17-Hydroxylase | F or A | M | + | - | - | - | - | - | Infantile Infantile/gynecomastia | Autosomal recessive | Hypertension hypokalemic alkalosis |
| 17,20-Desmolase | A | M | N | N | N | N | - | - | Infantile | X-linked | |
| 17-Ketosteroid reductase | F or A | M | N | N | N | N | N | +Estrone +Androstenedione -Estradiol -Testosterone | Partial virilization ±gynecomastia | Autosomal recessive | ++Androstenedione ++Estrone -Testosterone -Estradiol |

[a] Information based on patients reported in the literature.

[b] Abbreviations: F, female; M, male; A, ambiguous; N, normal amount; -, decreased to absent; +, increased.

tion. Therefore, inborn errors are in this way indistinguishable from the other causes of male pseudohermaphroditism. On the other hand, in some mutations in which adrenal function is defective the phenotypes may overlap those seen in female pseudohermaphrodites with virilizing adrenal hyperplasia.

In the text, reference is made to complete or partial enzyme deficiencies. These distinctions are not based on enzyme assays, but on clinical phenotype and relative quantities of metabolites. At times the degree of masculinization provides the most sensitive assay for enzyme activity.

None of the enzymes involved in testosterone synthesis has been assigned to a human chromosome. The small number of affected individuals with each defect has precluded discriminating between autosomal recessive and X-linked inheritance (see Genetic Considerations).

**Defects in Steroidogenesis Involving Both the Adrenal Glands and the Testes.** The early steps of the steroidogenic pathway take place in the adrenal glands and testes. Therefore, deficiencies of enzymes required for these reactions result in manifestations of adrenocortical insufficiency as well as defective masculinization of the external genitalia. The phenotype depends on the nature of the mutation, i.e., whether it interferes with adrenal as well as testicular function and whether it results in a partial or complete deficiency of the pertinent product. It should be noted that production of müllerian inhibiting factor is not affected, and therefore none of the affected individuals has remnants of female internal ducts. Furthermore, the complete absence of androgen secretion results in the presence of a vaginal–utricular pouch with separate urethral and vaginal orifices. In cases of partial enzyme deficiency, there is incomplete masculinization with a utricular pouch of variable size and, in most cases, a urogenital sinus. Gynecomastia is frequently observed at puberty in males with partial deficiencies with an abnormal testosterone to estrogen ratio.

Deficiencies in enzymes involved in the early pathways (20-hydroxylase, 22-hydroxylase, 20,22-desmolase, 3β-hydroxysteroid dehydrogenase) will result in a life-threatening insufficiency of both mineralocorticoids and glucocorticoids. In contrast, a deficiency in 17-hydroxylase, the enzyme in the subsequent step, results in the accumulation of precursors with glucocortocoid and mineralo-corticoid activity and consequently is not as lethal; but in this case the excess of precursors produces hypertension. In each of these enzyme deficiencies, the production of cortisol is decreased, resulting in increased secretion of ACTH by the anterior pituitary. The excessive ACTH secretion is responsible for the accumulation of steroid precursors prior to the enzymatic defect.

*Deficiency of 20-Hydroxylase, 22-Hydroxylase or 20,22-Desmolase (202171).* Some inborn errors resulting from mutations involving an early step in the pathway have been termed "congenital lipoid adrenal hyperplasia" because of the accumulation of lipoid material within the cells of the adrenal cortex and gonad.[25,30,74,120] The synthesis of pregnenolone from cholesterol involves two hydroxylating enzymes, the 20-hydroxylase and the 22-hydroxylase, as well as a desmolase which catalyzes the subsequent cleavage of the side chain between carbons 20 and 22. Because these conditions are rare, frequently fatal in the neonatal period, and because sophisticated techniques in steroid chemistry are required for diagnosis, it is often impossible to determine which of the three enzymes is lacking. A deficiency of any one of these enzymes results in the same spectrum of clinical findings.

Although these mutations occur in both sexes, females do not have any abnormality of sexual differentiation but frequently succumb to adrenal insufficiency. On the other hand, the affected XY patients have female-like external genitalia, a shallow vagina, inguinal gonads, and male internal ducts. Even males, unless they have obviously ambiguous genitalia, are usually ascertained because of severe electrolyte imbalance. The urinary 17-ketosteroids and 17-hydroxycorticoids are low or undetectable.[25,30] Adrenal tissue, obtained from one affected male at autopsy was incubated with labeled cholesterol and showed impaired conversion of cholesterol to 20α-hydroxycholesterol; when 20α-hydroxycholesterol was supplied, the conversion to pregnenolone proceeded normally.[30]

Because the product resulting from the activity of these three enzymes is so essential it is not surprising that the affected individuals who survive excrete small amounts of androgen and glucocorticoid metabolites. The presence of the male internal duct system in the male survivors also indicates some degree of testosterone synthesis. In others whose genitalia are partially masculinized the symptoms of hypoadrenalism occur later, consistent with a less severe deficiency of the pertinent enzyme.[25]

Consanguinity has been observed among parents of affected males consistent with autosomal recessive transmission for at least one of the three enzyme deficiencies.[120]

*Deficiency of 3β-Hydroxysteroid Dehydrogenase (20181).* The next step in steroid biosynthesis is the conversion of pregnenolone to progesterone by the transfer of the 5,6-double bond to a 4,5-double bond and oxygenation of the $C_3$-hydroxyl group to a ketone. This reaction is mediated by an enzyme complex which includes a dehydrogenase and an isomerase. Pregnenolone also can be hydroxylated at $C_{17}$ and then undergo cleavage of the side chain to form dehydroepiandrosterone. The conversion of dehydroepiandrosterone (DHEA) to androstenedione, the immediate precursor of testosterone, is also mediated by 3β-hydroxysteroid dehydrogenase. As with the previous enzymes, a complete deficiency results in severe salt loss in both males and females and female external genitalia in the males. More than a dozen patients have been described but few survive the neonatal period.[17,63,113,161] Frequently, more than one sib is affected or there is a history of sibs who died in infancy with symptoms suggesting salt loss.

The enzyme deficiency is inferred by the pattern of steroid metabolites measured in urine and plasma. Specifically, the 17-ketosteroids are elevated, primarily because of an excess of dehydroepiandrosterone and its hydroxylated derivatives. Another abnormal urinary metabolite is pregn-5-ene-3,17,20-triol the result of alternate routes of pregnenolone metabolism.[63] In one instance, adrenal tissue obtained at autopsy was found to be deficient in 3β-hydroxysteroid dehydrogenase activity by histochemical methods.[161] This has been the most direct evidence supporting the proposed defect. There is preliminary evidence that the dehydrogenase and isomerase components of the enzyme complex are separable.[34,44]

Because of early enough initiation of cortisone therapy, one patient has survived to puberty, while his affected sib died in infancy.[113] Under treatment with cortisone, his pubertal development proceeded at the appropriate time, and although his plasma testosterone was in the normal pubertal range, dehydroepiandrosterone was abnormally elevated. When therapy was withdrawn, 3β-hydroxy-5-ene steroids reappeared in large amounts in both plasma and urine. Most likely, this patient has a partial enzyme deficiency; however, enzymatic activity might have been induced in the testes at puberty. Alternatively, the observed 3-keto-4-ene steroids such as testosterone may have been produced in the liver where it has been suggested that the enzyme is not deficient.[113]

*Deficiency of 17α-Hydroxylase (20211).* Figure 1 shows that both progesterone and pregnenolone can be hydroxylated in the 17α-position to produce steroids that are precursors for androgen or cortisol. If this hydroxylation cannot occur, cortisol secretion is low or absent with a resulting increase in ACTH secretion. Excessive ACTH, in turn, activates the 11-desoxycorticosterone–corticosterone pathway. The large amounts of corticosterone substitute for cortisol in providing normal glucocorticoid activity. However, the excessive 11-desoxycorticosterone is responsible for the hypertension and hypokalemic alkalosis characteristic of the syndrome and for the reduced secretion of renin and aldosterone.[15,20,90,104]

Clinical findings in males include lack of virilization if the deficiency is complete[57,73] or variable degrees of hypospadias and a utriculo-vaginal pouch if it is partial. The development of wolffian structures may be incomplete in those males with the most severe enzyme deficiency.[102]

Although affected females have normal müllerian ducts and external genitalia, they do not enter puberty because they fail to produce ovarian estrogens as a consequence of lacking the necessary precursor androgens for estrogen synthesis[50,90] (see Production of Testosterone).

The disorder is presumably transmitted as an autosomal recessive. Affected sibships have been identified; however, consanguinity has not been noted.

**Deficiencies of Enzymes of Testicular Origin.** Two inborn errors of testosterone biosynthesis involve steps that take place primarily in the testes. As expected, cortisol synthesis is not impaired but affected males fail to masculinize.

*Deficiency of 17,20-Desmolase.* The deficiency of the enzyme necessary for the cleavage of the side chain of 17-hydroxyprogesterone results in impaired production of androstenedione, the immediate precursor of testosterone. In the only reported family with this enzyme deficiency, the males had ambiguous genitalia characterized by labioscrotal fusion and a small phallus with hypospadias. In addition, there was incomplete development of the internal male ducts and inguinal gonads. The presence of some masculinization in these subjects is evidence that the enzyme deficiency is not complete. The urinary excretion of 17-ketosteroids was normal, but that of pregnenetriol was increased. Treatment with HCG did not stimulate testosterone secretion. ACTH administration did not affect dehydroepiandrosterone, but resulted in a normal increase in pregnanetriol and 17-hydroxycorticosteroids. The desmolase deficiency was further demonstrated by the inability to produce dehydroepiandrosterone and androstenedione from appropriate precursors in testicular tissue.

In this family, the enzyme deficiency had occurred in first cousins whose mothers were sisters. The proband's maternal aunt was also affected. The pattern suggests X-linkage of the pertinent enzyme.[160]

*Deficiency of 17-Ketosteroid Reductase (26430).* Production of testicular androgens is also impaired by a deficiency of the enzyme needed to form testosterone from androstenedione. Müllerian ducts regress as expected but wolffian ducts tend to be poorly developed. As in previously described inborn errors, the degree of masculinization of the external genitalia depends upon the extent of the enzyme deficiency. Usually the external genitalia appear nearly female at birth. At puberty, there is breast development as well as variable degrees of masculinization. The phenotype in adulthood is attributable to the plasma testosterone concentration which is greater than that of normal females, but less than that of adult males. Testicular specimens reveal leydig cell hyperplasia, consistent with chronic stimulation, and hyalinized seminiferous tubules with few spermatogonia. The most characteristic biochemical finding is the great increase in plasma androstenedione—up to ten times normal. There is also some increase in estrogens because of peripheral conversion from androgens.[3,48,49,127,128]

Most of the endogenous testosterone in these males is derived from androstenedione by extratesticular conversion.[49] Virtually no testosterone is obtained when testicular tissue is incubated with androstenedione, indicating the lack of the reductase activity in the testes.[49] However, fibroblasts and erythrocytes from the affected individuals form testosterone normally from androstenedione.[3] It is difficult to explain the lack of this enzyme activity in testicular cells but normal activity in other tissues such as skin fibroblasts, erythrocytes, and liver. It may be that the enzyme in leydig cells differs from that in extratesticular tissues or has been modified in some way. In the latter case, the mutation may involve the gene(s) specifying the modifiers, rather than the 17-ketosteroid reductase within the testes. Testicular tissue from rats with this deficiency manifest decreased testosterone production but can convert estrone to estradiol normally, which requires this enzyme activity. Perhaps the enzyme has a greater affinity for estrogens than androgens.[128]

The inheritance pattern has not been defined, because most of the cases have been sporadic, occurring in small families without a history of similarly affected relatives. Affected males do not reproduce because of azoospermia. In a few of the larger sibships more than one affected male has been found, but no affected females have been reported. In fact, females would not be expected to present any clinical abnormalities. Although ovarian cells in these females could not synthesize estradiol from testosterone, they could produce estrone, which is transformed into estradiol in the liver. As the parents of one affected male were first cousins, autosomal recessive transmission is likely.[49]

**Abnormalities of Androgen Target Cells.** Male pseudohermaphroditism may also result from abnormalities within the cells that respond to androgens. Among the disorders of target cells are a deficiency of the 5α-reductase enzyme and abnormalities related to androgen receptor activity.

*Deficiency of 5α-Reductase (26460).* Complete masculinization of the external genitalia depends upon the conversion of testosterone to a more potent metabolite, dihydrotestosterone (DHT). Target cells for androgens (see 5α-Reductase Activity) contain the enzyme 5α-reductase, which transforms testosterone to DHT.

The phenotype resulting from a deficiency of this enzyme depends upon the extent of the deficiency. At birth, the external genitalia of most affected males are so slightly masculinized that they are reared as females.[126] Wolffian ducts develop normally because internal duct differentiation depends upon testosterone rather than DHT.[154]

At puberty, the phenotype changes dramatically as certain male secondary sex characteristics appear (increase in muscle mass, enlargement of the phallus, and deepening of the voice) whereas others do not (development of facial and body hair, acne, hair-line recession, normal prostatic enlargement).[60,61,62,133]

Spermatogenesis has been documented, but insemination has not been reported, probably because of the severity of the hypospadias. None of the males has breast development, as testosterone levels are normal and estrogen levels are not elevated.[60,61,110,117]

Although incomplete, the masculinization at puberty is rather striking and contrasts with the relatively poor virilization which occurred in the fetus. It may be that DHT, although essential *in utero* for masculinization of the genitalia, is not essential for all of the secondary sex characteristics at puberty. It has been suggested that those secondary sex characteristics which develop at puberty are mediated by testosterone, whereas those that do not are mediated by DHT. As expected, there is no evidence of abnormal androgen receptors.[86] The relatively small amount of testosterone available *in utero* is probably insufficient for complete masculinization of the external genitalia. At puberty, however, the quantity of testosterone greatly exceeds that available to the fetus, and may be enough to promote masculinization.[86] Others have suggested that because some testosterone is diverted to estrogen in the fetus,[80] less is available for binding to the androgen receptor.

The diagnosis of 5α-reductase deficiency is confirmed by various laboratory studies. Diminished 5α-reductase activity can be demonstrated directly in cultured genital skin fibroblasts incubated with labeled testosterone.[100,118]

As expected, the ratio of plasma testosterone to DHT is increased.[60,61,118] However, the ratio of urinary 5α/5β steroids may provide a more sensitive test. In normals, testosterone is metabolized primarily in the liver yielding approximately equal amounts of 5α and 5β derivatives (Fig. 2), mainly androsterone (5α-androstan-3α-ol-17-one) and etiocholanolone (5β-androstan-3α-ol-17-one). Elevated ratios of urinary etiocholanolone to androsterone have been demonstrated in affected individuals and age-related values have been established.[62,118]

Most of the affected males belong to an inbred population in the southwestern Dominican Republic. Approximately 30 males have been ascertained among 17 related kindreds. Studies of these families indicate that the deficiency is transmitted as an autosomal recessive. The parents of affected males have ratios of urinary etiocholanolone to androsterone in a range intermediate between affected and normal. Some of the female relatives have ratios in the range of affected males and are believed to be homozygous for the mutation. These women are normal in all aspects of their sexual development including fertility and are identified only on the basis of their urinary metabolites.[118]

There is some evidence of genetic heterogeneity. Affected males ascertained in a Los Angeles family are phenotypically similar to those in the Dominican Republic kindreds, but have an enzyme with different characteristics.[78] In these male pseudohermaphrodites, the 5α-reductase activity was not detectable in homogenates of epididymal tissue but was normal in genital fibroblasts. The enzyme present in these fibroblasts had an increased $K_m$ for NADPH compared to the wild-type enzyme or to the residual enzyme from the Dominican Republic kindred. Other NADPH dependent enzymes in these males from Los Angeles exhibited normal kinetic properties.[78]

**Syndromes of Androgen Insensitivity.** A significant number of cases of male pseudohermaphroditism are related to androgen insensitivity. The lack of masculinization in this case is attributable not to an inadequate supply of androgens but to the inability of the target cell to respond to these hormones. The classification is based on the extent of the androgen insensitivity (complete or partial) and the presence (or absence) of androgen receptors.

*Complete Androgen Insensitivity with Absence of Androgen Receptor (31370).* This condition has been called the testicular feminization syndrome.[40,43,93,98,140] Characteristically the affected male has female external genitalia and is ascertained because of inguinal masses or at puberty because of primary amenorrhea and lack of pubic hair. Although the genitalia are unambiguously female and breast development occurs, the vagina ends in a blind pouch as müllerian inhibition has been complete. Frequently the wolffian ducts are hypoplastic. There is a maturation arrest in spermatogenesis and the leydig cells may be hyperplastic because of excessive LH stimulation.[37] The concentrations of testosterone and DHT in blood are often greater than those of normal adult males.[94,145,146] Characteristically there is a virtual absence of the receptor for DHT.[51,71,123,146] The feminization in these males is due to estrogens derived from the metabolism of androstenedione and testosterone in the liver. These individuals provide further evidence that receptors for androgens and estrogens are not identical.

This mutation is believed to be homologous with that at the testicular feminization (*Tfm*) locus in mouse mutants which lack the cytosol receptor protein.[84] The transmission is X-linked in the mouse and evidence from pedigrees supports the X-linkage in man. Studies of skin fibroblasts from an obligate heterozygote, the mother of three affected males, indicated that she had a significant number of DHT receptors and that there were two clonal populations with regard to DHT binding activity, one with normal activity and the other lacking activity, confirming the X-linkage of the mutation.[97]

Although it is clear that this X mutation results in the absence of androgen-binding activity, it remains to be determined if the binding protein is not made or is abnormal with respect to its ability to bind androgen (Fig. 3).

*Complete Androgen Insensitivity with Apparently Normal Androgen Receptor.* Not all individuals with the phenotype of androgen insensitivity lack androgen-binding activity.[69] Included among patients with normal androgen binding activity are families in which the segregation pattern suggests an X-linked disorder.[6] All affected members of a kindred are identical with regard to the presence or absence of androgen-binding activity.[6] The site of the mutation in these individuals has not been determined. There are several possible mutations that could result in androgen insensitivity (see Fig. 3). Although the receptor protein binds DHT, it is conceivable that it may not be able to be transferred to the nucleus, or the receptor may be altered so that it cannot bind to the acceptor. Alternatively, the acceptor may be modified so that it does not recognize the hormone receptor complex. Furthermore, mutations affecting other regulatory molecules needed for gene activation may produce the same effect. It is not yet clear if the hormone receptor complex interaction results in single or multiple androgen-dependent messages. If a single mRNA is produced, then mutations affecting processing and translation may also result in androgen insensitivity.

Studies of fibroblasts from two androgen insensitive males with normal binding activity indicated that translocation of the receptor complex to the nucleus was normal.[6] The mutation in these individuals therefore must affect the receptor protein's binding to the nuclear acceptor or subsequent steps.[5] Because of the lack of demonstrable biochemical abnormality at the level of cells in culture, it has not been possible to determine if this mutation is X-linked. If X-linked, the mutation may be allelic to the *Tfm* mutation with defective DHT-binding activity. It is important to recognize that there are two variants because prenatal diagnosis is feasible for affected males lacking the receptor, but not for those with normal binding activity (see Addendum).

*Partial Androgen Insensitivity (31380).* Other inborn errors have been described in which the insensitivity to androgens is not complete.[4,18,70,85,115,156] The syndrome described by Reifenstein[18] has been shown to represent partial androgen insensitivity.[4,70,115,156] These individuals have variable degrees of masculinization of the external genitalia and virilization at puberty is poor despite normal or elevated levels of androgens.[4] Gynecomastia is common and the testes are atrophic with tubular hyalinization and maturation arrest at the secondary spermatocyte stage.[4]

In the majority of the affected males, the binding capacity and affinity of the androgen receptor for DHT is normal so that these indivduals are most likely variants of the syndrome of androgen insensitivity with normal androgen binding activity. However, some affected males have a reduced number of binding sites for DHT and represent variants of the syndrome of androgen insensitivity with absent androgen-binding activity.[4]

There is familial aggregation of affected individuals. In several large pedigrees the pattern of transmission is compatible with X-linkage.[4]

In the case of "partial insensitivity," phenotypic expression is highly variable even within members of the same family. This variability has lead to multiple eponyms including Lubs syndrome,[83] Gilbert-Dreyfus syndrome,[46] and Rosewater syndrome[125] as well as Reifenstein syndrome (31230).

*Other Syndromes with Genital Abnormalities.* There are many disorders that include small or ambiguous genitalia as one of several congenital malformations. The etiology of the genital abnormality is usually related to maldevelopment of the genitourinary tract attributable to numerous insults, some no doubt, genetic. For instance, the association of Wilms' tumor with male pseudohermaphroditism is explained by a disruption of gonadal anlagen related to maldevelopment of the mesonephric structures.[7,11,33,142] (For a review of syndromes associated with abnormal external genitalia, the reader is referred to reference 24.)

## Heterozygote Detection

There has not been much success in detecting carriers of inborn errors of testosterone biosynthesis. This is primarily attributable to the fact that the phenotype being analyzed is usually not the pertinent enzyme, but an abnormal metabolite. It is unlikely that a 50% reduction in the activity of any enzyme will result in abnormal metabolism, at least under normal baseline circumstances. However, it is conceivable that under conditions of metabolic stress, it might be possible to detect even minimal deviations from normal. There has been some success in detecting carriers of 21-hydroxylase deficiency associated with adrenal hyperplasia. Although mean values of the increment of progesterone and 17-hydroxyprogesterone obtained for parents of affected children during an ACTH stimulation test differ from the mean in normal controls, individual values may be difficult to interpret.[54]

With regard to X-linked androgen insensitivity in which the DHT receptor protein is deficient, carriers have been identified as having both mutant and normal cells in fibroblast cultures.[97] Unfortunately, the assay is not a practical one for heterozygote detection as it is tedious requiring the examination of a sufficient number of clones.

Heterozygote detection would be feasible on the basis of association of the relevant locus with a closely linked polymorphic locus. For example, 21-hydroxylase deficiency associated with congenital adrenal hyperplasia has recently been shown to be linked to the *HLA-B* locus.[79]

## Prenatal Diagnosis

Recent advances in techniques suitable for prenatal diagnosis increase the possibility of diagnosis of male pseudohermaphroditism *in utero*. The combination of chromosome analysis in amniocytes and examination of the fetal genitalia using fetoscopy or refined sonography could determine if the genitalia are appropriate to the sex of the fetus. Specific etiologic diagnosis, expecially in regard to some of the inborn errors, is at least theoretically possible on the basis of the concentration of cortisol, testosterone, or the appropriate precursors and abnormal metabolites in the amniotic fluid.[103] However, normal values have not been established. The syndrome of androgen insensitivity with severe DHT-binding-protein deficiency is amenable to prenatal diagnosis based on the absence of DHT receptor activity in cultured amniocytes. Unfortunately, prenatal diagnosis is not possible for androgen insensitivity associated with androgen-binding activity.

ACKNOWLEDGMENTS. This work was supported by USPHS, National Institutes of Health Grant HD-05465, Grant AM-00180, Training Grant AM-07116, and Research Career Award AM-21855 (CJM).

## REFERENCES

1. Aarskog, D., Maternal progestins as a possible cause of hypospadias, *New Eng. J. Med.* **300**:75 (1979).
2. Abeyaratne, M., Aherne, W., and Scott, J., The vanishing testis, *Lancet* **ii**:822 (1969).
3. Akesode, F., Meyer, W., and Migeon, C., Male pseudohermaphroditism with gynecomastia due to testicular 17-ketosteroid reductase deficiency. *Clin. Endocrinol.* **7**:443 (1977).
4. Amrhein, J., Klingensmith, G., Walsh, P., McKusick, V., and Migeon, C., Partial androgen insensitivity—the Reifenstein syndrome revisited, *New Eng. J. Med.* **297**:350 (1977).
5. Amrhein, J., Meyer, W., Danish, R., and Migeon, C., Studies of androgen production and binding in 13 male pseudohermaphrodites and 13 males with micropenis, *J. Clin. Endocrinol. Metab.* **45**:732 (1977).

6. Amrhein, J., Meyer, W., Jones, H., and Migeon, C., Androgen insensitivity in man: Evidence for genetic heterogeneity, *Proc. Natl. Acad. Sci. USA* **73**:891 (1976).
7. Angstrom, T., Nephroblastoma in a case of agonadism, *Cancer* **18**:857 (1965).
8. Armendares, S., Buentello, L., and Frenk, S., Two male sibs with uterus and fallopian tubes, a rare, probably inherited disorder, *Clin. Genet.* **4**:291 (1973).
9. Axelrod, L., Neer, R., and Kilman, B., Hypogonadism in a male with immunologically active, biologically inactive luteinizing hormone: An exception to a venerable rule, *J. Clin. Endocrinol. Metab.* **48**:279 (1979).
10. Baghdassarian, A., Bayard, F., Borgaonkar, D., Arnold, E., Solez, K., and Migeon, C., Testicular function in XYY men, *Johns Hopkins Med. J.* **136**:15 (1975).
11. Barakat, Y., Papadopoulou, Z., Chandra, R., Hollerman, C., and Calcagno, P., Pseudohermaphroditism, nephron disorder and Wilms' tumor: A unifying concept. *Pediatrics* **54**:366 (1975).
12. Barr, M., Carr, D., Plunkett, E., Soltan, H., and Wiens, H., Male pseudohermaphroditism and pure gonadal dysgenesis in sisters, *Am. J. Obstet. Gynecol.* **89**:1047 (1964).
13. Baulieu, E., Atger, M., Best-Belpomme, M., Corval, P., Courvalen, J., Mester, J., Milgrom, E., Robel, P., Rochefort, H., and DeCatalogne, D., Steroid hormone receptors, *Vitam. Horm.* **33**:649 (1975).
14. Berthezene, F., Forest, M., Grimaud, J., Clasutrat, B., and Mornex, R., Leydig cell agenesis: A cause of male pseudohermaphroditism, *New Eng. J. Med.* **295**:969 (1976).
15. Biglieri, E., Herron, M., and Brust, N., 17-Hydroxylation deficiency in man, *J. Clin. Invest.* **45**:1946 (1966).
16. Blanchard, M., and Josso, N., Source of the anti-Mullerian hormone synthesized by the fetal testis:Mullerian-inhibiting activity of fetal bovine Sertoli cells in tissue culture, *Pediat. Res.* **8**:968 (1974).
17. Bongiovanni, A., The adrenogenital syndrome with deficiency of 3β-hydroxysteroid dehydrogenase, *J. Clin. Invest.* **41**:2086 (1962).
18. Bowen, P., Lee, C., Migeon, C., Kaplan, N., Whalley, P., McKusick, V., and Reifenstein, E., Hereditary male pseudohermaphroditism with hypogonadism, hypospadias and gynecomastia, *Ann. Intern. Med.* **62**:252 (1965).
19. Breg, W., Genel, M., Koo, G., Wachtel, S., Krupen-Brown, K., and Miller, O., H-Y antigen and human sex chromosomal abnormalities, in: *Genetic Mechanisms of Sexual Development* (L. Vallet and I. Porter, eds.), Academic Press, New York (1979).
20. Bricaire, H., Luton, J., Laudat, P., Legrand, J., Turpin, G., Corvol, P., and Lemmer, M., A new male pseudohermaphroditism associated with hypertension due to a block of 17α-hydroxylation, *J. Clin. Endocrinol Metab.* **35**:67 (1972).
21. Brook, C., Wagner, H., Zachman, M., Prader, A., Armendares, S., Frenk, S., Aleman, P., Najjar, S., Slim, M., Genton, N., and Bozic, C., Familial occurrence of persistent Mullerian structures in otherwise normal males, *Br. Med. J.* **1**:771 (1973).
22. Brown, D., Markland, C., and Dehner, L., Leydig cell hypoplasia: A cause of male pseudohermaphroditism, *J. Clin. Endocr. Metab.* **46**:1 (1978).
23. Bruchovsky, N. and Wilson, J., The conversion of testosterone to 5α-androstan-17β-ol-3-one by rat prostrate *in vivo* and *in vitro*, *J. Biol. Chem.* **213**:2012 (1968).
24. Buyser, M., and Feingold, M., Syndromes associated with abnormal external genital development, in: *Genetic Mechanisms of Sexual Development* (L. Vallet and I. Porter, eds.), Academic Press, New York (1979).
25. Camacho, A., Kowarski, A., Migeon, C., and Brough, A., "Congenital adrenal hyperplasia due to a deficiency of one of the enzymes involved in the biosynthesis of pregnenolone, *J. Clin. Endocr. Metab.* **28**:153 (1968).

26. Carr, D., Haggar, R., and Hart, A., Germ cells in the ovaries of XO female infants, *Clin. Path.* **49**:521 (1968).
27. Chemke, J., Carmichael, R., Stewart, J., Geer, R., and Robinson, A., Familial XY gonadal dysgenesis, *J. Med. Genet.* **7**:105 (1970).
28. Christian, J., Bixler, D., Dexter, R., and Donohue, J., Hypogonadotropic hypogonadism with anosmia: The Kallman syndrome, *Birth Defects Orig. Artic. Ser.* **VII**(6):166 (1971).
29. Cohen, M., and Shaw, M., Two XY siblings with gonadal dysgenesis and a female phenotype, *New Eng. J. Med.* **272**:1083 (1965).
30. Degenhart, H., Visser, H., Boon, H., and O'Doherty, N., Evidence for deficient 20α-cholesterol hydroxylase activity in adrenal tissue of a patient with lipoid adrenal hyperplasia, *Acta Endocrinol.* **71**:512 (1972).
31. de la Chapelle, A., Nature and origin of males with XX chromosomes, *Am. J. Hum. Genet.* **24**:71 (1972).
32. de la Chapelle, A., Koo, G., and Wachtel, S., Recessive sex-determining genes in human XX male syndrome, *Cell* **15**:837 (1978).
33. Drash, A., Sherman, F., Hartmann, W., and Blizzard, R., A syndrome of pseudohermaphroditism, Wilms' tumor, hypertension, and degenerative renal disease, *J. Pediatr.* **76**:585 (1970).
34. Edwards, D., O'Connor, J., Bransome, E., and Braselton, W., Human placental 3β-hydroxysteroid dehydrogenase: Δ5-isomerase, *J. Biol. Chem.* **251**:1632 (1976).
35. Fang, S., Anderson, K., and Liao, S., Receptor proteins for androgens, *J. Biol. Chem.* **244**:6584 (1969).
36. Ferenczy, A., and Richart, R., The fine structure of the gonads in the complete form of testicular feminization syndrome, *Am. J. Obstet. Gynecol.* **113**:399 (1972).
37. Ferguson-Smith, M., Karyotype-phenotype correlations in gonadal dysgenesis and their bearing on the pathogenesis of malformations, *J. Med. Genet.* **2**:142 (1965).
38. Ferguson-Smith, M., X-Y chromosomal interchange in the etiology of true hermaphroditism and of XX Klinefelter's syndrome, *Lancet* **ii**:475 (1966).
39. Fine, G., Mellinger, R., and Canton, J., Gonadoblastoma occurring in a patient with familial gonadal dysgenesis, *Am. J. Clin. Pathol.* **38**:615 (1962).
40. Forchielli, E., Rao, G., and Sarda, I., Testicular feminization: Clinical morphological and biochemical studies, *J. Clin. Endocrinol. Metab.* **25**:661 (1965).
41. Franks, R., Bunting, K., and Engel, E., Male pseudohermaphroditism with XYY sex chromosomes, *J. Clin. Endocr. Metab.* **27**:1623 (1967).
42. Frasier, S., Bashore, R., and Mosier, H., Gonadoblastoma associated with pure gonadal dysgenesis in monozygous twins, *J. Pediatr.* **64**:740 (1964).
43. French, F., Van Wyk, J., Baggett, B., Easterling, W., Talbert, L., Johnston, F., and Forchielli, E., Further evidence of a target organ defect in the syndrome of testicular feminization, *J. Clin. Endocrinol. Metab.* **26**:493 (1966).
44. Gallay, J., Vincent, M., DePaillerets, C., and Alfsen, A., Solubilization and separation of Δ5,3β-hydroxysteroid dehydrogenase and 3-oxosteroid-Δ4-Δ5-isomerase from bovine adrenal cortex microsomes, *Biochim. Biophys. Acta* **529**:79 (1978).
45. German, J., Simpson, J., and Chaganti, R., Genetically determined sex reversal in 46XY humans. *Science* **202**:53 (1978).
46. Gilbert-Dreyfus, S., Sebaoun, S., and Belaisch, J., Etude d'un cas familial d'androgynoidisme avec hypospadias grave, gynecomastie et hyperoestrogenie. *Ann. Endocrinol.* **18**:93 (1957).
47. Gillman, J., The development of the gonads in man with a consideration of the role

of fetal endocrines and histiogenesis of ovarian tumors, *Contrib. Embryol.* **32**:81 (1948).

48. Givens, J., Wiser, W., Summitt, R., Kerber, I., Andersen, R., Pittaway, D., and Fish, S., Familial male pseudohermaphroditism without gynecomastia due to deficient testicular 17-ketosteroid reductase activity, *New Eng. J. Med.* **291**:938 (1974).

49. Goebelsman, U., Horton, R., Mestman, J., Arce, J., Nagata, Y., Nakamura, R., Thorneycroft, I., and Mishell, D., Male pseudohermaphroditism due to testicular 17β-hydroxysteroid dehydrogenase deficiency, *J. Clin. Endocrinol. Metab.* **36**:867 (1973).

50. Goldsmith, O., Solomon, D., and Horton, R., Hypogonadism and mineralocorticoid excess: 17-hydroxylase deficiency, *New Eng. J. Med.* **277**:673 (1967).

51. Griffin, J., Punyashthiti, K., and Wilson, J., DHT binding by cultured human fibroblasts—comparison of cells from control subjects and from patients with hereditary male pseudohermaphroditism due to androgen insensitivity, *J. Clin. Invest.* **57**:1342 (1976).

52. Gruenwald, P., The development of the sex cords in the gonads of man and mammals, *Am. J. Anat.* **70**:359 (1942).

53. Grumbach, M. and Van Wyk, J., Disorders of sexual differentiation, in: *Textbook of Endocrinology* (R. Williams, ed.), W. B. Saunders, Philadelphia (1974).

54. Gutai, J., Lee, P., Johnsonbaugh, R., Gareis, F., Urban, M., and Migeon, C., Detection of the heterozygous state in siblings of patients with congenital adrenal hyperplasia due to 21-hydroxylase deficiency, *J. Pediatr.* **94**:770 (1979).

55. Hall, J., Morgan, A., and Blizzard, R., Familial congenital anorchia, in: *Genetic Forms of Hypogonadism* (D. Bergsma, ed.), p. 115, National Foundation March of Dimes, New York (1975).

56. Heller, G., and Clermont, Y., Kinetics of the germinal epithelium in man, *Rec. Prog. Horm. Res.* **20**:545 (1964).

57. Heremans, G., Moolenaar, A., and van Gelderen, H., Female phenotype in a male child due to 17α-hydroxylase deficiency, *Arch. Dis. Child.* **51**:721 (1976).

58. Hsu, L., Hirschhorn, K., Goldstein, A., and Barcinski, M., Familial chromosomal mosaicism, genetic aspects, *Ann. Hum. Genet.* **33**:343 (1970).

59. Hulten, M., and Pearson, P., Fluorescent evidence for spermatocytes with two Y chromosomes in an XYY male, *Ann. Hum. Genet.* **34**:273 (1971).

60. Imperato-McGinley, J., Guerrero, L., Gautier, T., German, J., and Peterson, R., Steroid 5α-reductase deficiency in man. An inherited form of male pseudohermaphroditism, in: *Genetic Forms of Hypogonadism* (D. Bergsma, ed.), p. 91, National Foundation March of Dimes, *Stratton*, New York, (1975).

61. Imperato-McGinley, J., Guerrero, L., Gautier, T., and Peterson, R., Steroid 5α-reductase deficiency in man: an inherited form of male pseudohermaphroditism, *Science* **186**:1213 (1974).

62. Imperato-McGinley, J., and Peterson, R., Male pseudohermaphroditism: The complexities of male phenotypic development, *Am. J. Med.* **61**:251 (1976).

63. Janne, O., Perheentupa, J., and Vihko, R., Plasma and urinary steroids in an eight year old boy with 3β-hydroxysteroid dehydrogenase deficiency, *J. Clin. Endocrinol. Metab.* **31**:162 (1970).

64. Jirasek, J., *Development of the Genital System and Male Pseudohermaphroditism*, Johns Hopkins Press, Baltimore (1971).

65. Josso, N., Picard, J., and Tran, D., The anti-Mullerian hormone, *Birth Defects Orig. Artic. Ser.* **XIII**(2):159 (1977).

66. Jost, A., A new look at the mechanisms controlling sex differentiation in mammals, *Johns Hopkins Med. J.* **130**:38 (1971).

67. Kaplan, S., and Grumbach, M., The ontogenesis of human foetal hormones. II. LH and FSH, *Acta Endocrinol.* **81**:808 (1976).
68. Kasdan, R., Nankin, H., Troen, P., Wald, N., Pan, S., and Yanaihara, T., Paternal transmission of maleness in XX human beings, *New Eng. J. Med.* **288**:539 (1973).
69. Kauffman, M., Straisfeld, C., and Pinsky, L., Male pseudohermaphroditism presumably due to target organ unresponsiveness to androgens, *J. Clin. Invest.* **58**:345 (1976).
70. Keenan, B., Kirkland, J., Kirkland, R., and Clayton, G., Male pseudohermaphroditism with partial androgen insensitivity, *Pediatrics* **59**:224 (1977).
71. Keenan, B., Meyer, W., Hadjian, A., Jones, H., and Migeon, C., Syndrome of androgen insensitivity in man: Absence of 5α-dihydrotestosterone binding protein in skin fibroblasts, *J. Clin. Endocrinol. Metab.* **38**:1143 (1974).
72. Keenan, B., Meyer, W., Hadjian, A., and Migeon, C., Androgen receptor in human skin fibroblasts—characterization of a specific 17β-hydroxy-5α-androstan-3-one protein complex in cell sonicates and nuclei, *Steroids* **25**:535 (1975).
73. Kershnar, A., Bornt, D., Kogut, M., Biglieri, E., and Schambelan, M., Studies in a phenotypic female with 17α-hydroxylase deficiency, *J. Pediatr.* **891**:395 (1976).
74. Kirkland, R., Kirkland, J., Johnson, C., Horning, M., Librik, L., and Clayton, G., Congenital lipoid adrenal hyperplasia in an eight year old phenotypic female, *J. Clin. Endocr. Metab.* **36**:488 (1973).
75. Kirschner, M., Jacobs, J., and Fraley, E., Bilateral anorchia with persistent testosterone production, *New Eng. J. Med.* **282**:240 (1970).
76. Koo, G., Wachtel, S., Krupen-Brown, K., Mittl, L., Breg, W., Genel, M., Rosenthal, I., Borgoankar, D., Miller, D., Tantravahi, R., Schreck, R., Erlanger, B., and Miller, O., Mapping the locus of the *H-Y* gene on the human Y chromosome, *Science* **198**:940 (1977).
77. Leonard, J., Paulsen, C., Ospina, L., and Burgess, E., The classification of Klinefelter's syndrome, in: *Genetic Mechanisms of Sexual Development* (L. Vallet and I. Porter, ed.), Academic Press, New York (1979).
78. Leshin, M., Griffin, J., and Wilson, J., Hereditary male pseudohermaphroditism associated with an unstable form of 5α-reductase, *J. Clin. Invest.* **60**:685 (1978).
79. Levine, L., Zachman, M., New, M., Prader, A., Pollack, M., O'Neill, G., Yang, S., Oberfield, S., and Dupont, B., Genetic Mapping of the 21-hydroxylase deficiency gene within the HLA linkage group, *New Eng. J. Med.* **299**:911 (1978).
80. Lieberburg, I. and McEwen, B., Estradiol-17β—a metabolite of testosterone recovered in cell nuclei from limbic areas of neonatal rat brain, *Brain Res.* **85**:165 (1975).
81. Lovinger, R., Kaplan, S., and Grumbach, M., Congenital hypopituitarism associated with neonatal hypoglycemia and microphallus: four cases secondary to hypothalamic hormone deficiencies, *J. Pediatr.* **87**:1171 (1975).
82. Lowry, R., Honore, L., Arnold, W., Johnson, H., Kliman, M., and Marshall, R., Familial true hermaphroditism, in: *Genetic Forms of Hypogonadism* (D. Bergsma, ed.), p. 105, National Foundation March of Dimes, New York (1975).
83. Lubs, H., Jr., Vilar, O., and Bergenstal, D., Familial male pseudohermaphroditism with labial testes and partial feminization: Endocrine studies and genetic aspects, *J. Clin. Endocrinol. Metab.* **19**:1110 (1959).
84. Lyon, M., and Hawkes, S., X-linked gene for testicular feminization in the mouse, *Nature* **225**:1217 (1970).
85. Madden, J., Walsh, P., MacDonald, P., and Wilson, J., Clinical and endocrinologic characterization of a patient with the syndrome of incomplete testicular feminization, *J. Clin. Endocrinol. Metab.* **41**:451 (1975).
86. Maes, M., Sultan, C., Zerhouni, N., Rothwell, S., and Migeon, C., Role of testosterone

binding to the androgen receptor in male sexual differentiation of patients with 5α-reductase deficiency, *J. Steroid Biochem.* **11**:1385 (1979).

87. Mainwaring, W., and Mangan, F., A study of the androgen receptors in a variety of androgen sensitive tissues, *J. Endocrinol.* **59**:121 (1973).

88. Mainwaring, W., and Milroy, E., Characterization of the specific androgen receptors in the human prostate gland, *J. Endocrinol.* **57**:371 (1973).

89. Mainwaring, W., and Peterken, B., A reconstituted cell free system for the specific transfer of steroid-receptor complexes into nuclear chromation isolated from rat ventral prostrate gland, *Biochem. J.* **125**:285 (1971).

90. Mallin, S., Cogenital adrenal hyperplasia secondary to 17-hydroxylase deficiency, *Ann. Intern. Med.* **70**:69 (1969).

91. Mancini, R., Narbaitz, R., and LaVieri, J., Origin and development of the germinative epithelium and sertoli cells in the human testis: Cytological, cytochemical, and quantitative study, *Anat. Rec.* **136**:477 (1960).

92. Manuel, M., Katayama, K., and Jones, H. The age of occurrence of gonadal tumors in intersex patients with a Y chromosome, *Am. J. Obstet. Gynecol.* **124**:293 (1976).

93. Marshall, H., and Harder, H., Testicular feminizing syndrome in male pseudohermaphrodite: report of two cases in identical twins, *Obstet. Gynecol.* **12**:284 (1958).

94. Mauvais-Jarvis, P., Bercovici, J., Crepy, O., and Gauthier, F., Studies on testosterone metabolism in subjects with testicular feminization syndrome, *J. Clin. Invest.* **49**:31 (1970).

95. McKusick, V., *Mendelian Inheritance in Man,* 5th Ed., Johns Hopkins University Press, Baltimore (1978).

96. Meyer, W., Keenan, B., DeLacerda, L., Park, I., Jones, H., and Migeon, C., Familial male pseudohermaphroditism with normal leydig cell function at puberty, *J. Clin. Endocrinol. Metab.* **46**:593 (1978).

97. Meyer, W., Migeon, B., and Migeon, C., Locus on human X chromosome for DHT receptor and androgen insensitivity, *Proc. Nat. Acad. Sci. USA* **72**:1469 (1975).

98. Migeon, C., Amrhein, J., Keenan B., Meyer, W., and Migeon, B., The syndrome of androgen insensitivity in man: Its relation to our understanding of male sex differentiation, in: *Genetic Mechanisms of Sexual Development* (L. Vallet and I. Porter, eds.), Academic Press, New York (1979).

99. Milner, W., Garlick, W., Fink, A., and Stein, A., True hermaphrodite siblings, *J. Urol.* **79**:1003 (1958).

100. Moore, R., Griffin, J., and Wilson, J., Diminished 5α-reductase activity in extracts of fibroblasts cultured from patients with familial incomplete male pseudohermaphroditism, type 2, *J. Biol. Chem.* **250**:7168 (1975).

101. Moore, R., and Wilson, J., Steroid 5α-reductase in cultured human fibroblasts. Biochemical and genetic evidence for two distinct enzyme activities, *J. Biol. Chem.* **251**:5895 (1976).

102. New, M., Male pseudohermaphroditism due to 17α-hydroxylase deficiency, *J. Clin. Invest.* **49**:1930 (1970).

103. New, M., Prenatal diagnosis of congenital adrenal hyperplasia, in: *Genetic Mechanisms of Sexual Development* (L. Vallet and I. Porter, eds.), Academic Press, New York (1979).

104. New, M., and Peterson, R., A new form of congenital adrenal hyperplasia, *J. Clin. Endocrinol. Metab.* **27**:300 (1967).

105. Niebuhr, E., Triploidy in man, *Humangenetik* **21**:103 (1974).

106. Nutting, P., and Schimke, R., The Kallman syndrome, *Birth Defects Orig. Artic. Ser.* **VII**(6):172 (1971).

107. Ohno, S., H-Y antigen and chromosomal determination of primary (gonadal) sex, in:

*Major Sex Determining Genes Monographs in Endocrinology,* Vol. II. Springer-Verlag. New York (1979).

108. O'Malley, B., Mechanisms of action of steroid hormones. *New Eng. J. Med.* **294**:370 (1971).

109. O'Malley, B., and Shrader, W., The receptors of steroid hormones, *Sci. Am.* **234**:32 (1976).

110. Opitz, J., Simpson, J., Sarto, G., Summit, R., New, M., and German, J., Pseudovaginal perineoscrotal hypospadias, *Clin. Genet.* **3**:1 (1971).

111. Park, J., Burnett, L., Jones, H., Migeon, C., and Blizzard, R., A case of male pseudohermaphroditism associated with elevated LH, normal FSH and low testosterone, possibly due to the secretion of an abnormal LH molecule, *Acta Endocrinol.* **83**:173 (1976).

112. Park, I., Jones, H., and Bias, W., True hermaphrodite with 46XX/46XY chromosome complement, *Obstet. Gynecol.* **36**:377 (1970).

113. Parks, G., Bermudez, J., Anast, C., Bongiovanni, A., and New, M., Pubertal boy with the 3β-hydroxysteroid dehydrogenase defect, *J. Clin. Endocrinol. Metab.* **33**:269 (1971).

114. Parks, G., Dumars, K., Limbeck, G., Quinlivan, L., and New, M., True agonadism: a misnomer?, *J. Pediatr.* **84**:375 (1974).

115. Perez-Palacios, G., Ortiz, S., Lopez-Amor, E., Morato, T., Febres, F., Lisker, R., and Scaglia, H., Familial incomplete virilization due to partial end organ insensitivity to androgen, *J. Clin. Endocrinol. Metab.* **41**:946 (1975).

116. Perez-Palacios, G., Scaglia, H., Kofman, S., Saavedra, D., Ochoa, S., Laroza, O., and Perez, A., Inherited deficiency of gonadotropin receptor in leydig cells: A new form of male pseudohermaphroditism, *Am. J. Hum. Genet.* **27**:71A (1975).

117. Peterson, R., Imperato-McGinley, J., Gautier, T., and Sturla, E., Male pseudohermaphroditism due to steroid 5α-reductase deficiency, *Am. J. Med.* **62**:170 (1977).

118. Pinsky, L., Kaufman, M., Straisfeld, C., Zilahi, B., and Hall, C., 5α-reductase activity of genital and nongenital skin fibroblasts from patients with 5α-reductase deficiency, androgen insensitivity, or unknown forms of male pseudohermaphroditism. *Am. J Med. Genet.* **1**:407 (1978).

119. Powers, H., New R., Sonulyan, H., and Gardner, L., An adult phenotypic male with a 46XX chromosome complement, *J. Clin. Endocrinol. Metab.* **31**:576 (1970).

120. Prader, V. and Siebenmann, R., Nebennlereninsuffizienz bei Kongenitaler Lipoidhyperplasie der Nebennieren. *Helv. Pediatr. Acta* **12**:569 (1957).

121. Rajfer, J., Mendelsohn, G., Amrhein, J., Jeffs, R., and Walsh, P., Dysgenetic male pseudohermaphroditism, *J. Urol.* **119**:525 (1978).

122. Rios, E., Herrera, J., Bermudez, J., Rocha, G., Lisker, R., Morato, T., and Perez-Palacios, G., Endocrine and metabolic studies in an XY patient with gonadal agenesis, *J. Clin. Endocrinol. Metab.* **39**:540 (1974).

123. Rivarola, M., Saez, J., Meyer, W., Kenny, F., and Migeon, C., Studies of androgens in the syndrome of male pseudohermaphroditism with testicular feminization, *J. Clin. Endocrinol. Metab.* **27**:371 (1967).

124. Rosenberg, H., Clayton, G., and Hsu, T., Familial true hermaphrodism, *J. Clin. Endocrinol. Metab.* **23**:203 (1963).

125. Rosewater, S., Gwinup, G., and Hamwi, G., Familial gynecomastia, *Ann. Intern. Med.* **63**:377 (1965).

126. Saenger, P., Goldman, A., Levine, L., Korthschutz, S., Muecke, E., Katsumata, M., Doberne, Y., and New, M., Prepubertal diagnosis of steroid 5α-reductase deficiency, *J. Clin. Endocrinol. Metab.* **46**:627 (1978).

127. Saez, J., dePeretti, E., Morera, A., David, M., and Bertrand, J., Familial male pseu-

dohermaphroditism with gynecomastia due to a testicular 17-ketosteroid reductase defect, studies *in vivo, J. Clin. Endocrinol. Metab.* **32**:604 (1971).

128. Saez, J., Morera, A., dePeretti, E., and Bertrand, J., Further *in vivo* studies in male pseudohermaphroditism with gynecomastia due to a testicular 17-ketosteroid reductase defect, *J. Clin. Endocrinol. Metab.* **34**:598 (1972).

129. Schultz, F. and Wilson, J., Virilization of the Wolffian duct in the rat fetus by various androgens, *Endocrinology* **94**:979 (1974).

130. Shanies, D., Hirschhorn, K., and New, M., Metabolism of testosterone $C^{14}$ by cultured human cells, *J. Clin. Invest.* **51**:1459 (1972).

131. Shapiro, L., Mohandes, T., Weiss, R., and Romeo, G., Non activation of an X chromosome locus in man, *Science* **204**:1224 (1979).

132. Siiteri, P. and Wilson, J., Testosterone formation and metabolism during male sexual differentiation in the human embryo, *J. Clin. Endocrinol. Metab.* **38**:113 (1974).

133. Simpson, J., *Disorders of Sexual Differentiation,* Academic Press, New York (1976).

134. Simpson, J., Gonadal dysgenesis and sex chromosome abnormalities, phenotype-karyotypic correlations, in: *Genetic Mechanisms of Sexual Development* (L. Vallet and I. Porter, eds.), Academic Press, New York (1979).

135. Simpson, J., True hermaphroditism: etiology and phentypic considerations in: *Sex Differentiation and Chromosomal Abnormalities, Birth Defects Orig. Artic. Ser.* **XIV** (6C):9 (1978).

136. Singh, R., and Carr, D., The anatomy and histology of XO human embryos and fetuses, *Anat. Rec.* **155**:369 (1966).

137. Shakkebaek, N., Philip, J., Mikkelsen, M., Hammen, R., Nielsen, J., Perboll, O., and Yde, H., Studies on spermatogenesis, meiotic chromosomes and sperm morphology in two males with 47XYY chromosome complement, *Fertil. Steril.* **21**:645 (1970).

138. Sloan, W., and Walsh, P., Familial persistent Mullerian duct syndrome, *J. Urol.* **115**:459 (1976).

139. Spaulding, M., The Development of the external genitalia in the human embryo, *Contrib. Embryol.* **13**:67 (1921).

140. Stenchever, M., Ng, A., Jones, G., and Jarvis, J., Testicular feminization syndrome. Chromosomal, histologic, and genetic studies in a large kindred, *J. Obstet. Gynecol.* **33**:649 (1969).

141. Sternberg, W., Barclay, D., and Kloepfer, H., Familial XY gonadal dysgenesis, *New Eng. J. Med.* **278**:695 (1972).

142. Stump, T., and Garret, R., Bilateral Wilms' tumor in a male pseudohermaphrodite, *J. Urol.* **72**:1146 (1964).

142a. Sultan, C., Migeon, B., Rothwell, S., Maes, M., Zerhouni, N., and Migeon, C., Androgen receptors in cultured human fetal fibroblasts, *Pediatr. Res.* **14** (1980).

143. Sundequist, U., and Hellstrom, E., Transmission of 47XYY karyotype?, *Lancet* **ii**:1367 (1969).

144. Thompson, H., Melnyk, J., and Hecht, F., Reproduction and meiosis in XYY, *Lancet* **ii**:831 (1967).

145. Tremblay, R., Kowarski, A., Park, I., and Migeon, C., Blood production rate of dihydrotestosterone in the syndrome of male pseudohermaphroditism with testicular feminization, *J. Clin. Endocrinol. Metab.* **35**:101 (1972).

146. Tremblay, R., Foley, T., Corvol, P., Park, I., Kowarski, A., Blizzard, R., Jones, H., and Migeon, C., Plasma concentration of testosterone, DHT, testosterone-oestradiol binding globulin and pituitary gonadotropins in the syndrome of male pseudohermaphroditism with testicular feminization, *Acta Endocrinol.* **70**:331 (1972).

147. von Seemen, H., Pseudohermaphroditismus masculinis internus-kryptorchismus hernia inguinalis congenita, *Bruns. Beitr. Klin. Chir.* **141**:370 (1927).

148. Wachtel, S., H-Y antigen and sexual development in: *Genetic Mechanisms of Sexual Development* (L. Vallet and I. Porter, eds.), Academic Press, New York (1979).
149. Wachtel, S., Immunogenetic aspects of abnormal sexual differentiation, *Cell* **16**:691 (1979).
150. Wachtel, S., Koo, G., Breg, W., Elias, S., Boyse, E., and Miller, O., Expression of H-Y antigen in humans with two Y chromosomes, *New Eng. J. Med.* **293**:1070 (1975).
151. Walsh, P., Madden, J., Harrod, M., Goldstein, J., MacDonald, P., and Wilson, J., Familial incomplete male pseudohermaphroditism, type 2. Decreased dihydrotestosterone formation in pseudovaginal perineoscrotal hypospadias, *New Eng. J. Med.* **291**:944 (1974).
152. Wartenberg, H., Human testicular development and the role of the mesonephros in the origin of the dual Sertoli cell system, *Andrologia* **10**(1):1 (1978).
153. Weiss, E., Kiefer, J., Rowlatt, U., and Rosenthal, I., Persistent Mullerian duct syndrome in male identical twins, *Pediatrics* **61**:797 (1978).
154. Wilson, J., Recent studies on the mechanism of action of testosterone, *New Eng. J. Med.* **287**:1284 (1972).
155. Wilson, J., Sexual differentiation, *Ann. Rev. Physiol.* **40**:279 (1978).
156. Wilson, J., Harrod, M., Goldstein, J., Hemsell, D., and MacDonald, P., Familial incomplete male pseudohermaphroditism type 1. Evidence for androgen resistance in a family with the Reifenstein syndrome, *New Eng. J. Med.* **290**:1097 (1974).
157. Wilson, J., and Walker, J., The conversion of testosterone to dihydrotestosterone by skin slices of man, *J. Clin. Invest.* **48**:371 (1969).
158. Winter, J., Faiman, C., and Reyes, R., Sex steroid production by the human fetus: Its role in morphogenesis and control by gonadotropins, *Birth Defects Orig. Artic. Ser.* **XIII**(2):41 (1977).
159. Witschi, E., Migrations of germ cells of human embryos from the yolk sac to the primitive gonadal folds, *Contrib. Embryol.* **32**:67 (1948).
160. Zachman, M., Vollman, J., Hamilton, W., and Prader, A., Steroid 17.20-desmolase deficiency. A new cause of male pseudohermaphroditism, *Clin. Endocrinol.* **1**:369 (1972).
161. Zachman, M., Vollmin, J., Murset, G., Curtius, H., and Prader, A., Unusual type of congenital adrenal hyperplasia probably due to a deficiency of 3β-hydroxysteroid dehydrogenase. Case report of a surviving girl and steroid studies, *J. Clin. Endocrinol. Metab.* **30**:719 (1970).

Patrick, S., et al. Illustrated hand... and computer control of the...

Rosenblum, J., Image Internetwork... Interferation and Computation Index...

Rosenblum, S., Image representation and...

# Addenda

## CHAPTER 1: BIOCHEMISTRY AND GENETICS OF THE ABO, LEWIS, AND P BLOOD GROUP SYSTEMS

Winifred M. Watkins

**THE ABO SYSTEM**

*Chemistry of A, B, and H Substances*

*Glycolipids.* A ganglioside with blood group H activity was isolated from human erythrocyte membranes and identified as a monosialosyl ceramide decasaccharide (Watanabe *et al.*, 1978). The structure of this compound was determined as

α-Fuc(1→2)β-Gal(1→4)β-GlcNAc(1

$$\searrow 6)$$

β-Gal(1→4)β-GlcNAc(1→3)
β-Gal(1→4)β-Glc-CER

$$\nearrow 3)$$

α-NeuNAc(2→3)β-Gal(1→4)β-GlcNAc(1

and it represents one of a new molecular species containing both fucosyl and sialosyl substitution (fucoganglioside) which has been found recently in various animal tissues. Structural studies on both glycolipids and glycoproteins with this complexity of carbohydrate chains have been greatly facilitated by the discovery of bacterial *endo*-glycosidases which split off

379

intact oligosaccharide fragments by breaking internal linkages in the carbohydrate chains (Kobata and Takasaki, 1978; Fukuda *et al.*, 1978).

Human meconium has for many years been known as a rich source of ABH blood group substances (Buchanan and Rapoport, 1951), and highly purified specimens of blood-group-active glycoproteins have been isolated from this material (Côté and Valet, 1976). The occurrence in meconium of glycolipids with blood group activity was also noted by Côté (1970), and more recently Karlsson and Larson (1978) started a systematic investigation of meconium as a source of epithelial blood-group-active glycolipids. Lacto-*N*-tetraosylceramide, β-Gal(1→3)β-GlcNAc(1→3)β-Gal(1→4)Glc-CER, which was postulated as the precursor of the Lewis active glycolipids and of the ABH glycolipids with a Type I saccharide chain (see p. 86), has been isolated for the first time from human meconium and structurally characterized (Karlsson and Larson, 1979). A more remarkable glycolipid isolated from the same source, α-Fuc(1→2)β-Gal(1→3)β-GalNAc(1→3)α-Gal(1→4)β-Gal(1→4)Glc-CER has a terminal H-structure attached to globoside (Larson, 1979). The existence of such a compound emphasizes the interrelationship between the precursor glycolipids of the ABH and P systems (see p. 109) and the fact that the *H*-gene-specified α-2-L-fucosyltransferase appears to be able to utilize a variety of acceptor substrates provided they contain a terminal nonreducing β-D-galactosyl residue (see p. 38).

A glycolipid based on lacto-*N*-tetraosylceramide has been isolated from the small intestine of a blood group B person (Briemer, 1979) and characterized as

$$\alpha\text{-Gal}(1\to3)\beta\text{-Gal}(1\to3)\beta\text{-GlcNAc}(1\to3)\beta\text{-Gal}(1\to4)\text{Glc-CER}$$

$$\uparrow 1,2 \qquad\quad \uparrow 1,4$$
$$\alpha\text{-Fuc} \qquad \alpha\text{-Fuc}$$

This compound lacks either B or Le[b] activity, but presumably the grouping at the nonreducing end comprises the structure reacting with those cytotoxic sera exhibiting anti-BLe[b] specificity (see p. 85).

*Ii Specificity and Structures of Ii Determinants.* Work culminating in the last year has largely unraveled the specificities of anti-I sera and clarified the relationships between I and i. Immunochemical inhibition experiments with a family of related glycosphingolipids (Feizi *et al.*, 1979; Watanabe *et al.*, 1979) established that most of the monoclonal anti-I reagents react with domains within the branched glycolipid lacto-*N*-*iso*-octaosylceramide:

Gal-β(1→4)-GlcNAc(1  
           ↘β  
           6)  
               Gal-β(1→4)GlcNAc-β(1→3)Gal-β(1→1)Glc-CER  
           3)  
           ↗β  
Gal-β(1→4)-GlcNAc(1

and the majority of i specificities are determined by the straight-chain glycolipid lacto-*N*-norhexaosylceramide (see p. 32). None of the anti-I sera was identical in its inhibition pattern with nine glycosphingolipid analogues, thus reinforcing earlier views on the heterogeneity of these monoclonal antibodies (see p. 31). Nevertheless fourteen out of sixteen anti-I reagents could be classified into three main types (Feizi *et al.*, 1979). The first type required the intact branch β-Gal(1→4)β-GlcNAc(1→6)Gal, the second type required β-Gal(1→4)β-GlcNAc(1→3)Gal with the branch point and the third type required both branches to be intact. The anti-I antibodies varied in their ability to react with their antigenic determinants when the terminal β-galactosyl residue was substituted with other sugars but removal of both the terminal β-galactosyl residues from the branched structure gave a glycosphingolipid which failed to react with any of the anti-I sera. This result thus does not agree with one of the inferences arrived at earlier on the basis of enzyme degradation experiments (see p. 30) that some anti-I reagents react with structures lacking terminal β-galactosyl residues.

    The finding that i specificity is associated with an unbranched chain supports the view that a progressive branching process is associated with development of fetal into adult erythrocyte membranes:

                        Gal-β(1→4)GlcNAc(1  
                                    ↘β  
                                 3)  
Gal-β(1→4)GlcNAc-β(1→3)Gal→R →          Gal→R  
                                   6)  
                                 ↗β  
                    Gal-β(1→4)GlcNAc(1

and that i reactivity is suppressed as branching occurs (Hakomori, 1979). Investigations on the complex glycosphingolipids of the red cell membrane support this hypothesis. Fractions of complex glycosphingolipids prepared from adult I, cord, and adult i red cells by the methods elaborated for the isolation of poly(glycosyl)ceramides revealed that the highly branched and complex poly(glycosyl)ceramides with an average of 30 glycosyl units can be obtained only from adult-I-active cells (Koscielak et al., 1979). Complex glycosphingolipids from cord and i red cells comprised 6 and 15 glycosyl units, respectively, and exhibited high i activity which is not detectable in the polyglycosyl ceramides. Whereas the poly(glycosyl)ceramides averaged about 5 branching points per molecule, the materials isolated from cord and adult i red cells averaged only 0.7 branching points per molecule. The association of I specificities with branched oligosaccharide chains accords with the view expressed earlier by Koscielak et al. (see p. 14) that the I gene can be considered to be the structural gene coding for the formation of the β-6-N-acetylglucosaminyltransferase that catalyzes the formation of the branch point. This enzyme has yet to be characterized, but it is to be anticipated that the enzyme will be absent, or poorly active, in newborn infants and in adults with the i phenotype.

The carbohydrate sequences associated with both i and I specificities occur as core structures in the ABH antigens on the red cells; hence the Ii antigenic sites available for reactivity with anti-I and anti-i reagents can be regarded as incomplete blood-group-active chains.

### Glycosyltransferase Products of the A and B Genes

*Allelic Status of the A and B Genes.* Further evidence in support of the concept that the expression of A and B transferases is controlled by genes located at a common locus has come from experiments on the donor substrate specificity of the B-gene-specified α-3-D-galactosyltransferase. It has been found that at higher pH values the B transferase has the capacity to transfer small amounts of N-acetyl[$^{14}$C]galactosamine to H-active structures to form compounds indistinguishable from the A-active oligosaccharides synthesized by the A-gene-specified α-3-N-acetyl-D-galactosaminyltransferase (Greenwell et al., 1979). Although under normal circumstances the conditions in vivo presumably are such that this transfer does not occur, the fact that the B transferase has some capacity to add N-acetylgalactosamine onto H structures suggests that the difference in primary structure between the active sites of the A-gene-specified transferase and the B-gene-specified enzyme must be relatively small and hence compatible with that to be expected of alternative forms at one genetic locus. The findings are also consistent with the view that a mutant allele at the *ABO* locus coding for an enzyme capable of transferring both *N*-acetylgalactosamine and D-galactose to *H* structures may account for the rare *cis AB* phenotypes in which both *A* and *B* genes appear to be inherited from one parent (see p. 65).

Independent immunological evidence in support of the allelic status of the *A* and *B* genes has come from the studies of Yoshida *et al.* (1979). Rabbits immunized with purified human *A* transferase produced antibodies which not only completely neutralized the activity of the homologous *A* enzyme but also inactivated the *B* transferase. Control globulin preparations obtained from preimmune rabbit serum had no such neutralization capacity. Moreover, protein isolated from O plasma similarly combined with the antibody as evidenced by its diminished capacity to neutralize the *A* transferase. These results point to the immunological similarity of the *A* and *B* transferase proteins and the existence of an enzymically inactive, but immunologically cross-reactive, protein in the plasma of group O individuals.

The demonstration of overlapping donor substrate specificity of the *A* and *B* transferases, together with the evidence for immunological cross-reactivity of the enzyme proteins, therefore lends support to the belief that the two enzymes are the primary protein products of alternative forms at a single locus and militate against the possibility that the *A, B,* and *O* alleles are normally involved in the regulation of ubiquitous genes situated at other loci (see p. 78).

## THE P SYSTEM

More detailed analyses of the antigens and antibodies in the *P* system have thrown further light on the complex interrelationships in this system although the biosynthetic pathways are still not clarified. Naiki and Kato (1979) demonstrated that the $P^k$ antigen on normal $P_2$ red cells is not "cryptic" as was formerly thought. They used serum from individuals of *p* phenotype (anti-$P_1$, *P*, $P^k$) from which *P* antibodies were removed by absorption with the *P*-active glycolipid, globoside (see p. 103); the remaining antibodies reacted with both $P_1$ and $P_2$ red cells. Earlier failure to demonstrate the $P^k$ activity of $P_2$ cells was attributed to the fact that the anti-$P^k$ reagents were prepared by absorption of *p* sera with $P_1$ red cells which themselves contain small amounts of ceramide trihexoside

($P^k$ antigen). The $P^k$ antibodies left after such an absorption would be those requiring a higher density of $P^k$ antigenic sites than is found in normal $P^k$ red cells.

A quantitative measure of the amount of ceramide trihexoside and other neutral glycosphingolipids in $P_1$ and $P_2$ cells has been achieved by Fletcher et al. (1979). These authors analyzed the glycosphingolipid content of erythrocytes by a method utilizing high-performance liquid chromatography which enabled them to measure accurately the amounts of the individual neutral glycolipids in extracts from samples of blood as small as 0.05 ml. By this method they established that the erythrocytes of $P_1$ individuals have a higher content of ceramide trihexoside ($P^k$ antigen) than lactosyl ceramide whereas the opposite is true for the cells of $P_2$ individuals. Moreover, the total amount of ceramide trihexoside was higher in the $P_1$ cells, and the authors considered that this finding was compatible with the idea that $P^k$ and $P_1$ genes code for separate $\alpha$-4-galactosyltransferases (see p. 105). The $P^k$-gene-specified transferase was considered to catalyze the formation of ceramide trihexoside from lactosyl ceramide in both the $P_1$ and $P_2$ phenotypes, and the elevated level of ceramide trihexoside which occurs when the $P_1$ gene is expressed was attributed to the ability of the $P_1$-gene-specified transferase to use as substrate both paragloboside, to form $P_1$ antigen, and lactosyl ceramide, to make $P^k$ antigen. This hypothesis is similar to that put forward by others (see p. 108) except that the $P^k$ and $P_1$ genes are not necessarily thought to be allelic. The overlapping function of the $P^k$ and $P_1$ enzymes would mean that only in potentially $P_2$ individuals would the inheritance of a double dose of mutated $P^k$ genes be expressed as the $p$ phenotype.

## REFERENCES

Breimer, M. E., 1979, Glycosphingolipids of human small intestine. Structural characterisation of some novel difucosyl compounds based on Type 1 carbohydrate chains, in: *27th IUPAC Congress, Helsinki, 1979* (Abstracts) (J. Larinkari and J. Oksanen, eds.), p. 383.

Buchanan, D. J., and Rapoport, S., 1951, Composition of meconium. Serological study of blood group specific substances found in individual meconiums, *J. Biol. Chem.* **192:**251–260.

Côté, R. H., 1970, Human sources of blood group substances, in: *Blood and Tissue Antigens* (D. Aminoff, ed.), pp. 249–259, Academic Press, New York.

Côté, R. H., and Valet, J. P., 1976, Isolation, composition and reactivity of the neutral glycoproteins from human meconiums with specificities of the ABO and Lewis systems, *Biochem. J.* **153:**63–73.

Feizi, T., Childs, R. A., Watanabe, K., and Hakomori, S.-I., 1979, Three types of blood group I specificity among monoclonal anti-I autoantibodies revealed by analogues of a branched erythrocyte glycolipid, *J. Exp. Med.* **149:**975–980.

Fletcher, K. S., Bremer, E. G., and Schwarting, G. A., 1979, P blood group regulation of glycosphingolipid levels in human erythrocytes, *J. Biol. Chem.* **254:**11196–11198.

Fukuda, M., Watanabe, K., and Hakomori, S., 1978, Release of oligosaccharides from various glycosphingolipids by *endo*-β-galactosidase, *J. Biol. Chem.* **253:**6814–6819.

Greenwell, P., Yates, A. D., and Watkins, W. M., 1979, Blood group *A* synthesising activity of the blood group *B* gene specified α-3-D-galactosyl transferase, in: *Glycoconjugates* (R. Schauer, P. Boer, E. Buddecke, M. F. Kramer, J. F. G. Vliegenthart, and H. Wiegandt, eds.), pp. 268–269, Thieme, Stuttgart.

Hakomori, S., 1979, Developmental changes in carbohydrate structures of human erythrocyte membranes, in: *27th IUPAC Congress, Helsinki, 1979* (Abstracts) (J. Larinkari and J. Oksanen, eds.), p. 314.

Karlsson, K.-A., and Larson, G., 1978, Molecular characterisation of cell-surface antigens of human fetal tissue. Meconium a rich source of epithelial blood-group glycolipids, *FEBS Lett.* **87:**283–287.

Karlsson, K.-A., and Larson, G., 1979, Structural characterisation of lactotetraosyl ceramide, a novel glycosphingolipid isolated from human meconium, *J. Biol. Chem.* **254:**9311–9316.

Kobata, A., and Takasaki, S., 1978, *endo*-β-Galactosidase and *endo*-α-N-acetylgalactosaminidase from *Diplococcus pneumoniae*, *Methods Enzymol.* **50:**560–567.

Koscielak, J., Zdebska, E., Wilcznska, Z., Miller-Podraza, H., and Dzierzkowa-Borodej, W., 1979, Immunochemistry of Ii-active glycosphingolipids of erythrocytes, *Eur. J. Biochem.* **96:**331–337.

Larson, G., 1979, A novel fucolipid isolated from human meconium, in: *27th IUPAC Congress, Helsinki 1979* (Abstracts) (J. Larinkari and J. Oksanen, eds.), p. 382.

Naiki, M., and Kato, M., 1979, Immunological identification of blood group $P^k$ antigen on normal erythrocytes and isolation of anti-$P^k$ with different affinity, *Vox Sang.* **37:**30–38.

Watanabe, K., Powell, M., and Hakomori, S., 1978, Isolation and characterisation of a novel fucoganglioside of human erythrocyte membranes, *J. Biol. Chem.* **253:**8962–8967.

Watanabe, K., Hakomori, S.-I., Childs, R. A., and Feizi, T., 1979, Characterisation of a blood group I-active ganglioside, *J. Biol. Chem.* **254:**3221–3228.

Yoshida, A., Yamaguchi, Y. F., and Davé, V., 1979, Immunologic homology of human blood group glycosyltransferases and genetic background of blood group (ABO) determination, *Blood* **54:**344–350.

# CHAPTER 2: HLA—A CENTRAL IMMUNOLOGICAL AGENCY OF MAN

D. Bernard Amos and D. D. Kostyu

The HLA nomenclature committee met after the 8th International Histocompatibility Testing Workshop in Los Angeles in February, 1980, to consider revisions of older HLA antigens and addition of new antigens. At the time of this addendum (March, 1980) these changes include the following:

HLA-B:    Nine new antigens, Bw55–Bw63.
HLA-C:    Two new antigens, Cw7 and Cw8.
HLA-D:    One new antigen, Dw12
HLA-DR:   Three new antigens, DRw8, DRw9, and DRw10.

Several antigens have been upgraded (the w preceding the number eliminated).

The new HLA antigens and the previous local designations for them are listed below. We would also like to mention the possible appearance of two new loci determining B-cell antigens. MB(1,2,3) and MT(1,2,3) are detectable serologically and are not identical with known DR antigens.*

---

* A third series of antigens designated SB (SB 1–5) are only detectable at this time by PLT and CML. They are not identical with D or DR antigens but segregate with HLA and map between HLA-B and GLO.

**New HLA Antigens**

| HLA | Old designation |
| --- | --- |
| Bw55 | Bw22.1 |
| Bw56 | Bw22.2 |
| Bw57 | B17.1, 17A, 17 long |
| Bw58 | B17.2, 17B, 17 short |
| Bw59 | Hoki, 8.2 |
| Bw60 | B40.1 |
| Bw61 | B40.2 |
| Bw62 | B15.1, 15B |
| Bw63 | B15.2, 15A |
| Cw7 | Cve, TOK |
| Cw8 | T8, T9 |
| Dw12 | |
| DRw8 | WIA 8 |
| DRw9 | WIA $4 \times 7$ |
| DRw10 | STI, LTM |

# CHAPTER 5: GENETIC DISORDERS OF MALE SEXUAL DIFFERENTIATION

Kaye R. Fichman, Barbara R. Migeon, and Claude J. Migeon

Since the preparation of this review, Evans *et al.* (1979) have studied the karyotype of 46, *XX* males by *G* and *R* banding, and their data suggest that many cases of 46, *XX* males may be attributable to a paternally derived *X-Y* interchange. In blind trials a heteromorphic *X* chromosome with an additional portion, $X_p+$, has been identified in 8 of 12 such males studied. The addition to the short arm represents an increase in size of the *X* chromosome varying from 4% to 23%, which the authors believe to be the result of an $X_p$-$Y_p$ interchange of variable length occurring during spermatic meiosis. The hypothesis is supported by preliminary studies using DNA hybridization in one of their subjects.

## REFERENCE

Evans, H. J., Buckton, K. E., Sowart, G., and Carothers, A. D., 1979, Heteromorphic *X* chromosomes in 46, *XX* males: Evidence for the involvement of *X-Y* interchange, *Hum. Genet.* **49**:11.

# Index